AF412693

ADVANCES IN MULTIPLE SCLEROSIS CLINICAL RESEARCH AND THERAPY

ADVANCES IN MULTIPLE SCLEROSIS

CLINICAL RESEARCH AND THERAPY

Edited by

STEN FREDRIKSON MD PhD
HANS LINK MD PhD
Karolinska Institutet
Division of Neurology
Huddinge Hospital
Huddinge, Stockholm
Sweden

Published in Association with the European Committee for
Treatment and Research in Multiple Sclerosis

MARTIN DUNITZ

© Martin Dunitz Ltd 1999

First published in the United Kingdom in 1999 by
Martin Dunitz Ltd
The Livery House
7–9 Pratt Street
London NW1 0AE

Tel: +44–(0)20–7482–2202
Fax: +44–(0)20–7267–0159
E-mail: **info@mdunitz.globalnet.co.uk**
Website: http://www.dunitz.co.uk

A CIP catalogue record for this book is available from the British Library

ISBN 1–85317–871–3

Distributed in the United States by:
Blackwell Science Inc.
Commerce Place, 350 Main Street
Malden MA 02148, USA
Tel: 1-800-215-1000

Distributed in Canada by:
Login Brothers Book Company
324 Salteaux Crescent
Winnipeg, Manitoba R3J 3T2
Canada
Tel: 1-204-224-4068

Distributed in Brazil by:
Ernesto Reichmann Distribuidora de Livros, Ltda
Rua Coronel Marques 335, Tatuape 03440–000
Sao Paulo
Brazil

Composition by Wearset, Boldon, Tyne and Wear
Printed and bound in Great Britain by Biddles Ltd, Guildford and King's Lynn

Contents

List of contributors

Oluf Andersen MD DMSci
Institute of Clinical Neuroscience
Department of Neurology
Sahlgrenska University Hospital
Göteborg
Sweden

Moiz Bakhiet MD PhD
Department of Immunology, Microbiology
Pathology and Infectious Diseases
Karolinska Institute
Huddinge University Hospital (F-82)
Huddinge, Stockholm
Sweden

Frederik Barkhof MD
MR Center for MS Research
Department of Radiology
University Hospital
1007 MB Amsterdam
The Netherlands

Mario A Battaglia MD
Institute of Hygiene
University of Siena
Siena
Italy

Alessandra Bergami
Experimental Neuroimmunotherapy Unit
Department of Neurology
University of Milan
San Raffaele Scientific Institute DIBIT
Milano
Italy

Chris A Clark PhD
NMR Research Unit
Institute of Neurology
The National Hospital for Neurology and
Neurosurgery
Queen Square
London
UK

Giancarlo Comi MD
Clinical Trials Unit
Department of Neuroscience
University of Milan
Scientific Institute H San Raffaele
Milano
Italy

Gaetano Desina
Department of Neurology
"Casa Sollievo della Sofferenza"
Scientific Institute
San Giovanni Rotondo
Italy

Virginia Devonshire MD FRCPC
Division of Neurology
Vancouver Hospital and Health Sciences
Centre
The University of British Columbia
Vancouver, British Columbia
Canada

David A Dyment MSc
MS Clinic
University Hospital
London, Ontario
Canada

George C Ebers MD FRCP(C)
MS Clinic
University Hospital
London, Ontario
Canada

Nikos Evangelou MD MRCP
Centre for Functional Magnetic
Resonance Imaging of the Brain
Department of Clinical Neurology
University of Oxford
UK

Cesare Fieschi MD
Department of Neurological Science
University of Rome
"La Sapienza"
Rome
Italy

Massimo Filippi MD
Neuroimaging Research Unit
Department of Neuroscience
University of Milan
Scientific Institute H San Raffaele
Milano
Italy

Jette L Frederiksen MD
The MS Clinic
Department of Neurology
University of Copenhagen
Glostrup Hospital
Glostrup, Copenhagen
Denmark

Roberto Furlan MD
Experimental Neuroimmunotherapy Unit
Department of Neurology
University of Milan
San Raffaele Scientific Institute DIBIT
Milano
Italy

Kin Ho PhD
Division of Internal Medicine
Vancouver Hospital and Health Sciences
Centre
The University of British Columbia
Vancouver, British Columbia
Canada

Jeremy Hobart MD
Neurological Outcome Measures Unit
Institute of Neurology
Queen Square
London
UK

Rikard Holmdahl MD
Section for Medical Inflammation
Research, CMB
Lund University
Lund
Sweden

Jakob Jensen MD
The MS Clinic
Department of Neurology
University of Copenhagen
Glostrup Hospital
Glostrup, Copenhagen
Denmark

Jürg Kesselring MD
Department of Neurology
Rehabilitation Centre
Valens
Department of Clinical Neurology and
Neurorehabilitation
Universities of Bern and Zurich
Switzerland

Pia Kivisäkk MD PhD
Division of Neurology
Karolinska Institutet
Huddinge University Hospital
Huddinge
Sweden

Martin Lee MRCP
Centre for Functional Magnetic
Resonance Imaging of the Brain
Department of Clinical Neurology
University of Oxford
UK

Chuan-Zhen Lu MD
Institute of Neurology
Huasham Hospital
Shanghai Medical University
Shanghai
China

Peggy Marconi
Telethon Institute for Gene Therapy (TIGET)
San Raffaele Scientific Institute
Milano
Italy

Gianvito Martino MD
Experimental Neuroimmunotherapy Unit
Department of Neurology
University of Milan
San Raffaele Scientific Institute DIBIT
Milano
Italy

Paul M Matthews MD Dphil
Centre for Functional Magnetic
Resonance Imaging of the Brain
Department of Clinical Neurology
University of Oxford
UK

Rune Midgard MD
Department of Neurology
Molde County Hospital
Molde
Norway

David H Miller MD
NMR Research Unit
Institute of Neurology
Queen Square
London
UK

Deborah M Miller PhD
Mellen Center for Multiple Sclerosis Treatment
and Research
The Cleveland Clinic Foundation
Cleveland OH
USA

John H Noseworthy MD FRCPC
Department of Neurology
Mayo Clinic
Mayo Foundation
200 First Street SW
Rochester MN
USA

Lucia Palmisano MD
Italian Multiple Sclerosis Foundation
MS Day Center
Rome
Italy

Donald W Paty MD FRCPC FACP
Multiple Sclerosis Research Programs
Division of Neurology
Vancouver Hospital and Health Sciences
Centre
The University of British Columbia
Vancouver, British Columbia
Canada

Angela Pisani MD
Department of Neurological Science
University of Rome
"La Sapienza"
Rome
Italy

Pietro Luigi Poliani MD PhD
Experimental Neuroimmunotherapy Unit
Department of Neurology
University of Milan
San Raffaele Scientific Institute DIBIT
Milano
Italy

Carlo Pozzilli MD PhD
Department of Neurological Science
University of Rome
"La Sapienza"
Rome
Italy

Marco Rovaris MD
Neuroimaging Research Unit
University of Milan
Scientific Institute H San Raffaele
Milano
Italy

Neil J Scolding PhD FRCP
Institute of Clinical Neuroscience
Frenchay Hospital
Bristol
UK

Finn Sellebjerg MD PhD
The MS Clinic
Department of Neurology
University of Copenhagen
Glostrup Hospital
Glostrup, Copenhagen
Denmark

Steve Shindell PhD
Paralyzed Veterans of America
Washington DC
USA

Torben L Sørensen MD
The MS Clinic
Department of Neurology
University of Copenhagen
Glostrup Hospital
Glostrup, Copenhagen
Denmark

James L Steckley MSc
MS Clinic
University Hospital
London, Ontario
Canada

Donald Studney MD FRCP
Division of Internal Medicine
Vancouver Hospital and Health Sciences Centre
The University of British Columbia
Vancouver, British Columbia
Canada

Alan J Thompson MD FRCP FRCPI
Institute of Neurology
Queen Square
London
UK

Paul van der Valk MS
Department of Pathology
University Hospital
Amsterdam
The Netherlands

Marianne AA van Walderveen MD
MR Center for MS Research
Department of Radiology
University Hospital
Amsterdam
The Netherlands

David J Werring MRCP
NMR Research Unit
Institute of Neurology
Queen Square
London
UK

Michele Messmer Uccelli BA
The Italian Multiple Sclerosis Society (FISM)
Genoa
Italy

Bao-Guo Xiao PhD
Division of Neurology
Karolinska Institutet
Huddinge University Hospital
Huddinge
Sweden

Preface

Multiple sclerosis (MS) is an important disease. The World Health Organization (WHO) has placed MS on the 'Top 100' list of diseases that are of great importance and causing considerable 'loss of health' in a global perspective.

The increasing interest in MS has stimulated new and fruitful research in several areas. In the present volume we try to facilitate the mutual understanding between basic and clinically oriented research. Experts in various fields of MS—ranging from genetics and immunology to organization of a MS-clinic—present up-to-date reviews of their activities. By sharing knowledge it will be possible to continue along the exciting way to further improved treatment and management of MS. After the introduction of new treatments of MS, it is now a treatable, but still not a curable, disease.

We would like to thank all the contributors for excellent co-operation.

Sten Fredrikson
Hans Link

PART I

Genetics

1

What the specialist in multiple sclerosis needs to know about genetics

David A Dyment, James L Steckley and George C Ebers

INTRODUCTION

Multiple sclerosis (MS) provides an excellent framework for an investigator to study the genetics of a complex trait. The disorder is characterized by many of the hallmarks that define complex or multifactorial inheritance. There is a variable age of onset, a wide range of clinical expressivity, reduced penetrance as manifested by a low recurrence risk in the relatives of MS patients and a high prevalence in the general population. Though these factors contribute to the difficulty in dissecting the genetics of MS, it compels the researcher to use novel and creative methods to demonstrate the contribution of genes. Most notably, family studies using twin, half-sibling, adopted and conjugal data have contributed a great deal to our understanding of MS inheritance. Also, the Human Genome Project has made available to the geneticist thousands of mapped polymorphic markers, which facilitate extensive and exhaustive searches for susceptibility genes. This high throughput genotyping has been aided by advances in automation, statistical methods and, of course, the collection of large numbers of MS families by research groups in North America and Europe. With such a rapid increase in our understanding of genetics, and in particular the genetics of MS, it is important for the MS specialist to be aware of the context in which this information is being added, the current status of our knowledge and the problems facing geneticists in the future.

EVIDENCE IN SUPPORT OF A GENETIC CONTRIBUTION TO MS PATHOGENESIS

If it is hypothesized that a genetic contribution to the pathogenesis of a disease exists there should be an increased risk to the family members of patients, and this increased risk should decrease with decreased relatedness to the patients. MS has a rich history of family studies in the investigation of these expectations, beginning with the early case reports of Eichhorst[1] and the pioneering work of Curtius[2,3] in the 1930s. This MS literature has served to highlight the difficulty in demonstrating, convincingly, the two expectations of a genetic disease. Previous studies were often flawed in their ascertainment scheme, they made no allowance for unaffected individuals and they often lacked appropriate clinical criteria, confidence intervals and statistical tests.

However, since these early studies there have been a number of population-based family studies that satisfactorily address these shortcomings.[4–6] And indeed, the two expectations of

Table 1.1 Recurrence risks in three population-based MS studies.

Investigation	Age-adjusted recurrence risks (%)							
	Familial	Parents	Siblings	Children	Aunts or uncles	Nieces or nephews	Cousins	Population prevalence
Sadovnick et al[4]	19.9	1.94	3.56	2.69	0.96	1.85	2.04	0.093[7]
Robertson et al[5]	18.9	2.05	3.82	1.83	0.87	1.64	0.88	0.130[8]
Carton et al[6]	15.4	1.61	2.10	1.73	0.66	0.45	0.44	0.088[9]

a genetic disorder are observed (*Table 1.1*). These population-based studies screened a representative population of MS patients, using a large sample size from which the familial recurrence risks could be estimated. The risk that an MS patient has any affected family member is approximately 15–20%.[10] The specific age-corrected risks to the first-, second- and third-degree relatives of MS patients are 3.6%, 1.4% and 0.9% respectively.[4,5,11] The risk to third-degree relatives may still be subject to overestimation owing to an expected ascertainment bias in more distant relatives.

From these empiric risk estimates, geneticists have inferred possible modes of inheritance for MS.[5,6,12] It is readily apparent that simple Mendelian models of inheritance do not accommodate the familial recurrence risks. The similarity in risks between parents, sibs and children is inconsistent with an autosomal recessive mode of inheritance, while an autosomal dominant gene would require an extremely low penetrance (<10%) to account for the low risk in the first-degree relatives. X-linked models of inheritance cannot explain the preponderance of female patients nor the similarity in risk between the maternal and paternal relatives of male probands.[5] The inability of Mendelian inheritance to explain the relatively low risk estimates, the skewed sex ratio and the delayed age of onset support a complex or multifactorial inheritance.

This model assumes that there are many genes contributing to an individual's liability to develop MS. If enough liability genes are present, a critical threshold is attained, which is permissive, but not necessarily sufficient, for the development of MS. Further evidence in support of a multigenic inheritance model for susceptibility is the observation of an increased recurrence risk to the offspring of conjugal MS patients.[13] In this family structure the offspring may inherit liability genes from both the mother and father and hence are more likely to accrue the liability genes necessary to attain the threshold level for MS susceptibility. It has also been observed that the lifetime risk to the sisters of MS patients with an age of onset under 20 years of age and with an affected parent is as high as 23%.[14] This is, again, in keeping with a hypothesis of many operative liability genes and the possibility that there are families that are 'loaded' with these liability genes.

A term often used to describe the extent of familial clustering is the population relative risk of $\lambda_{\text{relative-type}}$.[15] This value is the risk to a relative of interest divided by the risk in the general population. In Canada the population prevalence of MS is 1 per 1000[7] with a lifetime cumulative risk estimate of 0.2% and a recurrence risk to a sibling of 3.6%.[4] Therefore the λ_{sibs} is roughly 18. It is important to note that the familial clustering observed in MS is consistent with either a genetic contribution or a shared environmental contribution, or both. In fact, before the twin studies of the 1980s, actual evidence that inheritance contributes significantly to familial clustering had been less than convincing.

Demonstrating the presence of genetic factors

The classic twin study was first proposed by Galton in 1876 as a method of separating the contribution of nature and nurture in studies of human disposition and intelligence.[16] The basic rationale for two studies involves a comparison of concordance rates between dizygotic twins and monozygotic twins, the concordance rate being the proportion of doubly affected twin pairs present in the total twin sample. A monozygotic concordance rate that is significantly greater than the dizygotic concordance rate suggests a genetic component to the trait being studied. In contrast, if the dizygotic concordance rate is not significantly different from the monozygotic concordance rate, a non-genetic or shared environmental component to aetiology is supported.

There are a few factors regarding twin studies that must be considered before the results of MS twin studies are discussed. The first is that the twin study rests upon a major, and not always valid, assumption regarding environmental sharing. This assumption states that a dizygotic twin shares the environment with his or her co-twin to the same extent as a monozygotic twin pair does. This is not always the case because monozygotic and dizygotic twins have differing prenatal environments.[17] Dizygotic twins, formed from the fertilization of two eggs, have separate chorionic and amniotic membranes. In contrast, monozygotic twins pair, formed from the fertilization of one egg and subsequent division of the zygote, have different prenatal environments depending on the time of zygote division. If the division of the zygote occurs during the blastocyst stage, the monozygotic pair shares a single chorionic membrane and has separate amniotic membranes.[18] In addition the environmental sharing assumption includes the rearing or household

environment. Dizygotic twins can be of different sex and as a result be expected to share their environment to a different extent than the always like-sexed monozygotic twins.[19] This is an important consideration in MS, especially given the evidence that suggests that a putative environmental component to MS acts by the time of adolescence.[20]

The twinning rate in North America and Europe is 1200 per 100 000 births.[21] This is equivalent to 1 twin pair per 83.3 births. It is therefore apparent that if twins are used to study a disease with 0.1% prevalence it will take considerable effort to amass a large, representative study sample. It could be expected that an individual would be both an MS patient and a twin once for every 100 000 individuals in the general population. This relative rarity is largely responsible for the major limitation of MS twin studies, which is ascertainment bias. In order to get enough twins to study, researchers have often advertised and accepted volunteers. This would not be a problem if monozygotic concordant twin pairs were ascertained in a representative manner; however, this is not the case and there is often an over-representation of concordant, monozygous and female twin pairs in any volunteer ascertainment scheme.[22]

To overcome ascertainment bias and low sample numbers, a number of population-based MS studies have been performed.[23–28] The consensus difference observed between monozygotic and dizygotic twin concordance rates reflects the involvement of genes in MS pathogenesis (*Table 1.2*). To address any potential differences caused by unlike-sex dizygotic twin pairs, like-sexed dizygotic pairs have been used for comparison, with similar results and conclusions.[27] A number of additional inferences can be made from these MS twin studies. The first is that 70% of monozygotic twins, who share the same genetic material, remain discordant for MS. This implies that the penetrance is indeed low and that stochastic factors involved in the development of the immune system or the central nervous system (or both) play an important role. Secondly, the high MZ:DZ ratio does not support a single acting gene, but rather that at least two and perhaps more epistatically acting

Table 1.2 Population-based twin studies.

Investigation	Monozygotic twin concordance	Dizygotic twin concordance
Bobowick et al[24]	1/5	0/4
Heltberg et al[25]	4/19	1/28
Mumford et al[23]	9/44	2/61
Sadovnick[27] (including the twin series of Ebers et al[26])	13/45	2/66
Kinnunen et al[28]	1/11	0/10
Total	28/124 **(22.58%)**	5/169 **(2.96%)**
Monozygotic/dizygotic ratio: 7.63		

genes are required to determine susceptibility. Thirdly, the similarity in risk between dizygotic twins and full siblings is suggestive of a lack of a significant in utero effect.

The relative contribution of genetics and environment

Twin studies prove a genetic component to MS susceptibility, and the relatively low concordance rates imply a major environmental and/or random-chance influence on susceptibility. Adoption studies provide a tool to assess the nature of the environmental contribution to disease pathogenesis. To date, this strategy has been applied only once in the field of autoimmune disease.[29] This is primarily due to the resources that are necessary to undertake an unbiased population-based adoption study. The study undertaken by the Canadian Collaborative Project on the Genetic Susceptibility to Multiple Sclerosis (CCPGSMS)[29] screened 15 000 MS patients attending regional MS clinics across Canada. The study identified 582 MS patients who lived with a non-genetically related relative (i.e. adoptive sib-

lings, adopted children and adopting parents). If the familial clustering observed in family studies ($\lambda_{sibs} = 18$) is due to a shared environmental factor (e.g. a transmissible virus) then the rate of MS in these non-genetically related individuals should be comparable to the risk in genetically-related first-degree relatives (see Table 1.1). In actuality, of the 1201 adoptive relatives of the patients, only one was identified with clinically definite MS. This is significantly different than the 25 expected if familial clustering is caused by the shared familial environment (Table 1.3). In addition, the rate of 1 per 1201 is very similar to the Canadian population prevalence of 1 per 1000. If there is allowance for the known assortative mating, the expected prevalence may be closer to 1 per 700 in the Caucasian population. This study provides convincing evidence that familial clustering is due primarily to genes.

One qualifier of the twin and the adoption data is that an environmental factor contributing to risk does not operate in utero. To test for a possible maternal effect and to confirm the findings of the twin and adoption studies, a half-sibling study was performed by the CCPGSMS.[11] Of the 15 000 MS patients ques-

Table 1.3 Expected versus observed number of non-biological relatives with MS (from Ebers et al[29]).

| Non-biological relatives | Number | Number of MS cases | | Poisson probability |
		Expected	Observed	
Parents	470	9.2	1	1.0×10^{-3}
Siblings	345	10.7	0	2.3×10^{-5}
Children	386	5.5	0	4.1×10^{-3}
Total	1201	25.4	1	2.5×10^{-10}

tioned in the original screen, 939 had at least one maternal or paternal half-sibling. There was found to be no significant difference in risk between maternal and paternal half-siblings. This argues against a major maternal effect operating to increase MS risk (e.g. in utero and perinatal factors, breast-feeding, genomic imprinting and mitochondrial inheritance). In addition, no difference in risk was observed between half-siblings who lived with the MS index case versus and half-siblings who did not live with the index case, supporting the results of the CCPGSMS adoption study. Lastly, a statistically significant difference in risk was observed between full-siblings who lived with the index case and half-siblings who also lived with the index case, recalling the steep drop in risk between monozygotic and dizygotic twins.

An attempt to identify novel MS susceptibility genes

To attempt to identify MS susceptibility genes, four research groups have performed genome-wide searches.[30–33] This strategy requires the collection of large numbers of MS sib pairs and the genotyping of hundreds of microsatellite markers throughout the genome. If the microsatellite markers are in close proximity (i.e. 'linked') to a susceptibility gene, it would be expected that two siblings with MS would share the same marker at that region more often than would be expected by chance.[34] To assess the significance of this genetic sharing between family members, a lod score is estimated. A lod score is the log of the odds ratio of obtaining the observed data if the marker and disease locus are linked versus the probability of obtaining the observed data if they are unlinked. A significant score is generally held to be a lod score of 3.0, which is equivalent to a conservative significance level of 0.001.[35] However, in a genome-wide screen many hundreds of markers are tested and, in order to compensate for the increased probability of false-positive results, the significance level of the lod score is increased to 3.6.[36] Within the four individual genome-wide MS screens, several regions were found to be mildly suggestive (i.e. lod score $\geqslant 1.0$) of linkage to an MS susceptibility gene (*Table 1.4*), but unfortunately there was little overlap between studies (*Table 1.5*).

From these results a number of conclusions can be made. The most obvious and important is that there is no single gene operating to increase risk in the majority of the MS families, a conclusion supported by the results of family and twin studies. In addition, the incomplete overlap among the studies suggests that there are differences in the susceptibility genes

Table 1.4   The markers (and maximum lod scores) from four genome-wide screens.

USA[32]		UK[31]		Canada[30]		Finland[33]	
D2S131	(1.71)	D1S199	(1.2)	D2S119	(1.24)	D4S3248	(1.35)
D3S1744	(1.00)	D1S236	(2.0)	D3S1309	(1.01)	D5S416	(3.40)
D5S815	(1.14)	D2S169	(1.2)	D5S406	(4.24)	HLA-DR	(1.54)
HLA-DR	(1.46)	D3S1289	(1.3)	D11S2000	(1.38)	D11S910	(1.1)
D7S489	(1.14)	D4S426	(1.2)	DXS1068	(1.85)	D17S807	(4.2)
D7S554	(2.86)	D5S427	(2.5)				
D7S523	(1.11)	D5S409	(1.0)				
D9S162	(1.24)	D6S276	(2.8)				
D9S66	(1.13)	D7S629	(1.9)				
D10S464	(1.39)	D12S364	(2.1)				
D11S922	(1.13)	D14S292	(1.7)				
D12S1052	(1.48)	NF1	(1.5)				
D12S392	(1.71)	D17S807	(2.5)				
D16S748	(1.75)	D19S246	(1.5)				
APOC2	(1.47)	CYP2D	(1.9)				
		DXS991	(1.9)				
		DXS1059	(1.5)				

Table 1.5   Regions of overlap of positive lod scores between genome screens.

USA[32]	UK[31]	Canada[30]	Finland[33]
2p16		2p16	
3q21–q25		3q21–q25	3q21–q25
	3p21–p14	3p14–p12	
5q14–q15	5q14–q15	5q14–q15	
6p21	6p21	6p21	6p21
	7p21–p15	7p21–p15	
7q11–q22		7q21–q22	
	17q22–q24		17q22–q24
19q13	19q13	19q13	19q13
	Xp21–p11	Xp21–Xp11	

between populations. If this is indeed the case, careful planning is required when deciding the composition of future study samples.

Implicated candidate genes

One suggestively linked region indicated by all four major investigations was a region on chromosome 6p21. The English, American, Canadian and Finnish maximum lod scores were 2.8, 3.57, 0.65 and 1.54 respectively. This mildly positive and consistent result was not a surprise because researchers have been aware of a susceptibility gene located within this region for over 25 years.[37–39] The major histocompatibility complex (MHC) resides within this chromosomal region. The MHC region contains genes that encode human leukocyte antigens (HLA). These antigens which are present on the surface of cells, are responsible for the recognition of 'self' versus 'non-self' and hence make attractive candidates for MS susceptibility genes. The first studies demonstrated an association with the HLA Class I antigens A3 and B7,[37–39] and following these initial reports an association with the Class II polymorphisms Dw2 and DR2.[40,41] This has been sub-typed into a strong and consistent association with the HLA DRB1*1501, DQA1*0102 and DQB1*0602 haplotypes.[42–44] The strong linkage disequilibrium present within this region makes elucidation of the specific susceptibility gene present on this haplotype difficult.[45] Additionally, the association with the DR/DQ haplotype does not exclude the possibility that there are other genes in the region playing a role in MS pathogenesis. For example, there have been observations that suggest the presence of HLA genes operating in *cis* and/or *trans* with DRB1*1501, DQA1*0102, DQB1*0602 to increase relative risk.[46–48] Similarly, the observation of genetic heterogeneity in non-Caucasian populations[49,50] and the presence of resistance alleles[51,52] indicate that one or more other genes in the region contribute to MS susceptibility. If these are the interactions and conditions thought to occur within one locus, the amount of complexity generated by susceptibility loci throughout the

genome could be staggering. More importantly, these loci need not be identical between families; for example, the HLA DR2 antigen is present in only 60% of MS patients.[53] Taken together, HLA is certainly involved in the process of susceptibility, yet given the relatively weak results of linkage analysis the locus can account for less than 10% of the increased risk to family members.[10]

Because of the strong circumstantial evidence that MS is an autoimmune disorder, other candidate genes involved in immune functions have been examined. Convincing negative results have been obtained for the T-cell receptor α genes, interleukin-1 receptor agonist gene, interferon-α, -β and -γ genes and a variety of complement and cytokine genes (*Table 1.6*). The results are less clear-cut for three reasonable candidates: the myelin basic protein gene (coding for the major myelin protein with which an animal model of MS can be induced), the T cell receptor β locus and the immunoglobulin variable gene.[69,71,73]

In order to implicate a candidate gene these association studies estimate the frequency of genetic polymorphisms in cases compared to controls. The relative risk is the measure used to assess the magnitude of the association. The strength of such a study design is that, in order to detect an association, the marker must be in close proximity to the disease gene or, better yet, be the disease gene itself. The weakness of such a study is that population stratification or a mismatching of cases and controls may yield false-positive results. In order to overcome this problem, geneticists often use controls derived from the patient's own family by use of the transmission disequilibrium test[75] or the affected family based control method,[76] a strategy recommended for complex traits with a history of non-reproducible results,[77] since these tests are not affected by the presence of population stratification.

PROBLEMS FACING THE MS GENETICIST

So how can geneticists overcome the difficulties posed by the complex inheritance of MS? There

Table 1.6 Selected findings using the candidate gene approach.

Negative results	Further investigation needed	Positive results
TCR α[54–56]	Immunoglobulin variable region[69,70]	DRB1*1501, DQA1*0102, DQB1*0602[42–44]
Interleukin-1 receptor agonist, interleukins 1 and 2 and interleukins 2 and 5 receptors[57]	MBP[71,72]	
INF α, β, γ[57]	TCR beta[73,74]	
Immunoglobulin constant region[58,59]		
Alpha-1-antitrypsin[60]		
C3, C4, Bf, C2[61,62]		
TNF[63]		
TAP, LMP[64,65]		
HLA DP polymorphisms[66,67]		
Mitochondrial genes[68]		

are a number of options available. One strategy is to use very rare but potentially valuable families with exceptional MS penetrance. This has met with success in Parkinson's disease and Alzheimer's disease.[78,79] In doing so, one hopes to be reducing the complexity of the study sample since patients are assumed to be affected because of the same alleles. This approach is limited by the number of such families that can realistically be identified given the delayed age of onset of MS, the low recurrence risk and the small size of most North American families. In keeping with the theme of reducing complexity, one can use founder populations, which are, in a sense, extended families. In North America, the French Canadian and any one of the Anabaptist populations have been essential in the identification of a number of disease genes.[80–82] However the

Sardinian, Icelandic, Irish and other populations could be adequate for this purpose. Lastly one can stratify sib pair samples in an attempt to reduce complexity, a strategy opted for by some researchers in insulin-dependent diabetes mellitus.[83,84] One should proceed with caution when stratifying a sample in the absence of positive results since the power to detect mild susceptibility gene decreases with decreasing sample size whereas the false-positive rate increases with the increased number of comparisons performed.[85] In addition, the locus being tested must have a significant difference in identical allele sharing by descent between sample subsets in order to be detected, a situation that is unlikely to occur given the mild to moderate effect of susceptibility genes.[86] Another strategy not concerned with the reduction of complexity is simply to collect, genotype and analyse more sib pair families. This may provide suggestive results that can be used for later hypothesis testing. In the future, these large sib pair collections may be used for genome-wide screens for disequilibrium using a genome-wide panel of single nucleotide polymorphisms and automated genotyping technology.

CONCLUSION

By understanding the current status of the genetics of multiple sclerosis, the MS specialist can take advantage of new opportunities for solving the inherent problems of this complex trait. These opportunities may involve novel technical and statistical methods or the collection of unique biological material in order to understand the genetic complexity problem better. The technological advances in high throughput genotyping, the collection of large extended families or a series of blood samples from monozygotic twins are a few such examples. Alternatively, new opportunities may arise from developments in other disciplines such as human immunology, biochemistry, animal models of autoimmunity and clinical trials. Wherever the ideas are derived, it is to be hoped that the application to MS genetic research will provide the clues to the identification of susceptibility genes and, more importantly, to the elucidation of the function of the gene products in the determination of susceptibility. With this information, MS patients may be able to be more successfully treated and it may be possible to devise methods for the prevention of MS in people at high risk of developing the condition.

REFERENCES

1. Eichorst H. Multiple Sklerose und spastische Spinalparalyse. *Med Klin* 1913; **9**: 1617–1619.
2. Curtius F, Speer H. Multiple Sklerose und Erbanlage. *Z Neurol Psychiatr* 1937; **160**: 226–245.
3. Curtius F. *Multiple Sklerose und Erbanlage.* Leipzig: Georg Thieme, 1933.
4. Sadovnick AD, Baird PA. Multiple sclerosis: updated risks for relatives. *Am J Med Gen* 1988; **29**: 533–541.
5. Robertson N, Fraser M, Deans J et al. Age-adjusted recurrence risks for relatives of patients with multiple sclerosis. *Brain* 1996; **119**: 449–455.
6. Carton H, Vlietink R, Debruyne J et al. Risks of multiple sclerosis in relatives of patients in Flanders, Belgium. *J Neurol Neurosurg Psych* 1997; **62**: 329–333.
7. Sweeney VP, Sadovnick AD, Brandejs V. Prevalence of multiple sclerosis in British Columbia. *Can J Neurol Sci* 1986; **13**: 47–51.
8. Robertson N, Deans J, Fraser M, Compston DAS. Multiple sclerosis in the north Cambridgeshire districts of East Anglia. *J Neurol Neurosurg Psychiatry* 1995; **59**: 71–76.
9. van Ooteghem P, D'Hooghe MB, Vlietinck R, Carton H. Prevalence of multiple sclerosis in Flanders, Belgium. *Neuroepidemiology* 1994; **13**: 220–225.
10. Sadovnick AD, Dyment D, Ebers GC. Genetic epidemiology of multiple sclerosis. *Epidemiol Rev* 1997; **19**: 99–106.
11. Sadovnick AD, Ebers GC, Dyment DA, Risch N, the Canadian Collaborative Group. A population-based halfsib study of multiple sclerosis. *Lancet* 1996; **347**: 1728–1730.
12. Sadovnick AD, Bulman D, Ebers G. Parent–child concordance in multiple sclerosis. *Ann Neurol* 1991; **29**: 252–255.
13. Robertson NP, O'Riordan JI, Chataway J et al. Offspring recurrence rates and clinical characteristics of conjugal multiple sclerosis. *Lancet* 1997; **349**: 1587–1590.
14. Sadovnick AD, Yee IML, Ebers GC, Risch NJ. Effect of age at onset and parental disease status on sibling risks for MS. *Neurology* 1998; **50**: 719–723.
15. Risch N. Linkage strategies for genetically complex traits. I. Multilocus models. *Am J Hum Genet* 1990; **46**: 222–228.
16. Blacker CP. *Galton and After.* London, Gerald Duckworth, 1952.
17. Vogel F, Motulsky A. *Human Genetics: Problems and Approaches.* Berlin, Springer-Verlag, 1979.
18. Emery A. *Methodology in Medical Genetics.* Edinburgh, Churchill Livingstone, 1976.
19. Susser M. Separating heredity and environment. *Am J Prev Med* 1985; **1**: 5–23.
20. Kurtzke JF. Epidemiological evidence for multiple sclerosis as an infection. *Clin Microbiol Rev* 1993; **6**: 382–427.

21. Hrubec Z, Robinette C. The study of human twins in medical research. *N Engl J Med* 1984; **310**: 435–441.

22. Lykken D, McGue M, Tellegen A. A recruitment bias in twin research: the rule of two-thirds reconsidered. *Behav Genet* 1987; **17**: 343–362.

23. Mumford CJ, Wood NW, Kellar-Wood H et al. The British Isles survey of multiple sclerosis in twins. *Neurology* 1994; **44**: 11–15.

24. Bobowick AR, Kurtzke JF, Brody JA et al. Twin study of multiple sclerosis: an epidemiological inquiry. *Neurology* 1978; **28**: 978–987.

25. Heltberg A, Holm N. Concordance in twins and recurrence in sibships in multiple sclerosis. *Lancet* 1982; **i**: 1068.

26. Ebers GC, Bulman DE, Sadovnick AD et al. A population-based study of multiple sclerosis in twins. *N Eng J Med* 1986; **315**: 1638–1642.

27. Sadovnick AD, Armstrong H, Rice GP et al. A population-based study of twins: update. *Ann Neurol* 1993; **33**: 281–285.

28. Kinnumen E, Koskenvuo M, Kaprio J, Aho K. Multiple sclerosis in a nationwide series of twins. *Neurology* 1987; **37**: 1627–1629.

29. Ebers GC, Sadovnick AD, Risch NJ, the Canadian Collaborative Study Group. A genetic basis for familial aggregation in multiple sclerosis. *Nature* 1995; **377**: 150–151.

30. Ebers G, Kukay K, Bulman D et al. A full genome search in multiple sclerosis. *Nat Genet* 1996; **13**: 472–476.

31. Sawcer S, Jones H, Feakes R et al. A genome screen in multiple sclerosis reveals susceptibility loci on chromosome 6p21 and 17q22. *Nat Genet* 1996; **13**: 464–468.

32. Haines J, Pericak-Vance M, Seboun E, Hauser S, the Multiple Sclerosis Genetics Group. A complete genomic screen for multiple sclerosis underscores a role for the major histocompatibility complex. *Nat Genet* 1996; **13**: 469–471.

33. Kuokkanen S, Gschwend M, Rioux J et al. Genomewide scan of multiple sclerosis in Finnish multiplex families. *Am J Hum Genet* 1997; **61**: 1379–1387.

34. Penrose LS. The detection of autosomal linkage in data which consists of pairs of brothers and sisters of unspecified parentage. *Ann Eugen* 1935; **6**: 133–138.

35. Ott J. *Analysis of Human Genetic Linkage*. Baltimore, Maryland: The Johns Hopkins University Press, 1991.

36. Ladner E, Kruglyak L. Genetic dissection of complex traits: guidelines for interpreting and reporting linkage results. *Nat Genet* 1995; **11**: 241–247.

37. Naito S, Namerow N, Mickey M, Teraski P. Multiple sclerosis: association with HL-A3. *Tissue Antigens* 1972; **2**: 1–4.

38. Jersild C, Svejgaard A, Fog T. HL-A antigens and multiple sclerosis. *Lancet* 1972; **i**: 1240–1241.

39. Bertrams J, Kuwert E, Liedtke U. HL-A antigens and multiple sclerosis. *Tissue Antigens* 1972; **2**: 405–408.

40. Jersild C, Hansen C, Svejgaard A et al. Histocompatibility determinants in multiple sclerosis with special reference to clinical course. *Lancet* 1973; **ii**: 1221–1225.

41. Winchester RJ, Ebers G, Fu SM et al. B-Cell alloantigen Ag7a in multiple sclerosis. *Lancet* 1975; **ii**: 814.

42. Hauser SL, Fleischnick E, Weiner H et al. Extended major histocompatibility complex haplotypes in patients with multiple sclerosis. *Neurology* 1989; **39**: 275–277.

43. Allen M, Sandberg-Wollheim M, Sjogren K et al. Association of susceptibility to multiple sclerosis in Sweden with HLA class II DRB1 and DQB1 alleles. *Hum Immunol* 1994; **39**: 41–48.

44. Haegert DG, Francis GS. HLA-DQ polymorphisms do not explain HLA class II associations with multiple sclerosis in two patient groups. *Neurology* 1993; **43**: 1207–1210.

45. Begovich AB, McClure GR, Suraj VC et al. Polymorphism, recombination, and linkage disequilibrium within the HLA class II region. *J Immunol* 1992; **148**: 249–258.

46. Spurkland A, Ronningen K, Vandvik B et al. HLA-DQA1 and HLA-DQB1 genes may jointly determine susceptibility to develop multiple sclerosis. *Hum Immunol* 1991; **30**: 69–75.

47. Madigand M, Oger J, Fauchet R et al. HLA profiles in multiple sclerosis suggest two forms of disease and the existence of protective haplotypes. *J Neurol Sci* 1982; **53**: 519–529.

48. Ghabanbasani MZ, Gu XX, Spaepen M et al. Importance of HLA-DRB1 and DQA1 genes and of the amino acid polymorphisms in the functional domain of DRB1 chain in multiple sclerosis. *J Immunol* 1995; **59**: 77–82.

49. Marrosu MG, Murru MR, Costa G et al. Multiple sclerosis in Sardinia is associated and in linkage-disequilibrium with HLA-DR3 and -DR4 alleles. *Am J Hum Genet* 1997; **61**: 454–457.

50. Marrosu MG, Muntoni F, Murro MR. Sardinian multiple sclerosis is associated with HLA-DR4: a serologic and molecular survey. *Neurology* 1988; **38**: 1749–1753.

51. Runmarker B, Martinsson T, Wahlstrom J, Andersen O. HLA and prognosis in multiple sclerosis. *J Neurol* 1994; **241**: 385–390.

52. Haegert DG, Swift F, Benedikz J. Evidence for a complex role of HLA class II genotypes in susceptibility to multiple sclerosis. *Neurology* 1996; **46**: 1107–1111.

53. Olerup O, Hillert J. HLA class II-associated genetic susceptibility in multiple sclerosis: a critical evaluation. *Tissue Antigens* 1991; **38**: 1–15.

54. Hashimoto LL, Mak TW, Ebers GC. T cell receptor alpha chain polymorphisms in multiple sclerosis. *J Multiple Sclerosis* 1992; **40**: 41–48.

55. Hillert J, Chummao L, Olerup O. T cell receptor alpha chain germline gene polymorphisms in multiple sclerosis. *Neurology* 1992; **42**: 80–84.

56. Lynch SG, Rose JW, Petajan JH et al. Discordance of T cell receptor alpha chain in familial multiple sclerosis. *Neurology* 1992; **42**: 839–844.

57. Epplen C, Jackel S, Santos E et al. Genetic predisposition to multiple sclerosis as revealed by immunoprinting. *Neurology* 1997; **41**: 341–352.

58. Hillert J. Immunoglobulin gamma constant gene region polymorphisms in multiple sclerosis. *J Neuroimmunol* 1993; **43**: 9–14.

59. Yu JS, Pandey JP, Massacesi L et al. Segregation of immunoglobulin heavy chain constant region genes in MS sibling pairs. *J Neuroimmunol* 1993; **42**: 113–116.

60. Francis D, Klouda P, Brazier D et al. Alpha-1-Antitrypsin (Pi) types in MS and lack of interaction with immunoglobulin markers. *J Immunogenet* 1988; **5**: 251–255.

61. Franciotta D, Dondi E, Bergamaschi R et al. HLA complement gene polymorphisms in multiple sclerosis. A study on 80 Italian patients. *J Neurol* 1995; **242**: 64–68.

62. Bulman D, Armstrong H, Ebers G. Allele frequency of the third component of the complement system (C3) in MS patients. *J Neurol Neurosurg Psychiatry* 1991; **54**: 554–555.

63. Fugger L, Morling N, Sandberg-Wolheim M et al. Tumor necrosis factor alpha gene polymorphism in multiple sclerosis and optic neuritis. *J Neuroimmunol* 1990; **27**: 85–88.

64. Liblau R, van Endert PM, Sandberg-Wollheim M et al. Antigen processing gene polymorphisms in HLA-DR2 multiple sclerosis. *Neurology* 1993; **43**: 1192–1197.

65. Spurkland A, Knutsen I, Undlien DE, Vardal F. No association of multiple sclerosis to alleles at the TAP2 locus. *Hum Immunol* 1994; **39**: 299–301.

66. Begovich AB, Helmuth RC, Oksenberg J et al. HLA-DPB and susceptibility to multiple sclerosis. An analysis of Caucasoid and Japanese patient populations. *Hum Immunol* 1990; **28**: 365–372.

67. Howell WM, Sage DA, Evans PR et al. No association between susceptibility to multiple sclerosis and HLA-DPB1 alleles in the French Canadian population. *Tissue Antigens* 1991; **37**: 156–160.

68. Kellar-Wood H, Robertson N, Govan GG et al. Leber's hereditary optic neuropathy mitochondrial DNA mutations in multiple sclerosis. *Ann Neurol* 1994; **36**: 109–112.

69. Hashimoto LL, Walter MA, Cox DW, Ebers GC. Immunoglobulin heavy chain variable region polymorphisms and multiple sclerosis susceptibility. *J Neuroimmunol* 1993; **44**: 77–84.

70. Walter MA, Gibson WT, Ebers GC, Cox DW. Susceptibility to multiple sclerosis is associated with the proximal immunoglobulin heavy chain variable region. *J Clin Invest* 1991; **87**: 1266–1273.

71. Tienari PJ, Wikstrom J, Sajantila A et al. Genetic susceptibility to multiple sclerosis linked to myelin basic protein gene. *Lancet* 1992; **340**: 987–991.

72. Tienari PJ, Tertwilliger JD, Ott J et al. Two-locus linkage analysis in multiple sclerosis (MS). *Genomics* 1994; **19**: 320–325.

73. Hockertz M, Paty D, Beall S. Susceptibility to relapsing-progressive multiple sclerosis is associated with inheritance of genes linked to the variable region of the TCR β locus: use of the affected family-based controls. *Am J Hum Genet* 1998; **62**: 373–385.

74. Beall S, Concannon P, Charmley P et al. The germline repertoire of T cell receptor B-chain genes in patients with chronic progressive multiple sclerosis. *J Neuroimmunol* 1989; **21**: 59–66.

75. Ebers GC, Sadovnick AD. Association studies in multiple sclerosis. *J Neuroimmunol* 1994; **53**: 117–122.

76. Spielman RS, McGinnis RE, Ewens WJ. Transmission test for linkage disequilibrium: the insulin gene region and insulin-dependent diabetes mellitus (IDDM). *Am J Hum Genet* 1993; **52**: 506–516.

77. Thomsen G. Mapping disease genes: family-based association studies. *Am J Hum Genet* 1995; **57**: 487–498.

78. Polymeropoulos MH, Higgens JJ, Golbe LI et al. Mapping of a gene for Parkinson's disease to chromosome 4q21-q23. *Science* 1996; **274**: 1197–1199.

79. Levy-Lahad E, Wijsman EM, Nemens E et al. A familial Alzheimer's disease locus on chromosome 1. *Science* 1995; **269**: 970–973.

80. Kibar Z, Kaloustian VM, Brais B et al. The gene responsible for Clouston hidrotic ectodermal dysplasia maps to the pericentromeric region of chromosome 13q. *Hum Mol Genet* 1996; **5**: 543–547.

81. Lim LE, Duclos F, Brous O et al. Beta-sarcoglycan: characterization and role in limb-girdle muscular dystrophy linked to 4q12. *Nat Genet* 1995; **11**: 257–267.

82. Puffenberger EG, Hosoda K, Washington SS et al. A missense mutation of the endothelin-B receptor gene in multigenic Hirschsprung's disease. *Cell* 1994; **79**: 1257–1266.

83. Hashimoto LL, Habita C, Beressi JP et al. Genetic mapping of a susceptibility locus for insulin-dependent diabetes mellitus on chromosome 11q. *Nature* 1994; **371**: 161–164.

84. Mein CA, Esposito L, Dunn MG et al. A search for type I diabetes susceptibility genes in families from the United Kingdom. *Nat Genet* 1998; **19**: 297–300.

85. Lernmark A, Ott J. Sometimes it's hot, sometimes it's not. *Nat Genet* 1998; **19**: 213–214.

86. Concannon P, Gogolin-Ewens KJ, Hinds DA et al. A second-generation screen of the human genome for susceptibility to insulin-dependent diabetes mellitus. *Nat Genet* 1998; **19**: 292–296.

2

Genetic control of experimental models of multiple sclerosis

Rikard Holmdahl

INTRODUCTION

The recent development in genetic techniques and the development of more proper animal models for multiple sclerosis (MS) makes it possible to use a new approach for understanding this complex group of diseases. The major histocompatibility complex (MHC) harbours the most important genes but their definite identity and biological role is not fully understood. Circumstantial evidence suggest that the class II genes are of importance but there may also be other contributing genes in the MHC. There is also an important contribution from non-MHC genes. Several new loci outside the MHC region have recently been identified. Some of these are shared between several autoimmune diseases; e.g. on mouse chromosome 3 (experimental allergic encephalomyelitis (EAE), Theiler's encephalomyelitis, diabetes mellitus and collagen-induced arthritis) and rat chromosome 4 (collagen-induced arthritis and myelin oligodendrocytic glycoprotein (MOG)-induced EAE). In addition, some of the loci found in the murine models have also been indicated in human MS. The identification of these new loci is likely to make a major contribution to the understanding of the basic mechanisms that lead to MS.

The genetic influence on MS is significant but weak, as seen in monozygotic twin studies. Studies of children adopted to families with MS[1] indicate a stronger genetic component. An important common genetic factor seems to be the MHC locus, and circumstantial evidence indicates a role for MHC class II genes. This finding has fuelled the hypothesis that these diseases are autoimmune in the sense that self-peptides are bound to the class II molecules and recognized by pathogenic T lymphocytes. However, such peptides or T cells have so far not been identified, and the basic mechanisms that cause and drive MS are not known. It is not only MHC that is responsible for the genetic influence: the diseases are most likely controlled by a large number of genes that have not yet been defined. If these genes could be isolated, new clues to the pathogenesis would most likely be forthcoming. However, it has so far been difficult to obtain significant evidence of linkage to genes outside MHC. Large genome screens have obtained some possible linkages of several loci, which may demonstrate a polygenic control.[2,3] Animal models would in this case provide a way of studying genes in a genetically and environmentally more controlled way.

Obviously, animal models will never be identical to the human disease and their main advantage is that they enable species-common biological pathways of critical pathological importance to be defined and studied. To be useful, the models should be selected to mimic critical features of MS. Thus, they should be induced rather than spontaneous, although we do not know the relevant inducing agents. They should also involve a chronic development of tissue-specific inflammation and be associated with MHC class II genes. Considerable efforts over the years have been undertaken to establish such models and they are used today as tools to dissect and understand the genetics of MS.[4–6]

EXPERIMENTAL ALLERGIC ENCEPHALOMYELITIS

EAE is induced after immunization with myelin proteins or myelin protein peptides, which triggers attack on the central nervous system by pathogenic T cells. The disease is controlled by the MHC region, and strong circumstantial evidence show that MHC class II genes are of importance.[7] The disease-susceptible allele varies with the inducing peptide, but association is also found after induction with homologous spinal cord homogenate in mineral oil only.[8,9] A gene coding for a MHC class II molecule with a capacity to bind certain myelin protein peptides explains the MHC association of the various EAE models. Such MHC class II molecule–peptide complexes are recognized by encephalitogenic T cells. However, the most important questions remain to be solved. One of these is how and why the T cell is activated into aggressiveness, as occurs in the pathological situation, and not into a 'tolerant' state, as occurs in the physiological situation. 'Tolerance' is used here in its broadest sense to mean any type of state that does not involve an uncontrolled inflammatory-inducing T-cell activity. The current dogma of how autoreactive T cells are selected has been challenged by the recent demonstration of expression of myelin basic protein in the thymus of adult and EAE-susceptible mice.[10] Another important issue is whether there are other genes in the

MHC region, which may control disease susceptibility. For example, it has been reported that MHC class I genes, and even certain MHC class II genes, also protect against disease by controlling activation of cytokine-secreting, regulatory T cells.[11–13]

Thus, despite the important role for MHC in both MS and in the EAE model, it is still not known which gene or genes are operating and what their exact role in the disease process is. The role of MHC class II genes in the further progression of the disease and the role of MHC class II and other MHC genes as regulatory genes are important issues for further studies.

For further genetic studies, variants of the models have been used in which a chronic or relapsing disease develops, as seen in MS. Animal strains that vary in disease susceptibility but that share the MHC region have been selected. The first crosses to be mapped were chronic relapsing EAE (CREAE) induced in the B10. RIII mouse strain by immunization with the myelin basic protein (MBP) peptide 89–101,[14] in the SJL strain with the proteolipoprotein (PLP) peptide 139–151[15] and in the Biozzi ABH strain with mouse spinal cord homogenate.[16] In a more recent study using a cross between Biozzi ABH and BALB/c, which differ in the MHC region, no loci reach significance but synergy effects between loci on chr 4, 8 and 17 demonstrate the complexity of the genetic influence.[17] In an alternative approach to compare substrains of BALB/c differing dramatically in EAE susceptibility, it was found that this difference was most likely controlled by only one locus.[18] The loci that have been reported as reaching significance on a genome-wide level[19] or confirmed in additional crosses or congenic experiments are listed in *Table 2.1*. Some of the loci were found in several of the crosses, in spite of the usage of different strain combinations and different induction protocols. Thus, the Eae2 locus was identified in the B10.RIII × RIIIS/J cross and was reproduced in the B10.S × SJL cross in spite of the usage of a different strain combination and a different induction protocol.[15]

In addition, the same region has been found to control susceptibility to murine leishmania-

Table 2.1 Significant loci of importance in MS models.

Locus*	Model	Cross	Other diseases	Candidates/homologies
Eae1 (chr 17)	EAE and CREAE	MHC congenic strains[7]	CIA[29]	MHC class II Homologous region in MS on chr 6[39]
Eae2 (chr 15)	CREAE	B10.RIII × RIIIS/J[14] B10.S × SJL[15]	Leishmaniasis in B10.D2 × BALB/c[30]	Homologous region in MS on chr 5[40]
Eae3 (chr 3)	CREAE	B10.RIII × RIIIS/J[14] B10.S × SJL[15]	CIA (Cia2) in B10.RIII × RIIIS/J,[31] NOD diabetes (Idd 10 or Idd17) in NOD × B6,[32] TMEVD (Tmevd2) in DBA/2 × BALB/c[24]	
Eae4 (chr 7)	CREAE	B10.S × SJL[20]	EAE in NOD × ABH[16]	
Eae5 (chr 17)	CREAE	B10.S × SJL[20]		Close to but different from MHC
Eae6 (chr 11)	CREAE	B10.S × SJL[20]		
Eae7 (chr 11)	CREAE	B10.S × SJL[20]	Diabetes in NOD × B6 (Idd4)[33] autoimmune orchitis in Balb/c × DBA/2 (Orch3)[34]	
Eae8 (chr 2)	CREAE	B10.S × SJL[20]		
Eae9 (chr 9)	CREAE	B10.S × SJL[20]	NOD diabetes (Idd2) in NOD × NON[35]	
Eae10 (chr 3)	CREAE	B10.S × SJL[20]		
Lpr (chr 19) and gld (chr 1)		Congenic strains[21]	Murine lupus[36]	Fas and Fas ligand
Tmevd1 (chr 17)	TMEVD	Recombinant inbred strains[22,23]		D-region of MHC[22]
Tmevd2 (chr 3)	TMEVD	DBA/2 × BALB/c[24,25]	CREAE (Eae3)[14] and CIA (Mcia2)[31]	
Tmevd3† (chr 6)	TMEVD	SJL × BALB/c[26] SJL × C57L[27]	CIA (Cia3)[37] and MOG-induced EAE[38] in rats	Close to but not involving TCRb locus[27]
Tmevd4† (chr 10)	TMEVD	SJL × B10.S[28] Congenic strains[6]		Interferon γ?[6]

*Only reported loci reaching significance on a genome-wide level,[19] or confirmed in additional crosses or congenic experiments.
†The designation has not been suggested in the original publications and is therefore used here only in a preliminary way.
chr, chromosome.

sis.[30] The Eae3 locus has also been observed in the B10. S × SJL cross. In addition this locus has been observed in several other autoimmune models such as Theiler's virus-induced encephalomyelitis (TMEVD),[24] spontaneous diabetes mellitus in the NOD mouse and in collagen-induced arthritis.[31] This could very well be explained by several susceptibility genes within this region but also by a shared autoimmune gene of importance in different diseases occurring in different mouse strains. Another potentially interesting quantitative trait locus that controls both arthritis and encephalomyelitis was recently reported in rats in which EAE was induced with MOG.[38] Most recently, several new loci associated with development of EAE was identified in a cross between the highly susceptible SJL and the resistant B10.S strains. Interestingly some of the loci preferentially controlled disease onset whereas other were more related to severity.

The homologous regions corresponding to the loci identified in the B10.RIII × RIIIS/J cross experiment were tested for an association with MS in a population isolate with high frequency of MS in Finland. Interestingly, the homologous region to Eae2, located on human 5p, showed significant association with MS[40] and some suggestive indications in this region was also found in genome screens of other populations.[2,3]

of CREAE and TMEVD are different in many aspects. The TMEVD disease is controlled by the MHC region, however, not by class II genes but by classical class I coded from the D region.[22] Other loci have subsequently been identified (see *Table 2.1*).[6,28,42] Of interest is the finding that the Tmevd2 locus on chromosome 3 corresponds closely with Eae3,[21] showing that at least some aspects of the disease are shared with CREAE. In addition, a suggestive linkage in the model is found around the MBP gene on chromosome 18,[28] where a corresponding linkage have been noted in a MS study.[43]

CONCLUSIONS

Clearly, the genetic dissection of multiple sclerosis is in its infancy. However, the recent development in genetic techniques as well as the improvement of animal models gives the basis for clarification of the genetic contribution. During recent years, such efforts have been initiated. It is now known that MHC class II genes are of importance but their role in pathogenesis is not yet known. In addition, a number of non-MHC loci associated with disease development have been identified, although the responsible genes have not been identified.

THEILER'S MURINE ENCEPHALOMYELITIS VIRUS DISEASE

The Theiler virus (first discovered by Max Theiler in 1933) was found to persist in the central nervous system and to be responsible for demyelinating encephalomyelitis in mice. With the possibility that a corresponding virus also causes MS, the model has important implications for studies on MS pathogenesis. Interestingly, a comparison of mouse strains susceptible to TMEVD and CREAE show an obvious disconcordance (e.g. the RIIIS/J strain is more susceptible than the B10.RIII for TMEVD but more resistant for CREAE.[41] This confirms the observation that the pathogenesis

Polygenicity

The diseases are polygenic and it is expected that a very large number of genes of importance for disease development will be found. Different human families carry different sets of genes of importance for their increased susceptibility to disease. Similarly, animal models in different inbred strain combinations are expected to use different sets of genes. Accordingly it is expected that correspondences between strains, between models and between species will be exceptions, but once identified they will certainly be of particular importance.

Interactions

Genetic interaction is a rule rather than an exception. Clearly, sets of genes rather than individual genes produce pathogenicity. This means that powerful techniques are needed to study gene interactions. One such tool is the isolation of loci in congenic strains; another is knock-in techniques, in which specified alleles can be created. Such mouse strains can be crossed and their interactions studied in detail. Such work has shown to be potent for studies of other diseases.[44] and is in progress for studies of MS models.

Which genes do we expect?

The beauty of the genetic approach is that it can identify biological pathways that are not known to be of importance in the pathogenesis. No polymorphic disease-controlling genes has so far been identified, although one strong candidate is MHC class II. Hopes of identifying T-cell receptor genes as major loci for disease control have so far not been fulfilled. The development of MS, or the animal models, are clearly not physiological processes occurring according to a normal immune and inflammatory response to infectious agents or injected proteins. Rather, the diseases involve a pathological component that involves a lack of control of the response and an ensuing chronic development of inflammation. Thus, the most interesting genes may not be those controlling the normal inflammatory response, which presumably occur also in the central nervous system in response to infections, but rather genes that will not turn off the response properly. This is probably dependent on an immune response to persistent foreign pathogens or self-structures in the target organs, which needs to be defined in parallel as well.

ACKNOWLEDGEMENTS

The completion of this review was possible thanks to grants from the Kock and Österlund research foundations, the Swedish Medical Research Council and the EU (BMH4-CT97-2522 and ERBBIO4CT960562).

REFERENCES

1. Ebers GC, Sadovnick AD, Risch NJ, Group CCS. A genetic basis for familial aggregation in multiple sclerosis. *Nature* 1995; **377**: 150–151.
2. Sawcer S, Jones HB, Feakes R et al. A genome screen in multiple sclerosis reveals susceptibility loci on chromosome 6p21 and 17q22. *Nat Genet* 1996; **13**: 464–468.
3. Ebers GC, Kukay K, Bulman DE et al. A full genome search in multiple sclerosis. *Nat Genet* 1996; **13**: 472–476.
4. Holmdahl R, Jirholt J, Jansson L, Sundvall M. Genetic analysis of murine models for multiple sclerosis. In: Dragani TA, ed. *Human Polygenic Diseases: Animal Models.* Amsterdam: Harwood Academic Publisher, 1998; 131–146.
5. Martin R, McFarland HF, McFarlin DE. Immunological aspects of demyelinating diseases. *Annu Rev Immunol* 1992; **10**: 153–187.
6. Monteyne P, Bureau JF, Brahic M. The infection of mouse by Theiler's virus: from genetics to immunology. *Immunol Rev* 1997; **159**: 163–176.
7. Fritz RB, Skeen MJ, Chou CHJ et al. Major histocompatibility complex-linked control of the murine immune response to myelin basic protein. *J Immunol* 1985; **134**: 2328–2332.
8. Lorentzen JC, Andersson M, Issazadeh S et al. Genetic analysis of inflammation, cytokine mRNA expression and disease course of relapsing experimental autoimmune encephalomyelitis in DA rats. *J Neuroimmunol* 1997; **80**: 31–37.
9. Kjellén P, Issazadeh S, Olsson T, Holmdahl R. Genetic influence on disease course and cytokine response in relapsing experimental allergic encephalomyelitis. *Int Immunol* 1998; **10**: 333–340.
10. Fritz RB, Zhao ML. Thymic expression of myelin basic protein (MBP). Activation of MBP-specific T cells by thymic cells in the absence of exogenous MBP. *J Immunol* 1996; **157**: 5249–5253.
11. Mustafa M, Vingsbo C, Olsson T et al. Protective influences on experimental autoimmune encephalomyelitis by MHC class I and class II alleles. *J Immunol* 1994; **153**: 3337–3344.
12. Mustafa M, Vingsbo C, Olsson T et al. The major histocompatibility complex influences myelin

basic protetin 63-88-induced T cell cytokine profile and experimental autoimmune encephalomyelitis. *Eur J Immunol* 1993; **23**: 3089–3095.

13. Issazadeh S, Kjellén P, Olsson T et al. Major histocompatibility complex-controlled protective influences on experimental autoimmune encephalomyelitis are peptide specific. *Eur J Immunol* 1997; **27**: 1584–1587.

14. Sundvall M, Jirholt J, Yang HT et al. Identification of murine loci associated with susceptibility to chronic experimental autoimmune encephalomyelitis. *Nat Genet* 1995; **10**: 313–317.

15. Encinas JA, Lees MB, Sobel RA et al. Genetic analysis of susceptibility to experimental autoimmune encephalomyelitis in a cross between SJL/J and B10.S mice. *J Immunol* 1996; **157**: 2186–2192.

16. Baker D, Rosenwasser OA, O'Neill JK, Turk JL. Genetic analysis of experimental allergic encephalomyelitis in mice. *J Immunol* 1995; **155**: 4046–4051.

17. Croxford JL, O'Neill JK, Baker D. Polygenic control of experimental allergic encephalomyelitis in Biozzi ABH and BALB/c mice. *J Neuroimmunol* 1997; **74**: 205–211.

18. Teuscher C, Hickey WF, Grafer CM, Tung KS. A common immunoregulatory locus controls susceptibility to actively induced experimental allergic encephalomyelitis and experimental allergic orchitis in BALB/c mice. *J Immunol* 1998; **160**: 2751–2756.

19. Lander ES, Kruglyak L. Genetic dissection of complex traits: guidelines for interpreting and reporting linkage results. *Nat Genet* 1996; **11**: 241–247.

20. Butterfield RJ, Sudweeks JD, Blankenhorn EP et al. New genetic loci that control susceptibility and symptoms of experimental allergic encephalomyelitis in inbred mice. *J Immunol* 1998; **161**: 1860–1867.

21. Sabelko KA, Kelly KA, Nahm MH et al. Fas and Fas ligand enhance the pathogenesis of experimental allergic encephalomyelitis, but are not essential for immune privilege in the central nervous system. *J Immunol* 1997; **159**: 3096–3099.

22. Rodriguez M, Leibowitz J, David CS. Susceptibility to Theiler's virus-induced demyelination. Mapping of the gene within the H-2D region. *J Exp Med* 1986; **163**: 620–631.

23. Nicholson SM, Jokinen DM, Dal Canto MC et al. Genetic analysis of susceptibility to Theiler's murine encephalomyelitis virus-induced demyelinating disease in the SWR strain. *J Neuroimmunol* 1995; **59**: 19–28.

24. Teuscher C, Rhein DM, Livingstone KD et al. Evidence that Tmevd2 and eae3 may represent either a common locus or members of a gene complex controlling susceptibility to immunologically mediated demyelination in mice. *J Immunol* 1997; **159**: 4930–4934.

25. Melvold RW, Jokinen DM, Miller SD et al. Identification of a locus on mouse chromosome 3 involved in differential susceptibility to Theiler's murine encephalomyelitis virus-induced demyelinating disease. *J Virol* 1990; **64**: 686–690.

26. Melvold RW, Jokinen DM, Knobler RL, Lipton HL. Variations in genetic control of susceptibility to Theiler's murine encephalomyelitis virus (TMEV)-induced demyelinating disease. I. Differences between susceptible SJL/J and resistant BALB/c strains map near the T cell beta-chain constant gene on chromosome 6. *J Immunol* 1987; **138**: 1429–1433.

27. Bahk YY, Kappel CA, Rasmussen G, Kim BS. Association between susceptibility to Theiler's virus-induced demyelination and T-cell receptor Jbeta1-Cbeta1 polymorphism rather than Vbeta deletion. *J Virol* 1997; **71**: 4181–4185.

28. Bureau JF, Montagutelli X, Bihl F et al. Mapping loci influencing the persistence of Theiler's virus in the murine central nervous system. *Nat Genet* 1993; **5**: 87–91.

29. Brunsberg U, Gustafsson K, Jansson L et al. Expression of a transgenic class II Ab gene confers susceptibility to collagen-induced arthritis. *Eur J Immunol* 1994; **24**: 1698–1702.

30. Beebe AM, Mauze S, Schork NJ, Coffman RL. Serial backcross mapping of multiple loci associated with resistance to *Leishmania major* in mice. *Immunity* 1997; **6**: 551–557.

31. Jirholt J, Cook A, Sundvall M et al. Evidence for a susceptibility locus to collagen induced arthritis on mouse chromosome 3: a common susceptibility locus in multiple autoimmune disorders. *Eur J Immunol* 1998; **28**: 3321–3328.

32. Podolin PL, Denny P, Lord CJ et al. Congenic mapping of the insulin-dependent diabetes (Idd) gene, Idd10, localizes two genes mediating the Idd10 effect and eliminates the candidate Fcgr1. *J Immunol* 1997; **159**: 1835–1843.

33. Todd JA, Aitman T, Cornall R et al. Genetic analysis of autoimmune type 1 diabetes mellitus in mice. *Nature* 1991; **351**: 542–547.

34. Meeker ND, Hickey WF, Korngold R et al. Multiple loci govern the bone marrow-derived immunoregulatory mechanism controlling dom-

inant resistance to autoimmune orchitis. *Proc Natl Acad Sci USA* 1995; **92**: 5684–5688.

35. Prochazka M, Leiter EH, Serreze DV, Coleman DL. Three recessive loci required for insulin-dependent diabetes in nonobese diabetic mice [published erratum appears in *Science* 1988; **242**: 945]. *Science* 1987; **237**: 286–289.

36. Watanabe-Fukunaga R, Brannan C, Copeland N et al. Lymphoproliferation disorder in mice explained by defects in Fas antigen that mediates apoptosis. *Nature* 1992; **356**: 314–317.

37. Remmers EF, Longman RE, Du Y et al. A genome scan localizes five non-MHC loci controlling collagen-induced arthritis in rats. *Nat Genet* 1996; **14**: 82–85.

38. Dahlman I, Lorentzen JC, de Graaf KL et al. Quantitative trait loci disposing for both experimental arthritis and encephalomyelitis in the DA rat; impact on severity of myelin oligodendrocyte glycoprotein-induced experimental autoimmune encephalomyelitis and antibody isotype pattern. *Eur J Immunol* 1998; **28**: 2188–2196.

39. Haines JL, Pericak-Vance MA, Seboun E et al. A complete genomic screen for multiple sclerosis underscores a role for the major histocompatibility complex. *Nat Genet* 1996; **13**: 469–471.

40. Kuokkanen S, Sundvall M, Terwilliger JD et al. A putative vulnerability locus to multiple sclerosis maps to 5p14–p12 in a region syntenic to the murine locus Eae2. *Nat Genet* 1996; **13**: 477–480.

41. Rodriguez M, Patick AK, Pease LR, David CS. Role of T cell receptor V beta genes in Theiler's virus-induced demyelination of mice. *J Immunol* 1992; **148**: 921–927.

42. Bureau JF, Drescher KM, Pease LR et al. Chromosome 14 contains determinants that regulate susceptibility to Theiler's virus-induced demyelination in the mouse. *Genetics* 1998; **148**: 1941–1949.

43. Tienari PJ, Kuokkanen S, Pastinen T et al. Golli-MBP gene in multiple sclerosis susceptibility. *J Neuroimmunol* 1998; **81**: 158–167.

44. Morel L, Mohan C, Yu Y et al. Functional dissection of systemic lupus erythematosus using congenic mouse strains. *J Immunol* 1997; **158**: 6019–6028.

PART II

Immunology

3

Oligodendrocyte injury and the role of complement in multiple sclerosis

Neil J Scolding

INTRODUCTION

Complement was first implicated in the pathogenesis of tissue damage in multiple sclerosis (MS) almost 40 years ago, and it may therefore appear surprising to include this topic in a symposium concentrating on 'the *new* immunology of MS'. However, the precise mechanisms responsible for damaging oligodendrocytes remain—despite this long history—obscure. Recently, an increasing number of candidates have been proposed, but evidence pointing to a significant role for complement has also continued to accumulate, and it is timely and worthwhile to attempt a reassessment of these diverse observations.

A similar or indeed a greater degree of uncertainty surrounds the cause of MS and, in the absence of an aetiological understanding, treatments aimed at prevention or cure of the disease can only be wholly speculative.

At present, therefore, therapeutic efforts largely concentrate on immune manipulation and damage limitation, an approach that has produced only modest effects in MS, despite its considerable success in other neurological inflammatory disorders such as myasthenia gravis and demyelinating neuropathies. One reason for this must be the superior understanding of the mechanisms underlying immune damage in these other disorders, and this provides a yet more compelling reason to redirect attention to the oligodendrocyte–myelin unit, and to explore further the direct reasons for its demise in MS.

OLIGODENDROCYTE INJURY IN MULTIPLE SCLEROSIS

Classical descriptions of the histopathology of disseminated sclerosis, including those by both Dawson and Charcot, established myelin loss as the core feature. However, these studies antedated the discovery of the oligodendrocyte and recognition of its function as the central nervous system (CNS) glia responsible for myelin synthesis.[1] Del Rio Hortega[1] himself pointed out that oligodendrocytes were absent in Schilder's disease, perhaps the least well-defined of the 'multiple sclerosis variants', but soon after this it became clear that oligodendrocytes—as well as myelin—were conspicuously absent in chronic plaques.[2]

However, the precise timing of oligodendrocyte loss in acute lesions has remained a matter of some uncertainty and indeed controversy, with reports of increased, decreased or unchanged numbers.[3–6] This inconsistency has arisen for various reasons, some technical, including the difficulty of confident recognition of oligodendrocytes, the precise age and stage of lesions studied and the criteria adopted for this staging, and the type and mode of preservation of tissue. The issue of remyelination has also complicated matters: oligodendrocyte progenitors appear to migrate into lesions early in the course of inflammation and mature into myelinating oligodendrocytes, which therefore appear in increased numbers; whether this increase is accompanied by a parallel loss or a preservation of local oligodendrocytes is extremely difficult to determine. It is, however, suggested by some authors that there is indeed very early oligodendrocyte loss in lesions, which is very rapidly followed by repopulation by oligodendrocyte lineage cells.[2,7,8]

An additional aspect of cell damage—cell injury—must also be considered. Cell injury is a disturbance of cell function that may be reversible and does not necessarily lead to cell death. Myelin is a living membrane that is wholly dependent on its contacts with and support from the parent oligodendrocyte soma: it is, put simply, a highly specialized cellular extension of the oligodendrocyte. Myelin is, of course, temporarily injured in MS (perhaps best illustrated by the conduction delay apparent when visual evoked potentials are recorded) and it is therefore appropriate to consider which types of inflammatory mediator may be capable of reversibly injuring the myelin–oligodendrocyte unit.

Finally, despite the uncertainty surrounding the mediators of myelin–oligodendrocyte injury in MS, there is one clearly established and proven culprit: the phagocytic macrophage. Light and electron microscopic studies have consistently shown these cells to be responsible for engulfing myelin, stripping away lamellae from the myelin sheath.[9] It is unlikely that this process affects entirely normal myelin, however, so a third aspect of exploring myelin–oligodendrocyte damage is to consider the means by which myelin is opsonized, a prerequisite for macrophage–microgial attack.

Mediators of oligodendrocyte–myelin injury

Before considering the potential involvement of complement, it should first be emphasized that there is no reason whatsoever to suppose that complement—or indeed any other immune effector—might be *solely* responsible for oligodendrocyte–myelin injury. Although space prevents any detailed consideration here, there is extremely good evidence from in vitro studies that oligodendrocytes are unusually susceptible to injury by other mediators, including tumour necrosis factor borne on the surface of microglia,[10,11] nitric oxide[12] and perforin.[13] These molecules have variably also been implicated in experimental allergic encephalomyelitis (EAE) or shown to be present in MS lesions.[14]

It seems overwhelmingly likely that all these mediators may contribute to oligodendrocyte–myelin damage in MS. It may indeed be speculated that the extent to which each is involved may vary at different stages of the disease and between different patients, and that this variability in the mechanisms underlying cell damage may be one of the factors that underlies the pathological diversity or heterogeneity of lesions in MS.

COMPLEMENT AND OLIGODENDROCYTES

Complement is a group of serum proteins that circulate in an inactive form. Activation is initiated classically by antibody but also by an alternative pathway, and results in the formation of vasoactive and chemotactic peptides and terminal membrane attack complexes, which may injure or lyse target cells. It is important to recall that the effector functions of activated complement components include not only cell lysis, but also (among others) opsonization of target membranes triggering macrophage adhesion (*Fig. 3.1*). Both functions will be considered; first the unique relationship between oligodendrocytes and complement will be discussed.

Complement-dependent oligodendrocyte–myelin damage in vitro by serum from rodents with EAE was first demonstrated almost 40 years ago;[15] later ultrastructural studies

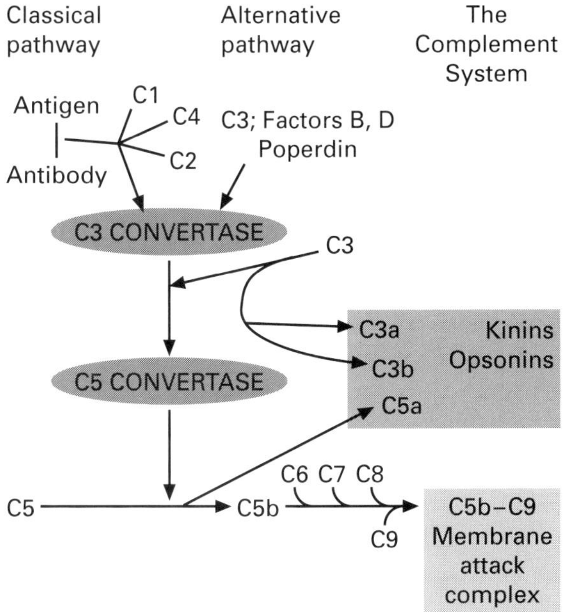

Figure 3.1 The complement cascade.

confirmed selective lysis of oligodendrocytes.[6,16] CNS myelin was subsequently shown to trigger antibody-independent classical pathway complement activation;[17–19] shortly after this, cultured rat oligodendrocytes were found to exhibit a unique sensitivity to complement: exposure to normal syngeneic serum also triggered classical pathway complement activation in the absence of antibody, leading to cell lysis.[16,20] The surface component responsible for activating complement remained elusive, but recent evidence that myelin oligodendrocyte glycoprotein (MOG) might bind native C1q has been presented.[21]

It appears, however, that many cell types exhibit a similar complement-activating capacity, but most are not lysed as a consequence. The explanation for this emerged from studies of the complement regulator CD59. This ubiquitously distributed surface protein, one of a number of complement regulatory molecules, inhibits membrane attack complex function, affording potent protection against homologous complement attack. Rat oligodendrocytes were found to lack CD59, resulting in an increased

susceptibility to injury by terminal complement membrane attack complexes.[22–24]

Attempts to extrapolate these findings to human glia proved complex. Human oligodendrocytes are not lysed when exposed to serum.[25,26] However, they do lack numerous surface complement regulatory proteins responsible for limiting activation and inhibiting membrane attack complex activity, including CR1 and MCP; a sub-population also lacks CD59 (*Fig. 3.2*),[27] suggesting they are likely to share with their rodent counterparts an increased susceptibility to complement. Purified CNS myelin shows a broadly comparable pattern of deficiency of complement regulatory proteins.[28] Furthermore, complement activation in vivo in the human CNS does occur when serum meets CNS parenchyma after blood–brain barrier breakdown.[29]

Complement and oligodendrocyte–myelin injury

Three aspects of oligodendrocyte–myelin injury and the potential involvement of complement will be considered: cell lysis, opsonization and, as mentioned above, reversible oligodendrocyte injury.

Oligodendrocyte lysis

Proving that oligodendrocyte lysis is caused by complement in vivo in MS may not be experimentally possible. Disclosing and indeed explaining a susceptibility in vitro is plainly insufficient. There is consistent evidence for intrathecal complement activation in MS, shown in spinal fluid samples by a decrease in native complement components and an increase in activation products.[30–34] Deposits of C9 and complement membrane attack complex within lesions have also been found,[35] but this too amounts only to circumstantial evidence. More recent careful immunohistochemical studies have demonstrated C9-neoantigen deposits in areas of active myelin destruction, accompanied by loss (albeit incomplete) of oligodendrocytes, perhaps the best evidence yet directly implicating complement.[36]

It is unknown whether or not complement

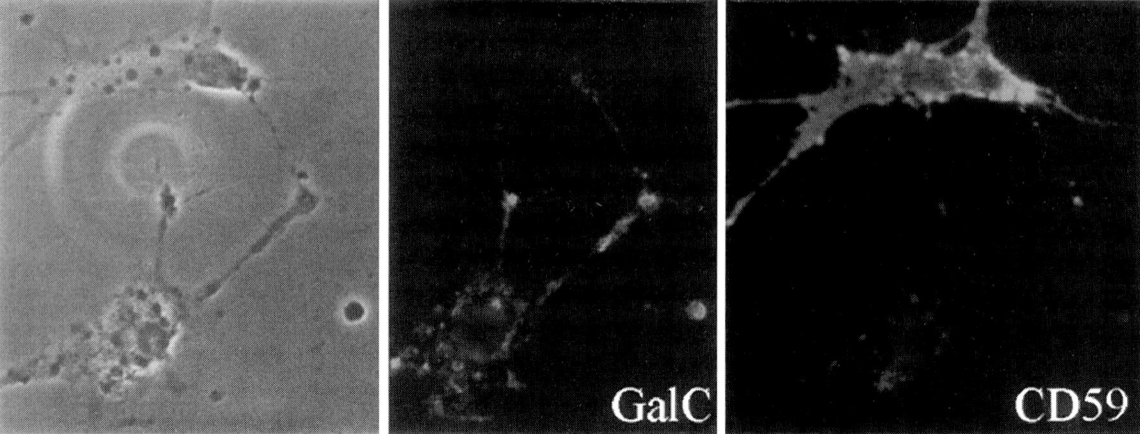

Figure 3.2 Heterogeneity of expression of CD59 by cultured human oligodendrocytes. Cultured human oligodendrocytes have been immunostained for surface CD59 (far right) and galactocerebroside (middle panel). The lower cell is an oligodendrocyte, and is CD59-negative; the GalC-negative upper cell, probably an astrocyte, serves as a useful positive control, staining clearly for CD59.

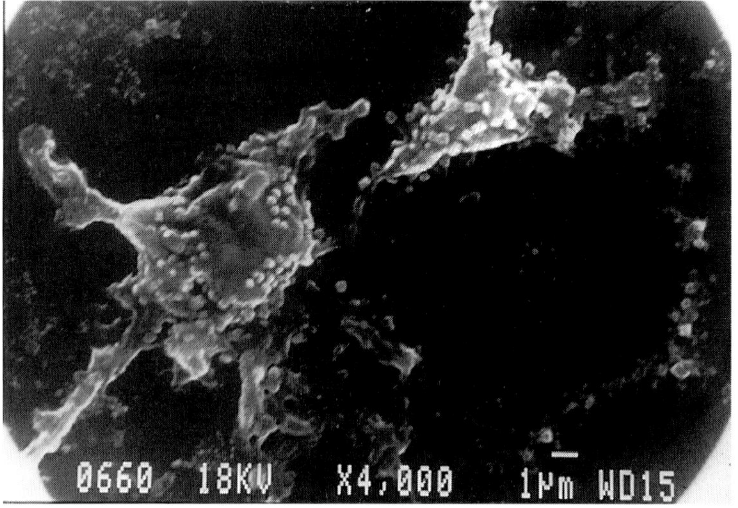

Figure 3.3 Reversible oligodendrocyte injury by complement. Cultured rat oligodendrocytes are illustrated by scanning electron microscopy. Minutes after exposure to low-level complement attack, the surface of the cells become covered by vesicles, which are subsequently shed. Similar oligodendrocyte-derived vesicles, rich in complement pore-forming membrane attack complexes, have been recovered from spinal fluid samples of patients with MS.

activation is direct, via surface contact with oligodendrocytes or mediated by antibody. The presence of antibodies to various myelin–oligo-dendrocyte antigens in the spinal fluid and blood of patients with MS[37] and the presence of immunoglobulin in lesions (again, particularly in areas of myelin destruction and, most clearly, on the surface of oligodendrocytes)[38,39] indicates that conventional classical pathway activation on the surface of oligodendrocytes in MS is very likely. Very recent studies have provided powerful evidence implicating myelin–oligo-dendrocyte–glycoprotein specific antibodies in MS (Cedric Raine, personal communication).

Oligodendrocyte–myelin opsonization

In vitro studies have also shed light on the opsonizing function of complement in relation to oligodendrocyte injury. Oligodendrocytes exposed to complement become coated with the opsonin C3b.[40] Co-culture of opsonized oligodendrocytes with resting macrophages or microglia triggers the adhesion of these phagocytic cells to the oligodendrocyte surface and the appearance of myelin components within the phagocytes—phenomena not seen when macrophages and oligodendrocytes are co-cultured without opsonins.[10,41]

As mentioned above, myelin stripping and phagocytosis by activated macrophages and microglia clearly accounts for much myelin removal in MS. Although antibody opsonization is apparent, it has also been demonstrated that complement fragment deposition contributes to opsonization of myelin in acute lesions.[42]

Reversible oligodendrocyte–myelin injury

Lysis is not the only possible consequence of complement attack: more subtle effects can also occur in response to both antibody-dependent and antibody-independent complement injury.[43] The first discernible event during cell injury by complement membrane attack complexes is the induction of a rapid rise in intracellular calcium.[44] This may be followed in oligodendrocytes by a series of calcium oscillations.[45] Calcium is an important second messenger, and the calcium transient(s) may precipitate a number of consequences. Perhaps the most important is the engagement of an effective cellular protective mechanism:[46] the injurious complement membrane attack complexes are gathered together in patches on the cell surface, and these are then extruded in the form of vesicles (*Fig. 3.3*).[47] In this way, oligodendrocytes that are exposed in vitro to concentrations of serum below a certain (lytic) threshold resist permanent damage or death by autologous complement attack.

The repair strategy appears energy dependent,[44] and the continuation of intracellular calcium transients for 30 minutes or more implies that complement-mediated cell injury may have significant, albeit temporary, consequences for oligodendrocyte function, and therefore for myelin function as well. Oligodendrocytes possess a number of calcium-dependent enzymes, including a neutral protease responsible for myelin breakdown[48] and a myelin protein kinase,[49] so that the complement-induced calcium changes might be predicted to disturb significantly the function of the oligodendrocyte–myelin unit. Indeed the calcium ionophore ionomycin induces CNS demyelination in vivo.[50]

Cultured oligodendrocytes have been shown to release pro-inflammatory leukotrienes from their cell surface as a consequence of sublethal complement attack;[51,52] enhanced degradation of messenger RNA encoding myelin proteins has also been demonstrated.[53] The immediate early gene *c-jun* becomes activated during sublytic injury, and this in turn induces the oligodendrocyte to enter the S-phase of the cell cycle[54] and, fascinatingly, confers protection against otherwise-mediated apoptoic cell death.

Furthermore, the presence in spinal fluid samples from patients with MS of vesicular membrane material rich in galactocerebroside (an oligodendrocyte membrane specific glycolipid) and bearing numerous membrane attack complexes (i.e. identical to the vesicles released by sublethally injured oligodendrocytes in vitro) provides more direct evidence of complement injury of oligodendrocytes in vivo in MS.[47]

CONCLUSIONS

In the past, the uncertainty concerning the fate of oligodendrocytes in acute MS lesions fuelled considerable speculation as to whether disease processes were targeted on oligodendrocytes or myelin. More recently, many have preferred simply to consider MS as a disease of the oligodendrocyte–myelin unit, which is, of course, a functional singularity. The spread of immune responses in the course of the disease[55] and increasing suspicion that different oligodendrocyte–myelin target antigens may be involved in initiating disease in different patients also diminishes the importance of this argument. In this brief review, the substantial body of information concerning the relationship of the oligodendrocyte–myelin unit and complement has been considered, and the various lines of experimental evidence independently implicating complement in oligodendrocyte lysis, opsonization of the oligodendrocyte–myelin unit and reversible injury have been rehearsed. Whether complement contributes equally to these different facets of immune damage, and the extent to which the role of complement varies between different patients, different lesions and at different stages of the disease, and whether this new information will yield a useful therapeutic dividend will, it is hoped, be revealed by the next few decades of complement research.

REFERENCES

1. Del Rio Hortega P. Tercera aportacia al conocimiento morfológico e interpretación funcional de la oligodendroglia. *Mem Real Soc Exp Hist Nat* 1928; **14**: 5–122.
2. Lumsden CE. Fundamental problems in the pathology of multiple sclerosis and allied demyelinating diseases. *Br Med J* 1951; **1**: 1035–1043.
3. Prineas JW. Pathology of the early lesion in multiple sclerosis. *Hum Pathol* 1975; **6**: 531–554.
4. Prineas JW, Kwon EE, Goldenberg PZ. Multiple sclerosis: oligodendrocyte proliferation and differentiation in fresh lesions. *Lab Invest* 1989; **61**: 489–503.
5. Raine CS, Scheinberg L, Waltz JM. Multiple sclerosis. Oligodendrocyte survival and proliferation in an active established lesion. *Lab Invest* 1981; **45**: 534–546.
6. Raine CS. The Norton Lecture: a review of the oligodendrocyte in the multiple sclerosis lesion. *J Neuroimmunol* 1997; **77**: 135–152.
7. Ozawa K, Suchanek G, Breitschopf H et al. Patterns of oligodendroglia pathology in multiple sclerosis. *Brain* 1994; **117**: 1311–1322.
8. Prineas JW, Barnard RO, Kwon EE et al. Multiple sclerosis: remyelination of nascent lesions. *Ann Neurol* 1993; **33**: 137–151.
9. Prineas JW. The neuropathology of multiple sclerosis. In: Vincken PJ, Bruyn GW, Klawans HL, eds. *Demyelinating Diseases.* Amsterdam: Elsevier Science, 1985; 213–257.
10. Zajicek JP, Wing M, Scolding NJ, Compston DAS. Interactions between oligodendrocytes and microglia. A major role for complement and tumour necrosis factor in oligodendrocyte adherence and killing. *Brain* 1992; **115**: 1611–1631.
11. Hofman FM, Hinton DR, Johnson K, Merrill JE. Tumor necrosis factor identified in multiple sclerosis brain. *J Exp Med* 1989; **170**: 607–612.
12. Parkinson JF, Mitrovic B, Merrill JE. The role of nitric oxide in multiple sclerosis. *J Mol Med* 1997; **75**: 174–186.
13. Scolding NJ, Jones J, Compston DAS, Morgan BP. Oligodendrocyte susceptibility to injury by T-cell perforin. *Immunology* 1990; **70**: 6–10.
14. Merril JE, Scolding NJ. Mechanisms of damage to myelin and oligodendrocytes and their relevance to disease. *Neuropathol Appl Neurobiol* 1999; in press.
15. Bornstein M, Appel SH. The application of tissue culture to the study of experimental allergic encephalomyelitis. I. Patterns of demyelination. *J Neuropathol Exp Neurol* 1961; **20**: 141–150.
16. Scolding NJ, Morgan BP, Houston A et al. Normal rat serum cytotoxicity against syngeneic oligodendrocytes. Complement activation and attack in the absence of anti-myelin antibodies. *J Neurol Sci* 1989; **89**: 289–300.
17. Cyong JC, Witkin SS, Rieger B et al. Antibody-independent complement activation by myelin via the classical complement pathway. *J Exp Med* 1982; **155**: 587–598.
18. Vanguri P, Koski CL, Silverman B, Shin ML. Complement activation by isolated myelin: activation of the classical pathway in the absence of myelin-specific antibodies. *Proc Natl Acad Sci USA* 1982; **79**: 3290–3294.
19. Vanguri P, Shin ML. Activation of complement by myelin: identification of C1-binding proteins of human myelin from central nervous tissue. *J Neurochem* 1986; **46**: 1535–1541.
20. Scolding NJ, Morgan BP, Campbell AK, Compston DAS. Complement mediated serum cytotoxicity against oligodendrocytes: a comparison with other cells of the oligodendrocyte-type 2 astrocyte lineage. *J Neurol Sci* 1990; **97**: 155–162.
21. Johns TG, Bernard CC. Binding of complement component C1q to myelin oligodendrocyte glycoprotein: a novel mechanism for regulating CNS inflammation. *Mol Immunol* 1997; **34**: 33–38.
22. Piddlesden SJ, Morgan BP. Killing of rat glial cells by complement: deficiency of the rat analogue of CD59 is the cause of oligodendrocyte susceptibility to lysis. *J Neuroimmunol* 1993; **48**: 169–176.

23. Wing MG, Zajicek J, Seilly DJ et al. Oligodendrocytes lack glycolipid anchored proteins which protect them against complement lysis. Restoration of resistance to lysis by incorporation of CD59. *Immunology* 1992; **76**: 140–145.

24. Zajicek J, Wing MG, Lachmann PJ, Compston DAS. Mechanisms of oligodendrocyte interaction with normal human serum—defining the role of complement. *J Neurol Sci* 1992; **108**: 65–72.

25. Ruijs TCG, Olivier A, Antel JP. Serum cytotoxicity to human and rat oligodendrocytes in culture. *Brain Res* 1990; **517**: 99–104.

26. Zajicek J, Wing M, Skepper J, Compston A. Human oligodendrocytes are not sensitive to complement: a study of CD59 expression in the human central nervous system. *Lab Invest* 1995; **73**: 128–138.

27. Scolding NJ, Morgan BP, Compston DA. The expression of complement regulatory proteins by adult human oligodendrocytes. *J Neuroimmunol* 1998; **84**: 69–75.

28. Koski CL, Estep AE, SawantMane S et al. Complement regulatory molecules on human myelin in glial cells: differential expression affects the deposition of activated complement proteins. *J Neurochem* 1996; **66**: 303–312.

29. Bellander BM, Von Holst H, Fredman P, Svensson M. Activation of the complement cascade and increase of clustering in the brain following a cortical contusion in the adult rat. *J Neurosurg* 1996; **85**: 468–475.

30. Compston DA, Morgan BP, Oleesky D et al. Cerebrospinal fluid C9 in demyelinating disease. *Neurology* 1986; **36**: 1503–1506.

31. Jans H, Heltberg A, Zeeberg I et al. Immune complexes and the complement factors C4 and C3 in cerebrospinal fluid and serum from patients with chronic progressive multiple sclerosis. *Acta Neurol Scand* 1984; **69**: 34–38.

32. Mollnes TE, Vandvik B, Lea T, Vartdal F. Intrathecal complement activation in neurological diseases evaluated by analysis of the terminal complement complex. *J Neurol Sci* 1987; **78**: 17–28.

33. Morgan BP, Campbell AK, Compston DA. Terminal component of complement (C9) in cerebrospinal fluid of patients with multiple sclerosis. *Lancet* 1984; **2**: 251–254.

34. Sanders ME, Koski CL, Robbins D et al. Activated terminal complement in cerebrospinal fluid in Guillain–Barré syndrome and multiple sclerosis. *J Immunol* 1986; **136**: 4456–4459.

35. Compston DAS, Morgan BP, Campbell AK et al. Immunocytochemical localization of the terminal complement complex in multiple sclerosis. *Neuropathol Appl Neurobiol* 1989; **15**: 307–316.

36. Storch MK, Piddlesden S, Haltia M et al. Multiple sclerosis: in situ evidence for antibody and complement-mediated demyelination. *Ann Neurol* 1998; **43**: 465–471.

37. Olsson T. Immunology of multiple sclerosis. *Curr Opin Neurol Neurosurg* 1992; **5**: 195–202.

38. Prineas JW, Graham JS. Multiple sclerosis: capping of surface immunoglobulin G on macrophages engaged in myelin breakdown. *Ann Neurol* 1981; **10**: 149–158.

39. Prineas JW, Raine CS. Electron microscopy and immunoperoxidase studies of early multiple sclerosis lesions. *Neurology* 1976; **26**: 29–32.

40. Agoropoulou C, Wing MG, Wood A. CD59 expression and complement susceptibility of human neuronal cell line (NTera2). *Neuroreport* 1996; **7**: 997–1004.

41. Scolding NJ, Compston DAS. Oligodendrocyte–macrophage interactions in vitro triggered by specific antibodies. *Immunology* 1991; **72**: 127–132.

42. Gay D, Esiri M. Blood–brain barrier damage in acute multiple sclerosis plaques. An immunocytological study. *Brain* 1991; **114**: 557–572.

43. Morgan BP. Complement membrane attack on nucleated cells: resistance, recovery and nonlethal effects. *Biochem J* 1989; **264**: 1–14.

44. Scolding NJ, Houston WAJ, Morgan BP et al. Reversible injury of cultured rat oligodendrocytes by complement. *Immunology* 1989; **67**: 441–446.

45. Wood A, Wing MG, Benham CD, Compston DA. Specific induction of intracellular calcium oscillations by complement membrane attack on oligodendroglia. *J Neurosci* 1993; **13**: 3319–3332.

46. Scolding NJ, Morgan BP, Campbell AK, Compston DA. The role of calcium in rat oligodendrocyte injury and repair. *Neurosci Lett* 1992; **135**: 95–98.

47. Scolding NJ, Morgan BP, Houston WAJ et al. Vesicular removal by oligodendrocytes of membrane attack complexes formed by activated complement. *Nature* 1989; **339**: 620–622.

48. Banik NL, McAlhaney WW, Hogan EL. Calcium-stimulated proteolysis in myelin: evidence for a Ca^{2+}-activated neutral proteinase associated with purified myelin of rat CNS. *J Neurochem* 1985; **45**: 581–588.

49. Turner RS, Chou CH, Kibler RF, Kuo JF. Basic protein in brain myelin is phosphorylated by endogenous phospholipid-sensitive Ca^{2+}-dependent protein kinase. *J Neurochem* 1982; **39**: 1397–1404.

50. Smith KJ, Hall SM. Central demyelination induced in vivo by the calcium ionophore ionomycin. *Brain* 1994; **117**: 1351–1356.

51. Shirazi Y, Imagawa DK, Shin ML. Release of leukotriene B4 from sublethally injured oligodendrocytes by terminal complement complexes. *J Neurochem* 1987; **48**: 271–278.

52. Shirazi Y, McMorris FA, Shin ML. Arachidonic acid mobilization and phosphoinositide turnover by the terminal complement complex, C5b-9, in rat oligodendrocyte C6 glioma cell hybrids. *J Immunol* 1989; **142**: 4385–4391.

53. Shirazi Y, Rus HG, Macklin WB, Shin ML. Enhanced degradation of messenger RNA encoding myelin proteins by terminal complement complexes in oligodendrocytes. *J Immunol* 1993; **150**: 4581–4590.

54. Rus HG, Niculescu F, Shin ML. Sublytic complement attack induces cell cycle in oligodendrocytes: S phase induction is dependent on c-jun activation. *J Immunol* 1996; **156**: 4892–4900.

55. Tuohy VK, Yu M, Weinstock Guttman B, Kinkel RP. Diversity and plasticity of self-recognition during the development of multiple sclerosis. *J Clin Invest* 1997; **99**: 1682–1690.

4

Cytokines and cerebrospinal fluid: methodology, findings and clinical relevance in multiple sclerosis

Pia Kivisäkk

INTRODUCTION

Cytokines are low-molecular weight proteins produced during the effector phases of natural or specific immunity. They serve to mediate and regulate immune and inflammatory responses. A wide range of cells in the immune system and the central nervous system (CNS) can produce cytokines, including T cells, macrophages, astrocytes, oligodendrocytes and microglia.[1,2] In multiple sclerosis (MS), a number of studies have demonstrated increased production of both pro-inflammatory and immune-response down-regulatory cytokines, not only systemically but also locally in the cerebrospinal fluid (CSF) and in MS brain lesions. A disequilibrium in the cytokine production is believed to play a major role in the process of activating or deactivating the immune system in MS, as well as mediating tissue damage.

CYTOKINE LEVELS IN THE CSF

Because MS is an organ-specific disease of the CNS, it could be anticipated that cytokines produced locally in relation to an MS lesion would be the most relevant for the disease process. For obvious reasons, the possibilities of obtaining tissue samples from the CNS of patients with MS during the course of the disease are highly limited. The CSF communicates freely with the interstitial fluid of the brain and contains both immunocompetent cells and their chemical products, making the CSF a suitable target for the study of intrathecal immune responses.

Several studies have addressed the question of cytokine levels in the CSF in MS, with partly conflicting results. There is evidence that patients with active MS have higher CSF levels of tumour necrosis factor-α (TNF-α) than patients examined during a more stable phase of the disease.[3–5] High TNF-α levels in CSF were also associated with disease progression, enhanced disability and disruption of the blood–brain barrier.[6] Furthermore, interleukin (IL)-1β, IL-2, IL-6 and the p40 subunit of IL-12 have been observed at higher levels in the CSF from patients with MS than in controls.[3,7–9] Other groups have, however, failed to detect elevated CSF levels of TNF-α, IL-1β, and IL-6 in patients with MS.[3,8,10–14]

Using an alternative approach, it has been shown that mononuclear cells in CSF from patients with MS respond to a variety of myelin autoantigens, including myelin basic protein (MBP), proteolipid protein (PLP), myelin oligodendrocyte glycoprotein (MOG) and myelin-associated glycoprotein (MAG), with increased secretion or expression of both pro- and anti-inflammatory cytokines as a result.[15–19] Furthermore, without antigen stimulation in vitro, higher numbers of CSF mononuclear cells expressing messenger RNA (mRNA) for interferon-γ (IFN-γ), TNF-α, transforming growth factor-β (TGF-β), IL-4 and IL-10 can be detected in patients with MS than in controls.[20–22]

Methodological aspects of cytokine detection

The contrasting results obtained when studying cytokines in the CSF in MS most probably reflect methodological dilemmas. Since cytokines are produced locally, act in an autocrine or paracrine fashion, usually exist in low concentrations and frequently have a short half-life, it is often difficult to detect cytokines in body fluids even with the most sensitive enzyme-linked immunosorbent assay (ELISA). Furthermore, cytokines are seldom found in free form in biological fluids; instead, they are almost always bound to soluble receptors, carrier proteins or autoantibodies (i.e. molecules that can block the antibody sandwich needed for cytokine detection).[23] As a result, only a fraction of the total amount of the cytokine present is usually measured. It should also be borne in mind that all binding assays have the restriction that they fail to provide any information on the bioactivity of the cytokine.

Determination of cytokine mRNA expression in CSF mononuclear cells by reverse transcriptase polymerase chain reaction (rt-PCR) or in situ hybridization constitute useful alternatives to ELISA. Both in situ hybridization and rt-PCR are highly sensitive and specific assays that can be used for the small number of cells usually obtained through routine lumbar puncture. A further advantage with in situ hybridization is the possibility of localizing the gene expression to a single cell. Cytokine mRNA expression is not, however, identical to translation and secretion of the protein. Consequently, cytokine mRNA expression may not necessarily parallel cytokine protein production. Nevertheless, for most cytokines, translational control does not seem to have a significant influence on the relative levels of cytokine produced. Several authors have reported a good correlation between cytokine mRNA expression and protein production for IFN-γ, TNF-α, TGF-β, IL-2, IL-3, IL-4, IL-8 and IL-10.[24–28]

A general problem related to cytokine determinations in CSF, irrespective of method adopted, is that it is not known to what extent the results reflect inflammatory and restorative processes occurring within the CNS. Great care is therefore required when interpreting cytokine data obtained from clinical studies performed on blood and CSF samples.

This report presents results from some recent studies on cytokine mRNA expression in CSF mononuclear cells from patients with MS, especially in relation to clinical parameters.

CYTOKINE EXPRESSION IN OPTIC NEURITIS

It has previously been shown that patients with an episode of acute monosymptomatic optic neuritis have increased numbers of mononuclear cells in the CSF that express mRNA for IFN-γ, TNF-α, IL-4, IL-10 and TGF-β compared to healthy persons, thereby resembling the pattern of cytokine expression seen in patients with clinically definite MS.[20–22] The presence of multiple lesions on brain magnetic resonance imaging (MRI) or oligoclonal IgG bands in the CSF is associated with a clearly elevated risk for the future development of MS in patients with acute monosymptomatic optic neuritis,[29–33] making it possible to discriminate between patients with a high risk and a low risk of developing MS in the future. In order to identify a possible relationship between the expression of certain cytokines and a high likelihood of progression to clinically definite MS, the numbers of mononuclear cells in the blood and CSF expressing cytokine mRNA were related to the presence or absence of MRI abnormalities and CSF oligoclonal bands in a group of patients with acute monosymptomatic optic neuritis who had never been treated with any immunomodulatory drugs.[34]

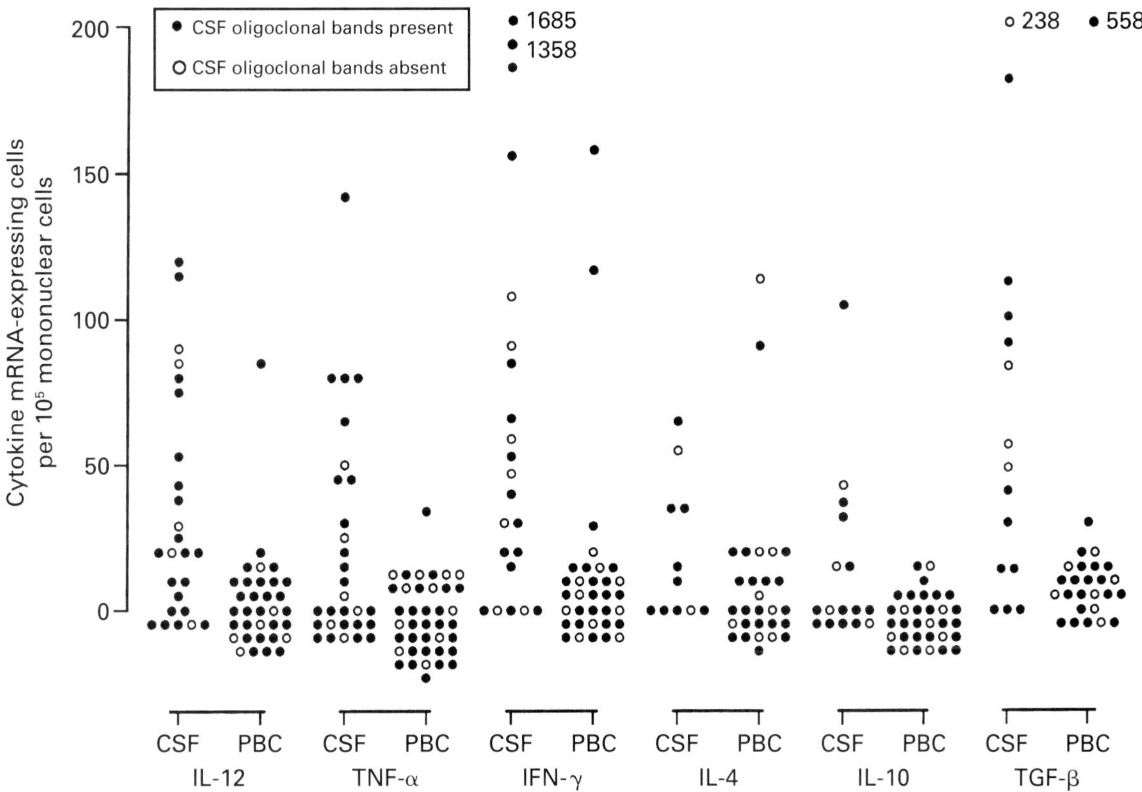

Figure 4.1 Numbers of cytokine mRNA-expressing cells per 10^5 peripheral blood mononuclear cells (PBC) or CSF mononuclear cells in patients with acute monosymptomatic optic neuritis subgrouped according to the presence or absence of CSF oligoclonal bands.

However, it was not possible to detect any predominance of the pro-inflammatory IFN-γ, TNF-α or IL-12 in CSF mononuclear cells from patients with acute monosymptomatic optic neuritis who had MRI lesions, oligoclonal bands or both (*Fig. 4.1*). Nor was there any clear tendency for elevated numbers of CSF mononuclear cells expressing mRNA for the immune-response down-regulatory TGF-β, IL-4 or IL-10 in patients lacking any of these laboratory abnormalities.

No controls with other diseases were included in this study, but the numbers of cytokine mRNA-expressing cells were similar to those previously reported from the author's laboratory in patients with optic neuritis and

MS.[20–22] Thus, increased numbers of mononuclear cells expressing mRNA for pro- and anti-inflammatory cytokines seem to be more related to the CNS inflammation per se, whether limited to the optic nerve or not, than to the process characteristic for MS. It has also been observed that patients with acute aseptic meningoencephalitis, a CNS inflammation that, in contrast to MS, is self-limiting and benign, have elevated numbers of mononuclear cells expressing cytokine mRNA in the CSF.[35] Furthermore, during the inflammatory response associated with acute cerebrovascular diseases, increased numbers of IFN-γ-secreting mononuclear cells and increased cytokine levels can be detected in the CSF.[36,37]

IL-12, IL-15 AND IL-17 mRNA EXPRESSING MONONUCLEAR CELLS IN MS AND ASEPTIC MENINGOENCEPHALITIS

Even though patients with MS and aseptic meningoencephalitis have mononuclear cells expressing mRNA for a number of cytokines in the CSF, differences in the cytokine pattern between these two diseases can be identified. Employing in situ hybridization, numbers of blood and CSF mononuclear cells expressing mRNA for IL-12, IL-15 and IL-17 were compared in patients with MS, aseptic meningoencephalitis and controls.[38–40]

Increased numbers of blood mononuclear cells expressing mRNA for all three cytokines under study (i.e. IL-12, IL-15 and IL-17) were detected in patients with MS and aseptic meningoencephalitis when compared to healthy persons. Numbers of IL-12 mRNA-expressing mononuclear cells were increased in CSF compared to blood to a similar extent in patients with MS and aseptic meningoencephalitis. In contrast, only patients with MS had elevated numbers of IL-15 and IL-17

mRNA-expressing cells in the CSF (*Fig. 4.2*). It has previously been demonstrated that there are higher numbers of TNF-α and lymphotoxin mRNA-expressing CSF mononuclear cells in MS patients than in aseptic meningoencephalitis patients, while no differences were observed between patients with these two diseases for numbers of IL-6 and IL-13 mRNA-expressing CSF mononuclear cells.[22,41–43]

Differences in cytokine patterns observed in MS compared to aseptic meningoencephalitis may reflect differences in disease pathogenesis and may in the end promote the understanding of differences in severity and outcome. TNF-α, lymphotoxin, IL-12, IL-15 and IL-17 all belong to the group of pro-inflammatory cytokines, but their biological effects vary. Differences in the production of individual cytokines may influence the outcome of an inflammatory event and lead to its decline or perpetuation.

IL-15 has biological functions resembling those of IL-2, of which induction of T-cell proliferation may be the most important. In addition, IL-15 can promote the induction of cytolytic effector cells (including natural killer

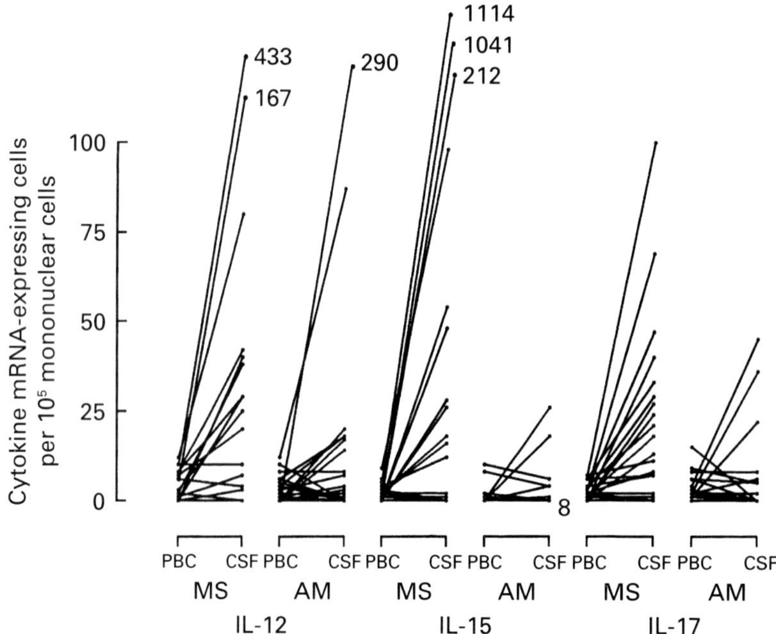

Figure 4.2 Numbers of cytokine mRNA-expressing cells per 10^5 peripheral blood mononuclear cells (PBC) or CSF mononuclear cells in paired blood and CSF samples from patients with MS and aseptic meningoencephalitis (AM).

cells and cytotoxic T cells), up-regulate the production of pro-inflammatory cytokines by natural killer cells and T cells and induce B-cell maturation and isotype switching.[44–47] In humans, IL-17 is almost exclusively produced by activated CD4[+] memory T cells.[48,49] Higher numbers of IL-17 mRNA-expressing mononuclear cells have been observed in blood from patients with MS who were examined during exacerbation compared to MS patients in remission.[40] Such an increase in the numbers of IL-17 mRNA-expressing mononuclear cells may reflect the activation of potentially harmful autoreactive memory T cells. Because IL-17 has been shown in vitro to enhance the expression of IL-1β, TNF-α, IL-6 and IL-8 in macrophages and adjacent parenchymal cells,[49,50] IL-17 can be speculated to have a triggering role in the development of new lesions in MS.

CYTOKINE mRNA EXPRESSION IN RELATION TO DISEASE ACTIVITY

A temporal profile in the pattern of cytokine expression in the CNS has been demonstrated in the acute experimental allergic encephalomyelitis model.[51,52] In the systemic circulation, shifts in the cytokine balance towards a predominance of certain cytokines have also been linked to clinical variables in MS. The expression of TNF-α and lymphotoxin was increased before exacerbations, whereas increased numbers of IL-10 mRNA-expressing blood mononuclear cells were observed in patients with optic neuritis in remission.[21,26,53] Patients with MS and no or only slight disability had higher numbers of TGF-β mRNA-expressing blood mononuclear cells than patients with moderate or severe disability.[20] In the CSF, it has been more difficult to demonstrate correlations between clinical variables and cytokine levels, often because of the small number of patients examined in many studies. The best evidence for a correlation between CSF cytokine levels and disease activity has come through the study of TNF-α (see above).

During the past few years it has become evident that serial MRI examinations reveal many active CNS lesions in patients without clinical symptoms.[54–57] It is thus difficult to estimate the extent of ongoing inflammation in MS based on clinical evaluation only and it may be more relevant to correlate CSF cytokine expression with disease activity as measured by MRI. TNF-α mRNA expression in blood mononuclear cells has, for instance, been shown to be increased in MS patients with non-enhancing T2-weighted brain MRI lesions,[26] and numbers of IL-2-secreting blood mononuclear cells correlates with numbers of gadolinium (Gd)-enhancing lesions.[58] However, it has not been possible to find any correlation between numbers of TNF-α, IL-10 or IL-12 mRNA-expressing CSF mononuclear cells and disease activity as measured by Gd-enhancing lesions in a number of untreated patients with MS (*Fig. 4.3*).[59] In a

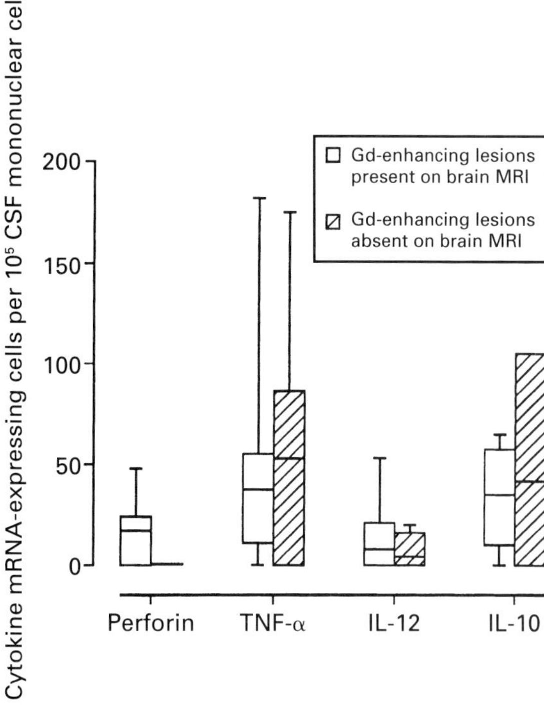

Figure 4.3 Numbers of cytokine mRNA-expressing cells per 10^5 CSF mononuclear cells in patients with MS subgrouped according to the presence or absence of Gd-enhancing lesions on brain MRI. Bars represent the 25th to 75th percentile.

recent longitudinal study, higher TNF-α secretion after phytohaemagglutinin stimulation in vitro was detected in blood mononuclear cells from MS patients before clinical exacerbations but not before episodes of disease activity as measured by the presence of Gd-enhancing brain MRI lesions.[60] Even though the presence of Gd-enhancing lesions on brain MRI is a sensitive marker for disease activity, it is a non-specific marker that provides no information about the degree of inflammation or the type of underlying pathological processes.[61]

Serial MRI examinations further demonstrate that MS lesions appear asynchronously (i.e. at the same time as some lesions are shrinking, other lesions may appear or expand).[62] When studying several cytokines in parallel in individual patients, it has been observed that many patients had mononuclear cells in their CSF expressing mRNA for a wide range of both pro- and anti-inflammatory cytokines simultaneously,[34,59] most probably reflecting a continuous process with inflammation and restoration occurring in parallel.

PERFORIN mRNA EXPRESSION IN MS

Perforin is a cytolytic effector molecule produced by killer lymphocytes such as natural killer cells, γδ T cells and cytotoxic T cells.[63] Using the presence of Gd-enhancing lesions on brain MRI as a surrogate marker for disease activity, high numbers of CSF mononuclear cells expressing mRNA for perforin in patients with active MS have been observed.[59] Six of nine patients with Gd-enhancing lesions on brain MRI had perforin mRNA positive cells in the CSF, whereas no perforin mRNA-expressing cells were detected in the CSF from any of the patients without disease activity on brain MRI (see *Fig. 4.3*).

An interesting discrepancy between MRI-positive and MRI-negative patients was observed when comparing paired blood and CSF samples from individual patients (*Fig. 4.4*). Patients with Gd-enhancing lesions on brain MRI had high numbers of perforin mRNA-expressing mononuclear cells in their

CSF, whereas there was a tendency for high numbers of perforin mRNA-positive cells in blood in patients without Gd-enhancing MRI lesions. Almost all other cytokines hitherto studied were expressed at higher levels in CSF than in blood in patients with MS. Perforin mRNA-expressing mononuclear cells have, however, also been previously demonstrated in higher numbers in CSF than in blood in some patients with MS while others had higher numbers of perforin mRNA-expressing mononuclear cells in blood than in CSF (see *Fig. 4.4*).[38] In this study no MRI scans were performed in parallel with the sampling of blood and CSF, but differences in disease activity could be one explanation for this varying distribution of perforin mRNA-positive cells between peripheral blood and CSF in MS.

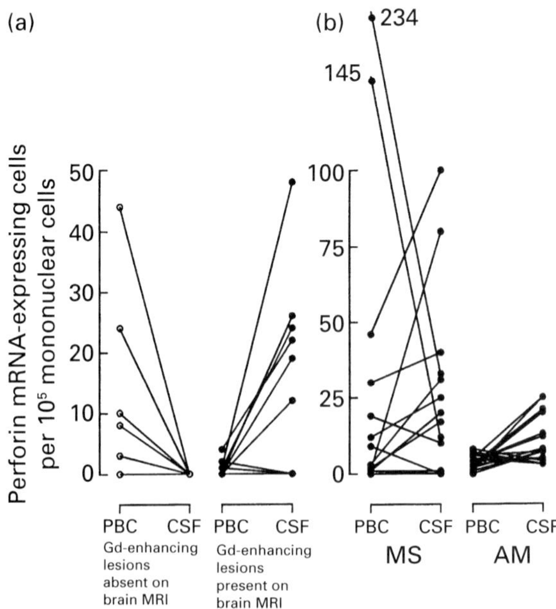

Figure 4.4 Numbers of perforin mRNA-expressing cells per 10⁵ peripheral blood mononuclear cells (PBC) or CSF mononuclear cells in (a) patients with MS subgrouped according to the presence or absence of Gd-enhancing lesions on brain MRI; and (b) patients with MS and aseptic meningoencephalitis (AM).

Cytotoxic T cells from patients with active MS can attack cerebral endothelial cells in vitro and, theoretically, damage the blood–brain barrier.[64] One possible pathway for this cell-mediated destruction could be perforin- mediated pore formation in synergy with other inflammatory mediators such as nitric oxide, hydrogenperoxide and proteases. Oligodendrocytes are highly susceptible to perforin, at least in vitro,[65] suggesting that perforin can be directly involved in demyelination. $\gamma\delta$ T cells, which are present in MS lesions,[66,67] have recently been demonstrated to kill oligodendrocytes through the perforin pathway.[68]

SUMMARY

Delineation of cytokine involvement could be essential for an understanding of MS and for improved therapies. Increased numbers of mononuclear cells expressing mRNA for both pro-inflammatory and immune-response down-regulatory cytokines in the CSF from patients with MS have been observed, reflecting the ongoing immune activation intrathecally. Furthermore, in patients with aseptic meningoencephalitis, elevated numbers of cytokine mRNA-expressing mononuclear cells in the CSF can be identified, suggesting that increased cytokine expression may be more related to an inflammatory process in the CNS per se than to the process characteristic for MS. Nevertheless, differences in the expression of individual cytokines exist between patients with MS and those with aseptic meningoencephalitis, indicating that the regulation of each cytokine is independent of each other. Some cytokines may vary in expression in parallel with disease activity. The factors that regulate the expression of cytokines are presently not completely known, but the net balance between cytokines most probably influences the course of MS.

ACKNOWLEDGEMENTS

The studies from the author's laboratory have been supported by the Swedish Medical Association, the Swedish Medical Research Council, the Swedish MS Society (NHR) and funds from Karolinska Institutet.

REFERENCES

1. Merrill JE, Benveniste EN. Cytokines in inflammatory brain lesions: helpful and harmful. *Trends Neurosci* 1996; **19**: 331–338.
2. Xiao BG, Link H. Immune regulation within the central nervous system. *J Neurol Sci* 1998; **157**: 1–12.
3. Hauser SL, Doolittle TH, Lincoln R et al. Cytokine accumulations in CSF of multiple sclerosis patients: frequent detection of interleukin-1 and tumor necrosis factor but not interleukin-6. *Neurology* 1990; **40**: 1735–1739.
4. Sharief MK, Hentges R. Association between tumor necrosis factor-α and disease progression in patients with multiple sclerosis. *N Engl J Med* 1991; **325**: 467–472.
5. Tsukada N, Miagi K, Matsuda M et al. Tumor necrosis factor and interleukin-1 in CSF and sera from patients with multiple sclerosis. *Ann Neurol* 1991; **104**: 230–234.
6. Sharief MK, Thompson EJ. In vivo relationship of tumor necrosis factor-α to blood–brain barrier damage in patients with active multiple sclerosis. *J Neuroimmunol* 1992; **38**: 27–34.
7. Gallo P, Piccinno M, Pagni S, Tavolato B. Interleukin-2 levels in serum and cerebrospinal fluid of multiple sclerosis patients. *Ann Neurol* 1988; **24**: 795–797.
8. Maimone D, Gregory S, Arnason BGW, Reder AT. Cytokine levels in the cerebrospinal fluid and serum of patients with multiple sclerosis. *J Neuroimmunol* 1991; **32**: 67–74.
9. Fassbender K, Ragoschke A, Rossol S et al. Increased release of interleukin-12p40 in MS. Association with intracerebral inflammation. *Neurology* 1998; **51**: 753–758.
10. Hossiau FA, Bukasa K, Sindic CJM et al. Elevated levels of the 26K human hybridoma growth factor (interleukin 6) in cerebrospinal fluid of patients with acute infection of the central nervous system. *Clin Exp Immunol* 1988; **71**: 320–323.
11. Franciotta DM, Grimaldi LME, Martino GV et al. Tumor necrosis factor in serum and cerebrospinal fluid of patients with multiple sclerosis. *Ann Neurol* 1989; **26**: 787–789.
12. Merrill JE, Strom SP, Ellison GW, Myers LW. In

vitro study of mediators of inflammation in multiple sclerosis. *J Clin Immunol* 1989; **9**: 84–96.

13. Gallo P, Piccinno MG, Krzalic L, Tavolato B. Tumor necrosis factor alpha (TNF-α) and neurological diseases. Failure in detecting TNF-α in the cerebrospinal fluid from patients with multiple sclerosis, AIDS dementia complex, and brain tumors. *J Neuroimmunol* 1989; **23**: 41–44.

14. Peter JB, Boctor FN, Tourtellotte WW. Serum and CSF levels of IL-2, IL-2R, TNF-α and IL-1β in chronic progressive multiple sclerosis: expected lack of clinical utility. *Neurology* 1991; **41**: 121–123.

15. Olsson T, Zhi WW, Höjeberg B et al. Autoreactive T lymphocytes in multiple sclerosis determined by antigen-induced secretion of interferon-gamma. *J Clin Invest* 1990; **86**: 981–985.

16. Sun JB, Link H, Olsson T et al. T and B cell responses to myelin–oligodendrocyte glycoprotein in multiple sclerosis. *J Immunol* 1991; **146**: 1490–1495.

17. Sun JB, Olsson T, Wang WZ et al. Autoreactive T and B cells responding to myelin proteolipid protein in multiple sclerosis and controls. *Eur J Immunol* 1991; **21**: 1461–1468.

18. Link J, Fredrikson S, Söderström M et al. Organ-specific autoantigens induce transforming growth factor-β mRNA expression in mononuclear cells in multiple sclerosis and myasthenia gravis. *Ann Neurol* 1994; **35**: 197–203.

19. Link J, Söderström M, Ljungdahl Å et al. Organ-specific autoantigens induce interferon-γ and interleukin-4 mRNA expression in mononuclear cells in multiple sclerosis and myasthenia gravis. *Neurology* 1994; **44**: 728–734.

20. Link J, Söderström M, Olsson T et al. Increased TGF-β, IL-4 and IFN-γ mRNA expression in mononuclear cells in multiple sclerosis. *Ann Neurol* 1994; **36**: 379–386.

21. Navikas V, Link J, Palasik W et al. Increased mRNA expression of IL-10 in mononuclear cells in multiple sclerosis and optic neuritis. *Scand J Immunol* 1995; **41**: 171–178.

22. Navikas V, He B, Link J et al. Augmented expression of tumor necrosis factor-α and lymphotoxin mRNA in mononuclear cells in multiple sclerosis and optic neuritis. *Brain* 1996; **119**: 213–223.

23. Barnes A. Measurement of serum cytokines. *Lancet* 1998; **352**: 324–325.

24. Cherwinski HM, Schumacher JH, Brown KD, Mosmann TR. Two types of mouse helper T cell clone. III. Further differences in lymphokine synthesis between Th1 and Th2 clones revealed by RNA hybridization, functionally monospecific bioassays, and monoclonal antibodies. *J Exp Med* 1987; **166**: 1229–1244.

25. Wingren AG, Dahlenborg K, Björklund M et al. Monocyte-regulated IFN-γ production in human T cells involves CD2 signaling. *J Immunol* 1993; **151**: 1328–1336.

26. Rieckmann P, Albrecht M, Kitze B et al. Tumor necrosis factor-α messenger RNA expression in patients with relapsing–remitting multiple sclerosis is associated with disease activity. *Ann Neurol* 1995; **37**: 82–88.

27. Rudick RA, Ransohoff RM, Peppler R et al. Interferon beta induces interleukin-10 expression: relevance to multiple sclerosis. *Ann Neurol* 1996; **40**: 618–627.

28. Kostulas N, Kivisäkk P, Huang Y et al. Ischemic stroke is associated with a systemic increase of blood mononuclear cells expressing interleukin-8 mRNA. *Stroke* 1998; **29**: 462–466.

29. Stendahl-Brodin L, Link H. Optic neuritis: oligoclonal bands increase the risk of multiple sclerosis. *Acta Neurol Scand* 1983; **67**: 301–304.

30. Morrissey SP, Miller DH, Kendall BE et al. The significance of brain magnetic resonance imaging abnormalities at presentation with clinically isolated syndromes suggestive of multiple sclerosis. *Brain* 1993; **116**: 135–146.

31. Jacobs LD, Kaba SE, Miller CM et al. Correlation of clinical, magnetic resonance imaging, and cerebrospinal fluid findings in optic neuritis. *Ann Neurol* 1997; **41**: 392–398.

32. Optic Neuritis Study Group. The 5-year risk of MS after optic neuritis. Experience of the Optic Neuritis Treatment Trial. *Neurology* 1997; **49**: 1404–1413.

33. Söderström M, Ya-Ping J, Hillert J, Link H. Optic neuritis. Prognosis for multiple sclerosis from MRI, CSF and HLA findings. *Neurology* 1998; **50**: 708–714.

34. Kivisäkk P, Tian W, Matusevicius D et al. Optic neuritis and cytokines: no relation to MRI abnormalities and oligoclonal bands. *Neurology* 1998; **50**: 217–223.

35. Navikas V, Haglund M, Link J et al. Cytokine mRNA profiles in mononuclear cells in acute aseptic meningo-encephalitis. *Infect Immun* 1995; **63**: 1581–1586.

36. Wang WZ, Olsson T, Kostulas V et al. Myelin antigen reactive T cells in cerebrovascular diseases. *Clin Exp Immunol* 1992; **88**: 157–162.

37. Tarkowski E, Rosengren L, Blomstrand C et al.

Intrathecal release of pro- and anti-inflammatory cytokines during stroke. *Clin Exp Med* 1997; **110**: 492–499.

38. Matusevicius D, Kivisäkk P, Navikas V et al. IL-12 and perforin mRNA expression is augmented in blood mononuclear cells in multiple sclerosis. *Scand J Immunol* 1998; **47**: 582–590.

39. Kivisäkk P, Matusevicius D, He B et al. Interleukin-15 mRNA expression is upregulated in blood and cerebrospinal fluid mononuclear cells in multiple sclerosis. *Clin Exp Immunol* 1998; **111**: 193–197.

40. Matusevicius D, Kivisäkk P, He B et al. Interleukin-17 mRNA expression is augmented in CSF mononuclear cells in multiple sclerosis. *Multiple Sclerosis* 1999; in press.

41. Navikas V, Matusevicius D, Söderström M et al. Increased interleukin-6 mRNA expression in blood and cerebrospinal fluid mononuclear cells in multiple sclerosis. *J Neuroimmunol* 1996; **64**: 63–69.

42. Matusevicius D, Navikas V, Söderström M et al. Multiple sclerosis: the proinflammatory cytokines lymphotoxin-α and tumor necrosis factor-α are upregulated in cerebrospinal fluid mononuclear cells. *J Neuroimmunol* 1996; **66**: 115–123.

43. Matusevicius D, Kivisäkk P, Navikas V et al. Autoantigen-induced IL-13 mRNA expression is increased in blood mononuclear cells in myasthenia gravis and multiple sclerosis. *Eur J Neurol* 1997; **4**: 468–475.

44. Grabstein K, Eisenman J, Shanebeck K et al. Cloning of a T cell growth factor that interacts with the β-chain of the interleukin-2 receptor. *Science* 1994; **264**: 965–968.

45. Carson W, Giri J, Lindmann M et al. Interleukin (IL) 15 is a novel cytokine that activates human natural killer cells via components of the IL-2 receptor. *J Exp Med* 1994; **180**: 1395–1403.

46. Armitage R, Macduff B, Eisenmann J et al. IL-15 has stimulatory activity for the induction of B cell proliferation and differentiation. *J Immunol* 1995; **154**: 483–490.

47. MacInnes I, Leung B, Sturrock R et al. Interleukin-15 mediated T cell-dependent regulation of tumor necrosis factor-α production in rheumatoid arthritis. *Nature Med* 1997; **2**: 189–195.

48. Yao Z, Painter SL, Fanslow WC et al. Human IL-17: a novel cytokine derived from T cells. *J Immunol* 1995; **115**: 5483–5486.

49. Fossiez F, Djossou O, Chomarat P et al. T cell interleukin-17 induces stromal cells to produce proinflammatory and hematopoetic cytokines. *J Exp Med* 1996; **183**: 2593–2603.

50. Jovanovic DV, Di Battista JA, Martel-Pelletier J et al. IL-17 stimulates the production and expression of proinflammatory cytokines, IL-1β and TNF-α, by human macrophages. *J Immunol* 1998; **160**: 3513–3521.

51. Issazadeh S, Mustafa M, Ljungdahl Å et al. Interferon-γ, interleukin-4 and transforming growth factor in experimental allergic encephalomyelitis in Lewis rats: dynamics of cellular mRNA expression in the central nervous system and lymphoid cells. *J Neurosci Res* 1995; **40**: 579–590.

52. Issazadeh S, Ljungdahl Å, Höjeberg B et al. Cytokine production in the central nervous system of Lewis rats with experimental autoimmune encephalomyelitis: dynamics of mRNA expression for interleukin-10, interleukin-12, cytolysin, tumor necrosis factor α and tumor necrosis factor β. *J Neuroimmunol* 1995; **61**: 205–212.

53. Rieckmann P, Albrecht M, Kitze B et al. Cytokine mRNA levels in mononuclear cells from patients with multiple sclerosis. *Neurology* 1994; **44**: 1523–1526.

54. Miller DH, Rudge P, Johnson G et al. Serial gadolinium enhanced magnetic resonance imaging in multiple sclerosis. *Brain* 1988; **111**: 927–939.

55. Willoughby EW, Grochowski E, Li DKB et al. Serial magnetic resonance scanning in multiple sclerosis: a second prospective study in relapsing patients. *Ann Neurol* 1989; **25**: 43–49.

56. Stone LA, Smith ME, Albert PS et al. Blood–brain barrier disruption on contrast-enhanced MRI in patients with mild relapsing–remitting multiple sclerosis: relationship to course, gender, and age. *Neurology* 1995; **45**: 1122–1126.

57. Thorpe JW, Kidd D, Moseley IF et al. Serial gadolinium-enhanced MRI of the brain and spinal cord in early relapsing–remitting multiple sclerosis. *Neurology* 1996; **46**: 373–378.

58. Calabresi PA, Tranquill LR, McFarland HF, Cowan EP. Cytokine gene expression in cells derived from CSF of multiple sclerosis patients. *J Neuroimmunol* 1998; **89**: 198–205.

59. Kivisäkk P, Stawiarz L, Matusevicius D et al. High numbers of perforin mRNA expressing CSF cells in multiple sclerosis patients with gadolinium-enhancing brain MRI lesions. *Acta Neurol Scand* 1999; in press.

60. Van Oosten BW, Barkhof F, Scholten PET et al. Increased production of tumor necrosis factor α, and not of interferon γ, preceding disease activity in patients with multiple sclerosis. *Arch Neurol* 1998; **55**: 793–798.

61. Giovannoni G, Kieseier B, Hartung HP. Correlating immunological and magnetic resonance imaging markers of disease activity in multiple sclerosis. *J Neurol Neurosurg Psych* 1998; **64**: S31–S36.

62. Smith ME, Stone LA, Albert PS et al. Clinical worsening in multiple sclerosis is associated with increased frequency and area of gadopentetate dimeglumine-enhancing magnetic resonance imaging lesions. *Ann Neurol* 1993; **33**: 480–489.

63. Liu CC, Walsh CM, Young JDE. Perforin: structure and function. *Immunol Today* 1995; **16**: 194–201.

64. Tsukada N, Matsuda M, Miyagi K, Yanagisawa N. Cytotoxicity of T cells for cerebral endothelium in multiple sclerosis. *J Neurol Sci* 1993; **117**: 140–147.

65. Scolding NJ, Jones J, Compston DAS, Morgan BP. Oligodendrocyte susceptibility to injury by T-cell perforin. *Immunology* 1990; **70**: 6–10.

66. Selmaj K, Brosnan CF, Raine CS. Colocalization of lymphocytes bearing γδ T-cell receptor and heat shock protein HSP65+ oligodendrocytes in multiple sclerosis. *Proc Natl Acad Sci USA* 1991; **88**: 5452–5456.

67. Wucherpfennig KW, Newcombe J, Li H, et al. γδ T-cell receptor repertoire in acute multiple sclerosis lesions. *Proc Natl Acad Sci USA* 1992; **89**: 4588–4592.

68. Zeine R, Pon R, Ladiwala U et al. Mechanism of γδ T cell-induced human oligodendrocyte cytotoxicity: relevance to multiple sclerosis. *J Neuroimmunol* 1998; **87**: 49–61.

5

Immunological findings in very early multiple sclerosis reflected by monosymptomatic optic neuritis or other isolated syndromes

Finn Sellebjerg, Jakob Jensen, Torben L Sørensen and Jette L Frederiksen

INTRODUCTION

An increasing burden of evidence suggests an immunologically mediated attack on central nervous system (CNS) myelin to be central in the pathogenesis of multiple sclerosis (MS).[1–3] Demyelination and oligodendrocyte loss with only incomplete and very variable remyelination is a hallmark of MS, but the underlying mechanisms are incompletely understood.[4] Axonal loss may lead to irreversible disability in MS.[5–7] In contrast, a reversible conduction block induced by inflammatory mediators may contribute to reversible or rapidly fluctuating neurological dysfunction in patients with MS.[8]

Most patients with MS initially have a relapsing–remitting disease course and a diagnosis of clinically definite MS can be established only after the patient has suffered two attacks affecting different parts of the white matter.[9,10] Studies of cerebrospinal fluid (CSF) changes in patients with possible symptoms of the onset of MS are important not only because they allow the identification of factors that confer an increased risk of future development of clinically definite disease;[11] they also provide information about immunological changes at the earliest stage of the disease that can be reliably identified in patient studies. In many cases the patient does not, however, seek medical atten-

tion during the acute stage of the initial attack and most studies addressing immunological changes in MS have been confined to patients with clinically definite disease. The present article reviews studies of immunological changes in patients with first attacks of MS and their implications for understanding the pathogenesis of MS.

T CELLS AND CYTOKINES

Myelin-reactive T cells are believed to orchestrate the inflammatory response in the CNS of patients with MS.[1–3] This is thought to be accomplished by a delicate balance between T cell secretion of pro-inflammatory cytokines such as interferon (IFN)-γ and tumor necrosis factor (TNF)-α and cytokines such as interleukin (IL)-4, IL-10, and transforming growth factor (TGF)-β, which tend to down-regulate the biological effects of pro-inflammatory cytokines.

In previous studies it was established that patients with acute optic neuritis have increased numbers of cells in the blood and cerebrospinal fluid (CSF) that express messenger RNA (mRNA) encoding both pro-inflammatory and immunoregulatory cytokines.[12–15] It was also shown that the number of cytokine-secreting or cytokine mRNA-expressing cells increased further after stimulation with myelin proteins or synthetic myelin peptides.[13,14,16–18] Previous studies of cytokine concentrations in CSF and serum or plasma have yielded highly variable results, most likely as a result of methodological difficulties in measuring these substances.[19] IL-2 and IL-6 was detected in CSF in only one out of three previous studies of patients with optic neuritis.[19–21] With the possible exception of several chemokines (see below), no other cytokines have been consistently detected at increased concentrations in CSF from patients with possible onset symptoms of MS.

The activation status of lymphocytes can be monitored by measuring the expression of activation and differentiation markers on individual cells by flow cytometry. The authors have recently completed a flow cytometry study of CD4[+] T cells from patients with possible onset symptoms of MS. In these patients, all of whom had intrathecal synthesis of IgG oligoclonal bands, increased expression of the CD26 molecule on CD4[+] T cells in peripheral blood was found (Sellebjerg et al, unpublished). CD26 is a co-stimulatory molecule that is involved in T-cell activation and is expressed on memory T cells.[22] An increase in peripheral blood lymphocyte expression of CD26 has previously been reported only in patients with chronic progressive MS.[23,24] The finding of increased expressed expression of CD26 and cytokine mRNA in peripheral blood even in patients with possible onset symptoms of MS is consistent with the notion that systemic T-cell activation is an important step in the pathogenesis of MS.

The authors have found that there is a decreased expression of the class II MHC molecule HLA-DR on CD4[+] T cells in CSF from patients with possible first attacks of MS (Sellebjerg et al, unpublished). No difference was found in CD4[+] T-cell expression of CD25 (IL-2 receptor α-chain), CD26, or CD45RA/R0 isoforms. In a separate study it was found that patients with possible onset symptoms of MS and intrathecal synthesis of IgG had a lower percentage of CD3[+] T cells in CSF that expressed the co-stimulatory molecule CD86 (B7-2) than did patients with possible onset symptoms of MS and no intrathecal synthesis of

IgG.[25] A decrease in HLA-DR expression on CD3[+] T cells in CSF was previously reported in active relapsing–remitting MS and correlated with clinical disease activity.[26–28]

It may seem paradoxical that T-cell surface marker studies of CSF cells from patients with onset symptoms of MS suggest no alterations or even a lower activation level in active disease whereas cytokine expression studies suggest increased CSF T-cell activation. Hypothetically, some of the observed changes could reflect alterations in immune regulation rather than hyperactivation in the T cells in CSF. Indeed, dysfunction of regulatory cells that normally maintain self-tolerance is increasingly recognized as an important mechanism in the pathogenesis of autoimmune disease.[29]

The importance of the balance between proinflammatory and immunoregulatory cytokines in the pathogenesis of MS is supported by studies of the effect of interferon-β and methylprednisolone on cytokine production in patients with MS.[30–35] Similarly, the relevance of the increased expression of CD26 on CD4[+] cells in the pathogenesis of MS is supported by the finding of a decrease in CD26 expression after treatment with high-dose oral methylprednisolone (Sellebjerg et al, unpublished).

B CELLS AND IMMUNOGLOBULINS

Intrathecal synthesis of IgG in the form of oligoclonal bands can be detected in approximately 95% of patients with clinically definite MS.[11] IgG oligoclonal bands are present in CSF from fewer patients with possible onset symptoms of MS, but those patients that have intrathecal synthesis of IgG have a markedly increased risk of developing clinically definite MS.[36–43] In addition, one should be very cautious when considering the diagnosis MS in patients without intrathecal synthesis of IgG because such patients frequently turn out to have other diseases.[44,45]

Numerous studies have addressed whether the intrathecally synthesized IgG in patients with MS includes autoantibody specificities. In contrast, only very few studies on autoantibody production have been conducted in patients with possible onset symptoms of MS. Myelin basic protein (MBP) and proteolipid protein (PLP) account for approximately 90% of the protein content of CNS myelin. A high prevalence of an anti-MBP antibody response in CSF from patients with optic neuritis as a possible onset symptom of MS was found using an antibody-dependent cellular cytotoxicity assay.[46] Cells secreting anti-MBP antibodies have also been detected in CSF from patients with optic neuritis.[47–49] Studies from a Canadian group suggest that the majority of patients with MS and optic neuritis as a possible onset symptom of MS have anti-MBP antibodies in CSF whereas anti-PLP antibodies are rare.[50] This finding is not supported by studies of anti-PLP antibody-secreting cells in CSF from patients with optic neuritis or clinically definite MS.[49,51]

Apart from their role as precursors of immunoglobulin-secreting plasma cells, B cells are increasingly recognized as antigen-presenting cells. When specific antibodies are present on their surface, they are able to ingest antibody-reactive antigens at much lower concentrations than other antigen presenting cells.[52,53] In addition, B cells have been shown in some models to be involved in the initial priming of naïve T cells and in the induction of autoreactive T cells.[52,54,55] There is very little knowledge about the possible role of B cells in antigen presentation in MS. The presence of an association between class II human leukocyte antigen (HLA) genes and the specificity of the antibody response against synthetic MBP peptides together with the presence of clonally expanded B cells in the CNS may, however, be taken as indirect evidence of interactions between T cells and B cells in vivo in patients with MS.[11,56,57]

Surface expression of co-stimulatory molecules such as CD80 (B7-1) and CD86 (B7-2) is important in the activation of T cells by antigen-presenting cells.[58,59] It has been suggested that MBP reactive T cells from patients with MS are relatively independent of co-stimulatory signals.[60,61] Studies in the animal model of MS experimental autoimmune encephalomyelitis (EAE) do, however, provide evidence for an important role of CD80 in the induction of disease, whereas co-stimulation by CD86 may confer protection from disease.[62–64] A flow cytometry study found that patients with possible onset symptoms of MS had a higher percentage of B cells in CSF with expression of CD80 than did neurological control subjects.[25] Importantly, the expression of CD80 on B cells in patients with possible onset symptoms of MS differed according to whether there was intrathecal synthesis of IgG or not. In contrast, there was no difference in B cell expression of CD86. This finding is consistent with the notion that B-cell antigen presentation in patients with MS may be altered. Interferon-β has been shown to decrease the antigen presentation function of activated B cells in vitro.[65] In addition, the B cell expression of CD80 decreases in patients with MS after treatment with interferon-β, lending further indirect support for the involvement of this molecule in the pathogenesis of MS.[66]

LEUKOCYTE RECRUITMENT TO THE CNS

The presence of myelin-reactive T cells is insufficient to induce demyelination even in mice that express a rearranged MBP-reactive T-cell receptor transgene on the majority of the T cells in peripheral blood. In these mice, the key element in the development of CNS inflammation is the ability of activated T cells that secrete pro-inflammatory cytokines to enter the CNS.[67]

Leukocyte recruitment is a complex multiple-step process. It is initiated by the binding of selectin or integrin molecules on leukocytes to counter receptors on endothelial cells.[68,69] This allows the slow 'rolling' of leukocytes on vessel walls. Rolling is followed by the activation or clustering of integrin molecules on the leukocyte.[68] This is induced by chemotactic factors produced by endothelial cells and parenchymal cells, bacterial products or complement split products.[70] The central role of members of the chemokine family of cytokines in this stage of leukocyte recruitment is increasingly being recognized.[71–73] Activated integrins mediate tight adhesion to immunoglobulin superfamily molecule members expressed on endothelial cells and to basement membrane and extracellular matrix molecules.[69] The subsequent migration across basement membranes and extracellular matrix is presumably guided by chemotactic factors and is facilitated by the activity of proteolytic enzymes (e.g. members of the matrix metalloproteinase (MMP) family).[74–76]

Based on conserved amino acid motifs, chemokines are divided into the CXC chemokines (α-chemokines), the CC chemokines (β-chemokines), a C chemokine and a CX_3C chemokine.[71–73] Patients with possible first attacks of MS and intrathecal synthesis of IgG have significantly increased CSF concentrations of the CXC chemokines IP-10 (interferon-inducible protein 10) and MIG (monocyte induced by γ-interferon) and of the CC chemokine RANTES (released on activation, normal T cell expressed and secreted).[77] The physiological role of IP-10 and MIG in leukocyte recruitment in possible first attacks of MS is supported by a significant correlation between the CSF concentration of these chemokines and the CSF leukocyte count.[77]

Intercellular adhesion molecule (ICAM)-1, a member of the immunoglobulin superfamily, is expressed on endothelial cells, some glia and mononuclear cells in active MS plaques.[78–80] ICAM-1 enables intercellular interactions with leukocytes that express β_2-integrins. The β_2-integrin leukocyte function antigen (LFA)-1 is abundantly expressed on mononuclear cells in active MS plaques.[78,80] Differential splicing of ICAM-1 mRNA and proteolytic cleavage of membrane-bound ICAM-1 can generate a soluble form of ICAM-1 (sICAM-1).[81,82] Although highly conflicting results regarding the serum concentration of sICAM-1 in patients with clinically definite MS have previously been reported, there is some agreement that changes in the concentration of sICAM-1 in CSF and serum may correlate with disease activity.[83–85] Intrathecal synthesis of sICAM-1 can be detected in patients with possible onset symptoms of MS at levels comparable to those seen in patients with clinically definite MS. Intrathecal synthesis of sICAM-1 correlates both with the CSF leukocyte count and with the CSF concentration of MBP in patients with possible onset symptoms of MS.[86]

Increased CSF activity of MMP-9 (gelatinase B) can be detected in patients with possible onset symptoms and in patients with clinically definite MS (Sellebjerg et al, unpublished).[21,87] MMP-9 appears to be mainly expressed by macrophages and glia in MS plaques.[88–90] MMP activity could facilitate leukocyte migration by degrading basement membrane proteins and extracellular matrix proteins and it may be involved in myelin degradation in MS.[74,75] The activity of MMP-9 in CSF correlates with intrathecal synthesis of IgG and the CSF leukocyte count in patients with possible onset symptoms of MS or clinically definite MS (Sellebjerg et al, unpublished).

Taken together, the available evidence suggests that chemokines, ICAM-1 and MMP-9 could be involved in leukocyte recruitment to the CNS even in patients presenting with possible onset symptoms of MS. Experiments with blocking antibodies in EAE have provided evidence for a role of ICAM-1 and the chemokines MIP-1α and monocyte chemotactic protein (MCP)-1 in the pathogenesis of CNS autoimmune disease.[91–92] It does, however, appear that the ICAM-1 molecule may be more important in the induction of autoreactive T cells than in the recruitment of T cells to the CNS.[91] The role of the chemokines MIP-1α and MCP-1 may differ in acute and relapsing EAE.[92,93] There is not yet conclusive evidence from clinical treatment trials in humans to substantiate the involvement of MMP-9 in MS but in vitro experiments have shown that the effects of interferon-β include suppression of MMP-9 activity in T cells.[94,95]

CONCLUSION

The complexity of chemokine signalling on cells of the immune system is only beginning to be appreciated. In addition to their role in leukocyte recruitment some chemokines provide co-stimulatory signals to T cells and influence the cytokine secretion pattern of activated

T cells.[95–97] Although the chemokine family consists of more than 40 different molecules with a dozen or so characterized receptors, the experiments discussed above suggest that some chemokines may nevertheless be pivotal in specific autoimmune diseases. Indeed, studies of a deletion allele in the CC chemokine receptor CCR5, which encodes a truncated protein that is not expressed on the cell surface, suggest that this allele confers protection from attacks of MS (Sellebjerg et al, unpublished).[99,100] As CCR5 binds the chemokines MIP-1α and RANTES, both of which are detected in increased concentrations in CSF of patients with MS, it is possible that the presence of the deletion allele leads to attenuated signalling by these chemokines (Sørensen et al, submitted).[71,73,101] Certainly, these findings suggest that studies of chemokines, chemokine receptors and the biological response to chemokines may increase our understanding of differential leukocyte recruitment and activation in patients with MS and hence may lead to the development of novel therapeutic strategies.

ACKNOWLEDGEMENTS

The studies were supported by grants from the Danish Eye Research Foundation, the Danish Multiple Sclerosis Society, the Danish Toyota Foundation, the Foundation for Neurological Research, the Johnsen Memorial Foundation, the Lily Benthine Lund Foundation and the Abrahamson Memorial Foundation. The technical assistance of Annetta Clausen and Karen Severin is acknowledged.

REFERENCES

1. Olsson T. Critical influences of the cytokine orchestration on the outcome of myelin antigen-specific T-cell autoimmunity in experimental autoimmune encephalomyelitis and multiple sclerosis. *Immunol Rev* 1995; **144**: 245–268.

2. Steinman L. Multiple sclerosis: a coordinated immunological attack against myelin in the central nervous system. *Cell* 1996; **85**: 299–302.

3. Weiner HL. A 21 point unifying hypothesis on the etiology and treatment of multiple sclerosis. *Can J Neurol Sci* 1998; **25**: 93–101.

4. Raine CS. The Norton Lecture: a review of the oligodendrocyte in the multiple sclerosis lesion. *J Neuroimmunol* 1997; **77**: 135–152.

5. Davie CA, Barker GJ, Webb S et al. Persistent functional deficit in multiple sclerosis and autosomal dominant cerebellar ataxia is associated with axon loss. *Brain* 1995; **118**: 1583–1592.

6. Ferguson B, Matyszak MK, Esiri MM, Perry VH. Axonal damage in acute multiple sclerosis lesions. *Brain* 1997; **120**: 393–399.

7. Trapp BD, Peterson J, Ransohoff RM et al. Axonal transection in the lesions of multiple sclerosis. *N Engl J Med* 1998; **338**: 278–285.

8. Moreau T, Coles A, Wing M et al. Transient increase in symptoms associated with cytokine release in patients with multiple sclerosis. *Brain* 1996; **119**: 225–237.

9. Poser CM, Paty DW, Scheinberg L et al. New diagnostic criteria for multiple sclerosis: guidelines for research protocols. *Ann Neurol* 1983; **13**: 227–231.

10. Lublin FD, Reingold SC. Defining the clinical course of multiple sclerosis: results of an international survey. *Neurology* 1996; **46**: 907–911.

11. Andersson M, Alvarez Cermeno J, Bernardi G et al. Cerebrospinal fluid in the diagnosis of multiple sclerosis: a consensus report. *J Neurol Neurosurg Psychiatry* 1994; **57**: 897–902.

12. Link J, Söderström M, Olsson T et al. Increased transforming growth factor-beta, interleukin-4, and interferon-gamma in multiple sclerosis. *Ann Neurol* 1993; **36**: 379–386.

13. Navikas V, Link J, Palasik W et al. Increased mRNA expression of IL-10 in mononuclear cells in multiple sclerosis and optic neuritis. *Scand J Immunol* 1995; **41**: 171–178.

14. Navikas V, He B, Link J et al. Augumented expression of tumour necrosis factor-alfa and lymphotoxin in mononuclear cells in multiple sclerosis and optic neuritis. *Brain* 1996; **119**: 219–223.

15. Kivisäkk P, Tian W, Matusevicius D et al. Optic neuritis and cytokines. No relation to MRI abnormalities and oligoclonal bands. *Neurology* 1998; **50**: 217–223.

16. Söderström M, Link H, Sun JB et al. Autoimmune T cell repertoire in optic neuritis and multiple sclerosis: T cells recognising multiple myelin proteins are accumulated in cerebrospinal fluid. *J Neurol Neurosurg Psychiatry* 1994; **57**: 544–551.

17. Söderström M, Link H, Fredrikson S, Sun J-B. Optic neuritis and multiple sclerosis: the T cell repertoires to myelin proteins and MBP peptides change with time. *Acta Neurol Scand* 1994; **90**: 10–18.

18. Link J, Söderström M, Kostulas V et al. Optic neuritis is associated with myelin basic protein and proteolipid protein reactive cells producing interferon-gamma, interleukin-4 and transforming growth factor-beta. *J Neuroimmunol* 1994; **49**: 9–18.

19. Sellebjerg F, Bendtzen K, Christiansen M, Frederiksen J. Cytokines and soluble IL-4 receptors in patients with acute optic neuritis and multiple sclerosis. *Eur J Neurol* 1997; **4**: 59–67.

20. Deckert-Schlüter M, Schlüter D, Schwendemann G. Evaluation of IL-2, sIL2R, IL-6, TNF-alpha, and IL-1beta in serum and CSF of patients with optic neuritis. *J Neurol Sci* 1992; **113**: 50–54.

21. Paemen L, Olsson T, Söderström M et al. Evaluation of gelatinases and IL-6 in the cerebrospinal fluid of patients with optic neuritis, multiple sclerosis and other inflammatory neurological diseases. *Eur J Neurol* 1994; **1**: 55–63.

22. Fleischer B. CD26: a surface protease involved in T-cell activation. *Immunol Today* 1994; **15**: 180–184.

23. Hafler DA, Fox DA, Manning ME et al. In vivo activated T lymphocytes in the peripheral blood and cerebrospinal fluid of patients with multiple sclerosis. *N Engl J Med* 1985; **312**: 1405–1411.

24. Constantinescu CS, Kamoun M, Dotti M et al. A longitudinal study of the T cell activation marker CD26 in chronic progressive multiple sclerosis. *J Neurol Sci* 1995; **130**: 178–182.

25. Sellebjerg F, Jensen J, Ryder LP. Costimulatory CD80 (B7-1) and CD86 (B7-2) on cerebrospinal fluid cells in multiple sclerosis. *J Neuroimmunol* 1998; **84**: 179–182.

26. Konttinen YT, Bergroth V, Kinnunen E et al. Activated T lymphocytes in patients with multiple sclerosis in clinical remission. *J Neurol Sci* 1987; **81**: 133–139.

27. Fredrikson S, Karlsson Parra A, Olsson T. Link H, HLA-DR antigen expression on T cells from cerebrospinal fluid in multiple sclerosis and aseptic meningo-encephalitis. *Clin Exp Immunol* 1987; **68**: 298–304.

28. Oksaranta O, Tarvonen S, Ilonen J et al. Influx of nonactivated T lymphocytes into the cerebrospinal fluid during relapse of multiple sclerosis. *Ann Neurol* 1995; **38**: 465–468.

29. Kumar V, Sercarz E. Dysregulation of potentially pathogenic self reactivity is crucial for the manifestation of clinical autoimmunity. *J Neurosci Res* 1996; **45**: 334–339.

30. Weinstock Guttman B, Ransohoff RM, Kinkel RP, Rudick RA. The interferons: biological effects, mechanisms of action, and use in multiple sclerosis. *Ann Neurol* 1995; **37**: 7–15.

31. Hall GL, Compston A, Scolding NJ. Beta-interferon and multiple sclerosis. *Trends Neurosci* 1997; **20**: 63–67.

32. Ossege LM, Sindern E, Voss B, Malin JP. Corticosteroids induce expression of transforming-growth-factor-beta1 mRNA in peripheral blood mononuclear cells of patients with multiple sclerosis. *J Neuroimmunol* 1998; **84**: 1–6.

33. Pitzalis C, Sharrack B, Gray IA et al. Comparison of the effects of oral versus intravenous methylprednisolone regimens on peripheral blood T lymphocyte adhesion molecule expression, T cell subsets distribution and TNF alpha concentrations in multiple sclerosis. *J Neuroimmunol* 1997; **74**: 62–68.

34. Smith DR, Balashov KE, Hafler DA et al. Immune deviation following pulse cyclophosphamide/methylprednisolone treatment of multiple sclerosis: increased interleukin-4 production and associated eosinophilia. *Ann Neurol* 1997; **42**: 313–318.

35. Gayo A, Mozo L, Suarez A et al. Glucocorticoids increase IL-10 expression in multiple sclerosis patients with acute relapse. *J Neuroimmunol* 1998; **85**: 122–130.

36. Paolino E, Fainardi E, Ruppi P et al. A prospective study on the predictive value of CSF oligoclonal bands and MRI in acute isolated neurological syndromes for subsequent progression to multiple sclerosis. *J Neurol Neurosurg Psychiatry* 1996; **60**: 572–575.

37. Sandberg Wollheim M, Bynke H, Cronqvist S et al. A long-term prospective study of optic neuritis: evaluation of risk factors. *Ann Neurol* 1990; **27**: 386–393.

38. Stendahl Brodin L, Link H. Relation between benign course of multiple sclerosis and low-grade humoral immune response in cerebrospinal fluid. *J Neurol Neurosurg Psychiatry* 1980; **43**: 102–105.

39. Kostulas VK, Henriksson A, Link H. Monosymptomatic sensory symptoms and

cerebrospinal fluid immunoglobulin levels in relation to multiple sclerosis. *Arch Neurol* 1986; **43**: 447–451.

40. Sharief MK, Thompson EJ. The predictive value of intrathecal immunoglobulin synthesis and magnetic resonance imaging in acute isolated syndromes for subsequent development of multiple sclerosis. *Ann Neurol* 1991; **29**: 147–151.
41. Söderström M, Lindqvist M, Hillert J et al. Optic neuritis: findings on MR, CSF examination and HLA class II typing in 60 patients and results of a short-term follow-up. *J Neurol* 1994; **241**: 391–397.
42. Jacobs LD, Kaba SE, Miller CM et al. Correlation of clinical, magnetic resonance imaging, and cerebrospinal fluid findings in optic neuritis. *Ann Neurol* 1997; **41**: 392–398.
43. Söderström M, Jin Y-P, Hillert J, Link H. Optic neuritis. Prognosis for multiple sclerosis from MRI, CSF, and HLA findings. *Neurology* 1998; **50**: 708–714.
44. Zeman AZ, Kidd D, McLean BN et al. A study of oligoclonal band negative multiple sclerosis. *J Neurol Neurosurg Psychiatry* 1996; **60**: 27–30.
45. Fieschi C, Gasperini C, Ristori G et al. Diagnostic problems in 'clinically definite' multiple sclerosis patients with normal CSF and multiple MRI abnormalities. *Eur J Neurol* 1994; **1**: 127–133.
46. Frick E, Stickl H. Optic neuritis and multiple sclerosis. An immunological study. *Neurology* 1980; **19**: 185–191.
47. Söderström M, Link H, Xu Z, Fredriksson S. Optic neuritis and multiple sclerosis: anti-MBP and anti-MBP peptide antibody-secreting cells are accumulated in CSF. *Neurology* 1993; **43**: 1215–1222.
48. Sellebjerg FT, Frederiksen JL, Olsson T. Anti-myelin basic protein and anti-proteolipid protein antibody-secreting cells in the cerebrospinal fluid of patients with acute optic neuritis. *Arch Neurol* 1994; **51**: 1032–1036.
49. Sellebjerg F, Madsen HO, Frederiksen JL et al. Acute optic neuritis: myelin basic protein and proteolipid protein antibodies, affinity, and the HLA system. *Ann Neurol* 1995; **38**: 943–950.
50. Warren KG, Catz I, Johnson E, Mielke B, Anti-myelin basic protein and anti-proteolipid protein specific forms of multiple sclerosis. *Ann Neurol* 1994; **35**: 280–289.
51. Sun JB, Olsson T, Wang WZ et al. Autoreactive T and B cells responding to myelin proteolipid protein in multiple sclerosis and controls. *Eur J Immunol* 1991; **21**: 1461–1468.
52. Constant S, Sant'Angelo D, Pasqualini T et al. Peptide and protein antigens require distinct antigen-presenting cell subsets for the priming of CD4+ T cells. *J Immunol* 1995; **154**: 4915–4923.
53. Constant S, Schweitzer N, West J et al. B lymphocytes can be competent antigen-presenting cells for priming CD4+ T cells to protein antigens in vivo. *J Immunol* 1995; **155**: 3734–3741.
54. Lin R-H, Mamula MJ, Hardin JA, Janeway CA. Induction of autoreactive B cells allows priming of autoreactive T cells. *J Exp Med* 1991; **173**: 1433–1439.
55. Mamula MJ, Fatenajad S, Craft J. B cells process and present lupus autoantigens that initiate autoimmune T cell responses. *J Immunol* 1994; **152**: 1453–1461.
56. Sellebjerg F, Frederiksen JL, Olsson T et al. Peptide specificity of anti-myelin basic protein antibodies in patients with acute optic neuritis and the HLA system. *Scand J Immunol* 1994; **39**: 575–580.
57. Owens GP, Kraus H, Burgoon MP et al. Restricted use of VH4 germline segments in an acute multiple sclerosis brain. *Ann Neurol* 1998; **43**: 236–243.
58. Chambers CA, Allison JP. Co-stimulation in T cell responses. *Curr Opin Immunol* 1997; **9**: 396–404.
59. Lenschow DJ, Walunas TL, Bluestone JA. CD28/B7 system of T cell costimulation. *Annu Rev Immunol* 1996; **14**: 233–258.
60. Scholz C, Patton KT, Anderson DE et al. Expansion of autoreactive T cells in multiple sclerosis is independent of exogenous B7 co-stimulation. *J Immunol* 1998; **160**: 1532–1538.
61. Lovett-Racke AE, Trotter J, Lauber J et al. Decreased dependence of myelin basic protein-reactive T cells on CD28-mediated costimulation in multiple sclerosis patients. *J Clin Invest* 1998; **101**: 725–730.
62. Racke MK, Scott DE, Quigley L et al. Distinct roles for B7-1 (CD-80) and B7-2 (CD-86) in the initiation of experimental allergic encephalomyelitis. *J Clin Invest* 1995; **96**: 2195–2203.
63. Kuchroo VK, Das MP, Brown JA et al. B7-1 and B7-2 costimulatory molecules activate differentially the Th1/Th2 developmental pathways: application to autoimmune disease therapy. *Cell* 1995; **80**: 707–718.

64. Freeman GJ, Boussiotis VA, Anumanthan A et al. B7-1 and B7-2 do not deliver identical co-stimulatory signals, since B7-2 but not B7-1 preferentially costimulates the initial production of IL-4. *Immunity* 1995; **2**: 523–532.

65. Jiang H, Milo R, Swoveland P et al. Interferon beta-1b reduces interferon gamma induced antigen-presenting capacity of human glial and B cells. *J Neuroimmunol* 1995; **61**: 17–25.

66. Genc K, Dona DL, Reder AT. Increased CD80+ B cells in active multiple sclerosis and reversal by interferon beta-1b therapy. *J Clin Invest* 1997; **99**: 2664–2671.

67. Brabb T, Goldrath AW, von Dassow P et al. Triggers of autoimmune disease in a murine TCR-transgenic model for multiple sclerosis. *J Immunol* 1997; **159**: 497–507.

68. Springer TA. Traffic signals for lymphocyte recirculation and leukocyte emigration: the multistep paradigm. *Cell* 1993; **76**: 301–314.

69. Berlin C, Bargatze RF, Campbell JJ et al. Alfa4 integrins mediate lymphocyte attachment and rolling under physiologic flow. *Cell* 1995; **80**: 413–433.

70. Murphy PM. The molecular biology of leukocyte chemoattractant receptors. *Annu Rev Immunol* 1994; **12**: 593–633.

71. Baggiolini M, Dewald B, Moser B. Human chemokines: an update. *Annu Rev Immunol* 1997; **15**: 675–705.

72. Rollins BJ. Chemokines. *Blood* 1997; **3**: 909–928.

73. Luster AD. Chemokines–chemotactic cytokines that mediate inflammation. *N Engl J Med* 1998; **338**: 436–445.

74. Romanic AM, Madri JA. Extracellular matrix-degrading proteinases in the nervous system. *Brain Pathol* 1994; **4**: 145–156.

75. Chandler S, Miller KM, Clements JM et al. Matrix metalloproteinases, tumor necrosis factor and multiple sclerosis: an overview. *J Neuroimmunol* 1997; **72**: 155–161.

76. Yong VW, Krekoski CA, Forsyth PA et al. Matrix metalloproteinases and diseases of the CNS. *Trends Neurosci* 1998; **21**: 75–80.

77. Sørensen TL, Tani M, Jensen J et al. Expression of specific chemokines and chemokine receptors in the central nervous system of multiple sclerosis patients. *J Clin Invest* 1999; **103**: 807–815.

78. Bö L, Peterson JW, Mørk S et al. Distribution of immunoglobulin superfamily members ICAM-1, -2, -3, and the beta2 integrin LFA-1 in multiple sclerosis lesions. *J Neuropathol Exp Neurol* 1996; **55**: 1060–1072.

79. Washington R, Burton J, Todd RF 3rd et al. Expression of immunologically relevant endothelial cell activation antigens on isolated central nervous system microvessels from patients with multiple sclerosis. *Ann Neurol* 1994; **35**: 89–97.

80. Sobel RA, Mitchell ME, Fondren G. Intercellular adhesion molecule-1 (ICAM-1) in cellular immune reactions in the human central nervous system. *Am J Pathol* 1990; **136**: 1309–1316.

81. Wakatsuki T, Kimura K, Kimura F et al. A distinct mRNA encoding a soluble form of ICAM-1 molecule expressed in human tissues. *Cell Adhesion Communication* 1995; **3**: 283–292.

82. Lyons PD, Benveniste EN. Cleavage of membrane-associated ICAM-1 from astrocytes. *Glia* 1998; **22**: 103–112.

83. Trojano M, Avolio C, Simone IL et al. Soluble intercellular adhesion molecule-1 in serum and cerebrospinal fluid of clinically active relapsing-remitting multiple sclerosis. *Neurology* 1996; **47**: 1535–1541.

84. Rieckmann P, Altenhofen B, Riegel A et al. Soluble adhesion molecules (sVCAM-1 and sICAM-1) in cerebrospinal fluid and serum correlate with MRI activity in multiple sclerosis. *Ann Neurol* 1997; **41**: 326–333.

85. Giovannoni G, Lai M, Thorpe J et al. Longitudinal study of soluble adhesion molecules in multiple sclerosis: correlation with gadolinium enhanced magnetic resonance imaging. *Neurology* 1997; **48**: 1557–1565.

86. Petersen AA, Sellebjerg F, Frederiksen J et al. Soluble ICAM-1, demyelination, and inflammation in multiple sclerosis and acute optic neuritis. *J Neuroimmunol* 1998; **88**: 120–127.

87. Gijbels K, Masure S, Carton H, Opdenakker G. Gelatinase in the cerebrospinal fluid of patients with multiple sclerosis and other inflammatory disorders. *J Neuroimmunol* 1992; **41**: 29–34.

88. Cuzner ML, Gveric D, Strand C et al. The expression of tissue-type plasminogen activator, matrix metalloproteases and endogenous inhibitors in the central nervous system in multiple sclerosis: comparison of stages in lesion evolution. *J Neuropathol Exp Neurol* 1996; **55**: 1194–1204.

89. Anthony DC, Ferguson B, Matyszak MK et al. Differential matrix metalloproteinase expression in cases of multiple sclerosis and stroke. *Neuropathol Appl Neurobiol* 1997; **23**: 406–415.

90. Cossins JA, Clements JM, Ford J et al. Enhanced expression of MMP-7 and MMP-9 in demyelinating multiple sclerosis lesions. *Acta Neuropathol (Berl)* 1997; **94**: 590–598.

91. Archelos JJ, Jung S, Maurer M et al. Inhibition of experimental autoimmune encephalomyelitis by an antibody to the intercellular adhesion molecule ICAM-1. *Ann Neurol* 1993; **34**: 145–154.

92. Karpus WJ, Lukacs NW, McRae BL et al. An important role for the chemokine macrophage inflammatory protein-1 alfa in the pathogenesis of the T cell mediated autoimmune disease, experimental autoimmune encephalomyelitis. *J Immunol* 1995; **155**: 5003–5010.

93. Karpus WJ, Kennedy KJ. MIP-1alpha and MCP-1 differentially regulate acute and relapsing autoimmune encephalomyelitis as well as Th1/Th2 lymphocyte differentiation. *J Leukoc Biol* 1997; **62**: 681–687.

94. Leppert D, Waubant E, Bürk MR et al. Interferon beta-1b inhibits gelatinase secretion and in vitro migration of human T cells: a possible mechanism for treatment efficacy in multiple sclerosis. *Ann Neurol* 1996; **40**: 846–852.

95. Stüve O, Dooley NP, Uhm JH et al. Interferon beta-1b decreases the migration of T lymphocytes in vitro: effects on matrix metalloproteinase-9. *Ann Neurol* 1996; **40**: 853–863.

96. Bacon KB, Premack BA, Gardner P, Schall TJ. Activation of dual T cell signalling pathways by the chemokine RANTES. *Science* 1995; **269**: 1727–1730.

97. Taub DD, Turcovski-Corrales SM, Key ML et al. Chemokines and T lymphocyte activation. I. Beta chemokines costimulate human T lymphocyte activation in vitro. *J Immunol* 1996; **156**: 2095–2103.

98. Karpus WJ, Lukacs NW, Kennedy KJ et al. Differential CC chemokine-induced enhancement of T helper cell cytokine production. *J Immunol* 1997; **158**: 4129–4136.

99. Liu R, Paxton WA, Choe S et al. Homozygous defect in HIV-1 coreceptor accounts for resistance of some multiply exposed individuals to HIV-1 infection. *Cell* 1996; **86**: 367–377.

100. Wu L, Paxton WA, Kassam N et al. CCR5 levels and expression pattern correlate with infectability by macrophage-tropic HIV-1, in vitro. *J Exp Med* 1997; **185**: 1681–1691.

101. Miyagishi R, Kikuchi S, Fukazawa T, Tashiro K. Macrophage inflammatory protein-1alpha in the cerebrospinal fluid of patients with multiple sclerosis and other inflammatory neurological diseases. *J Neurol Sci* 1995; **129**: 223–227.

6

Cross-talk between cells of the immune and nervous systems in health and in multiple sclerosis

Bao-Guo Xiao

INTRODUCTION

For a long time, the immune and nervous systems have been considered as two separate systems, incapable of meaningful cross-talk. Because the cerebrospinal fluid, the blood–brain barrier and the meninges effectively shield the central nervous system (CNS) from other tissues, it was proposed that the brain is an 'immunologically privileged organ' with recent evidence that both microglia and astrocytes secrete numerous cytokines, it is widely accepted that these cells participate actively in an integrative communication between resident immune cells of the CNS and those of the periphery. The CNS is not separated from the immune system, and can turn on, restrict and regulate the immune system.[1] These communications between cells of the immune and nervous systems occur via the co-ordinate use of surface structures (major histocompatibility complex (MHC) class II, costimulatory and adhesion molecules as well as receptors) and soluble mediators (hormones, cytokines, neurotrophic factors and synaptic transmitters).

The interactions between cells of the immune and nervous system are bi-directional in regulating immune reactivities within the CNS. Microglia and astrocytes may play distinct roles in the regulation of immune responses against pathogens and in immune dysregulation, leading to immune attack of CNS-related components. Our increasing understanding of the mechanisms by which microglia and astrocytes modulate immune responses within the CNS undoubtedly will contribute to the development of better immunotherapeutic strategies.

DOES THE CNS SHAPE IMMUNE RESPONSES?

A number of investigations have demonstrated that the CNS constitutes an environment that accommodates, regulates and shapes immune responses.[1-5] First, activated microglia and astrocytes have been observed in multiple sclerosis (MS). Virus, superantigens, lipopolysaccharide and heat shock protein or infiltrating autoreactive T cells can induce activation of microglia and astrocytes in inflammatory conditions. Activated microglia express MHC class II, CD40, B7 and intercellular adhesion molecule (ICAM)-1, while activated astrocytes express MHC class II, ICAM-1 and possibly B7. This contrasts with the situation in health, when the expression of MHC, co-stimulatory and adhesion molecules on glial cells is very low. Activated microglia also exhibit additional properties such as enlargement, increased proliferation, migration and phagocytosis.

Activated microglia and astrocytes not only express MHC, co-stimulatory and adhesion molecules, but produce cytokines. Both microglia and astrocytes secrete interleukin (IL)-1β, IL-3, IL-6, IL-10, interferon (IFN)-γ, tumour necrosis factor (TNF)-α, transforming growth factor (TGF)-β, macrophage colony stimulating factor (M-CSF) and granulocyte–macrophage CSF (GM-CSF). Microglia can also produce IL-2, IL-8 and IL-12. In health, the production of these cytokines within the CNS is low. However, in inflammatory states in the CNS, both infiltrating cells and resident glial cells produce cytokines. These CNS-derived cytokines affect different types of cells, including T cells, B cells, microglia and astrocytes, and constitute a cytokine-mediated network within the CNS (*Fig. 6.1*). For example, M-CSF and GM-CSF stimulate microglial proliferation; TGF-β induces selective microglial apoptosis; IL-1β or IL-6 promote astrocytes to produce glial-derived neurotrophic factor; IL-4 inhibits astrocytes to produce TNF-α and nitric oxide and promotes astrocytes to secrete nerve growth factor; IL-12 promotes the development of T-helper 1 (Th_1) cells; TNF-α triggers astrocytes to produce IFN-γ; and TGF-β or IL-10 inhibit microglia so that secretion of TNF-α and nitric oxide is reduced.

In general, microglia and astrocytes present antigen to T cells, thereby reactivating infiltrating T cells. After treatment with IFN-γ, microglia express high levels of MHC class II, CD40, B7 and ICAM-1, while astrocytes express MHC class II and ICAM-1. Some studies showed that astrocytes express B7, contradicting results from other studies. Both B7-1 and B7-2 can provide co-stimulatory signals to T cells for proliferation and IL-2 production.[6] Local blockage of B7 expression prevents the induction of T-cell-mediated inflammation.[7] It is clear that microglia constitute professional antigen-presenting cells within the CNS.

Immune responses within the CNS are rather weak compared to peripheral immune organs. Fas-ligand (FasL)-induced apoptosis may be a mechanism of immune privilege.[8] Inflammatory cells entering the anterior chamber of the eye in response to viral infection undergo apoptosis that is dependent on Fas–FasL, and produce no tissue damage.[8] The apoptosis of autoreactive T cells in the target organ of experimental allergic encephalomyelitis (EAE) represents activation-induced cell death through the Fas–FasL pathway.[9] However, it has been proposed that Fas–FasL interactions may be a common pathogenic mechanism in organ-specific autoimmunity.[10]

A MODEL OF INFLAMMATORY CNS DEMYELINATION IN MS

In MS, microglia activation factors such as virus, superantigens, lipopolysaccharide and heat shock protein induce activation of microglia. Activated microglia produce proteases, TNF-α and nitric oxide, resulting in damage to the oligodendrocyte–myelin unit. The expression of chemokines on glial cells contributes to the recruitment of autoreactive T cells, which results in reactivation of microglia. Based on such findings, the following statements can be made:

(a) An essential element in inflammatory demyelination is the expansion of autoreactive T cells targeting the CNS.
(b) Autoreactive T cells in the CNS are not directly involved in demyelinating processes, because neither myelin nor oligodendrocyte express MHC class II molecules that are the natural ligands for T cell receptor.
(c) Demyelination might result from secretion of microglial factors that directly induce damage of the oligodendrocyte–myelin unit. Whether these soluble factors produced by microglia are sufficient to induce damage of the oligodendrocyte myelin unit remains to be determined.

A model has been proposed that is not based on an autoimmune response, but is likely to explain the clinical presentation and disease course seen in MS. In this model, microglia

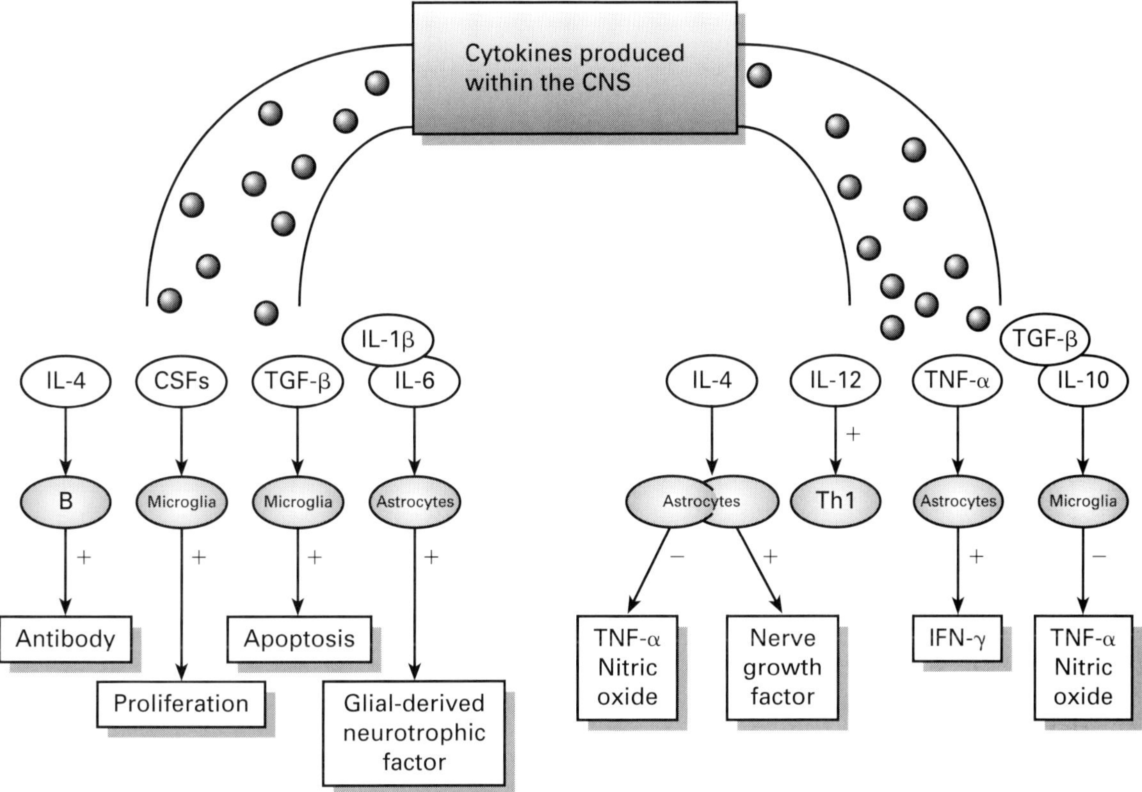

Figure 6.1 Cytokine-mediated network within the CNS. CNS-derived cytokines affect different types of cells (infiltrating cells and resident glial cells), and constitute a cytokine-mediated network.

activation is a central element in CNS demyelination.

Interactions between cells of immune and nervous systems

The interactions between cells of the immune and nervous systems are bi-directional and involve two principles:

(a) bi-directional interaction between cells of the immune and nervous systems.

(b) bi-directional events induced by interaction between cells of the immune and nervous system.

Bi-directional interaction between cells of the immune and nervous systems

In this interaction, autoreactive T cells induce activation of glial cells. Activated human T lymphocytes induce microglial production of TNF-α.[12] Conversely, activated glial cells also influence the functions of infiltrating T cells. Human microglia activate lymphoproliferative responses to recall viral antigen,[13] and non-activated rat astrocytes down-regulate T-cell expression, T-cell proliferation and TNF-α production.[14] The interactions were mediated by cell–cell contact or soluble factors. The author has found that T cells derived from EAE rats trigger astrocytes to produce nitric oxide, and that this interaction is specific antigen dependent (Xiao et al, unpublished). It has also been reported that conditioned medium from encephalitogenic myelin basic protein (MBP)-reactive lymphoid cells induced the expression of inducible nitric oxide synthase (iNOS) in primary cultures of murine astrocytes in a time-dependent and concentration-dependent manner.[15]

Bi-directional events induced by interaction between cells of the immune and nervous systems

The interaction between T cells and glial cells stimulates activation of microglia and astrocytes. Microglia can stimulate naïve T-cell proliferation, while astrocytes conversely inhibit microglia to stimulate T-cell proliferation.[16] The author has found that astrocytes not only inhibited antigen-specific T-cell proliferation and IFN-γ production, but reduced MBP-specific IgG production by B cells in vitro.[17] Double staining by the Tdt-mediated dUTP-biotin nick end labeling (TUNEL) method and immunocytochemistry for astrocytes and microglia revealed that astrocytes, rather than microglia, induce apoptosis of infiltrating cells.[18] Taken together, the bi-directional interactions play a much more active role in regulating immune reactivity within the CNS than was anticipated. Besides autoreactive T cells, glial cells also have an important role in communicating with antigen-specific T cells: they serve as antigen-presenting cells in the initial phase of the immune response and as accessory cells that amplify the effector phase of the immune response.

The balance between microglia and astrocytes

Mechanisms that regulate the balance of Th_1 and T-helper 2 (Th_2) cell responses are of great interest because they may determine the outcome of disease. Cytokines can regulate the balance of Th_1 and Th_2 cells. For example, IL-12 promotes the development of Th_1 cells whereas IL-4 leads to the expansion of Th_2 cells. In CNS inflammation, it is proposed that there may be a balance between microglia and astrocytes in regulating local immune responses (*Fig. 6.2*). Microglia not only induce the development of Th_1 cells via IL-12 production by microglia, but also damage the oligodendrocyte–myelin unit directly through secretion of proteases, TNF-α and nitric oxide. Astrocytes present antigen mainly to Th_2 cells and induce Th_2 cell responses, or contribute to remyelination by the production of neurotrophic factors such as nerve growth factor, glial-derived neurotrophic factor and basic fibroblast growth factor.

Recent studies provide much evidence for such a balance. Microglia produce IL-12 and promote the development of Th_1 cells.[19] Astrocytes mainly induce Th_2 cell responses.[20] Astrocytes also promote outgrowth by human oligodendrocytes in vitro through basic fibroblast growth factor or other neurotrophic factors.[21] MHC class II-positive microglia directly support an effector response in vivo by encephalitogenic MBP-reactive CD4[+] T cells, which in turn produce IFN-γ and TNF-α.[22] Astrocytic factors deactivate antigen-presenting cells that invade the CNS. For example, rat spleen activated macrophages were changed to resting state after co-culture with astrocytes. The resting state was accompanied by reduced expression of leukocyte function antigen, ICAM-1 and MHC class II.[23] Endotoxin-induced expression of iNOS in microglia is inhibited by astrocyte-derived TGF-β[24] and production of IL-12 by microglia is inhibited in the presence of astrocytes.[19] TGF-β also selectively induces microglial apoptosis,[25] and inhibits proliferation and expression of ICAM-1 on glial cells.[26] The balance between microglia and astrocytes seems thus to be important for regulating Th_1 and Th_2 cell responses and demyelinating processes.

The multiplicity of astrocyte functions

There is no doubt that astrocyte functions are complicated. Besides negative regulation (astrocytes present antigen to Th_2 cells, inhibit microglia reactivity, suppress T and B cell functions, and produce neurotrophic factors), many

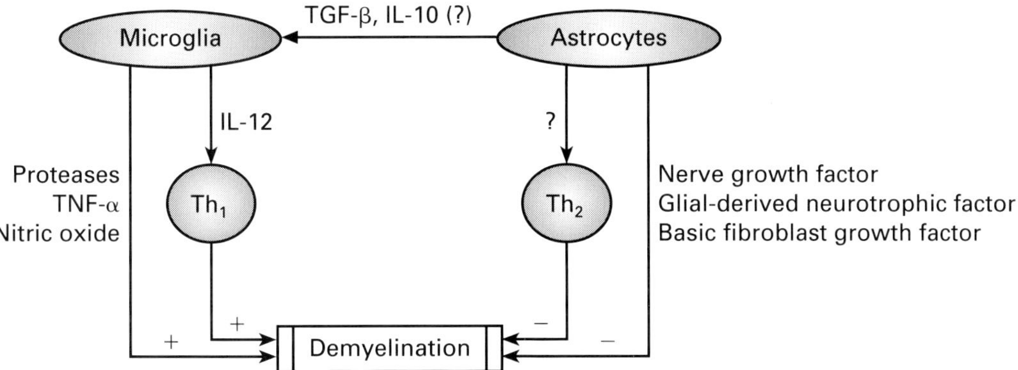

Figure 6.2 The balance of microglia and astrocytes in regulating Th$_1$ and Th$_2$ cell responses and demyelinating processes. The left panel represents positive regulation of microglia by promoting Th$_1$ cell responses and producing proteases, TNF-α and nitric oxide. The right panel demonstrates the negative regulation of astrocytes by inducing Th$_2$ cell responses and secreting nerve growth factor, glial-derived neurotrophic factor and basic fibroblast growth factor. The upper panel indicates that astrocytes also result in deactivation of microglia.

contrary results have also been reported (*Fig. 6.3*). IFN-γ-activated astrocytes in an inflammatory environment have the capacity to express the required MHC class II and B7 co-stimulatory molecules necessary for efficient activation of naïve T cells.[27] IL-1 stimulates human astrocyte iNOS messenger RNA expression and nitric oxide production via a NF-κB mechanism.[28] Astrocytes also express IFN-γ, TNF-α and β-family chemokines in vivo and in vitro.[29–32]

The multiplicity of astrocyte functions may have different origins:

(a) Different culture stage: after astrocytes are treated with IFN-γ, they express both B7-1 and B7-2 and induce mainly Th$_2$ cell responses at an early stage; at a later stage, however, astrocytes express only B7-2 and induce mainly Th$_2$ cell responses.

(b) Different culture conditions: when astrocytes are cultured alone, they produce only low levels of TGF-β, while IL-10 was not detectable; however when astrocytes are co-cultured with T cells, levels of TGF-β and IL-10 produced by astrocytes are increased.

(c) Different types of astrocytes: astrocytes are divided into type 1 and type 2 astrocytes, and different types of astrocytes may have different functions.

(d) Different regions of the brain: astrocytes derived from different brain regions may have different functions.

IMPORTANCE OF INTERACTIONS BETWEEN THE IMMUNE AND NERVOUS SYSTEMS

The migration of lymphocytes through the blood–brain barrier is not completely random. T cells have marked propensity to migrate towards the CNS. The selective infiltration by T cells seems to reflect some changes observed in inflammatory lesions within the CNS. The expression of MHC and cell adhesion molecules on microglia and astrocytes may provide some signals for the selective migration of T cells.

T cells activated in peripheral lymphoid organs can cross the blood–brain barrier and recognize target antigens within the CNS. In this scenario, resident CNS glial cells are likely

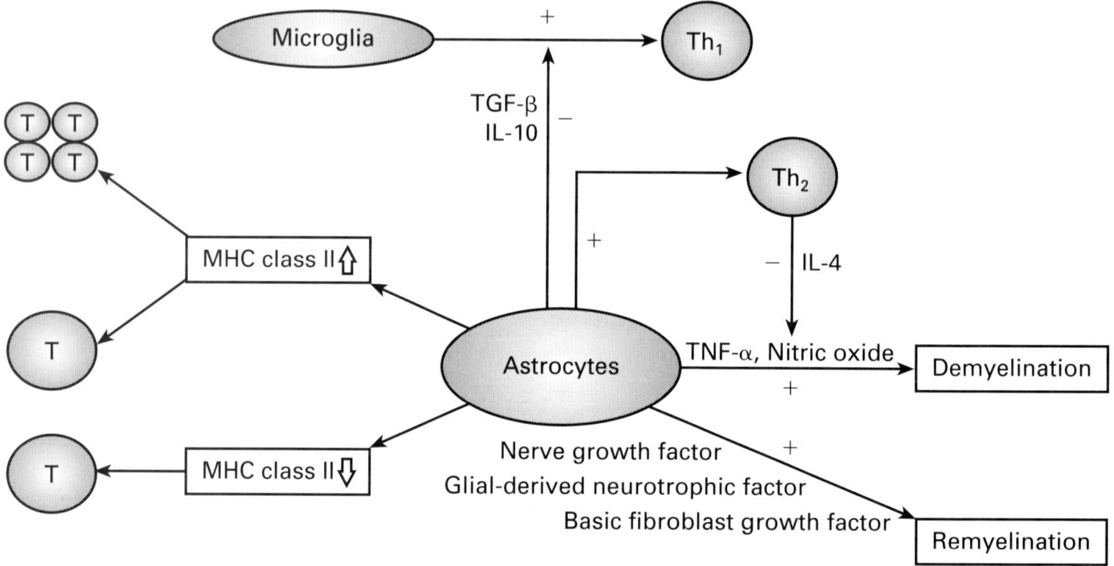

Figure 6.3 The multiplicity of astrocyte functions in regulating Th$_1$ and Th$_2$ cell responses and demyelinating processes. Astrocytes can induce Th$_2$ cell responses, inhibit microglia activity, suppress T cell functions and produce neurotrophic factors. Conversely, astrocytes also produce TNF-α and nitric oxide, and prime T cell activity when expression of MHC class II is increased.

to play a major role in cell reactivation and may contribute to the propagation and maintenance of immune responses in MS. T-cell activation within the CNS is still poorly understood and no information is yet available on the efficiency of CNS antigen-presenting cells to restimulate Th$_1$ and Th$_2$ responses in vivo. Microglia and astrocytes may play distinct roles in the regulation of immune responses against pathogens and in immune dysregulation, leading to an autoimmune attack against CNS-related components. One hypothesis would argue that immunotherapy based on reducing the activity of microglia is likely to bear greater dividends than immunotherapy targeted at T cells.[11]

The interaction between cells of the immune and nervous systems requires MHC expression on glial cells. However, MHC expression on glial cells is controlled by two signals. A positive signal is mediated by IFN-γ produced by T cells. A negative signal arises from functional neurons. For example, functional neurones pro-

duce glutamate, which suppresses MHC class II expression on microglia. Evidence supports the notion that immune cells can bind different neurotransmitters and neuropeptides. Immune responses in peripheral immune organs may also be regulated by the nervous system.

In the brain, immune responses are indeed down-regulated by cell–cell effects. In health, glial cells are under strict control by functional neurones that limit CNS immune responses to a necessary minimum. Under pathological condition, the interaction between cells of immune and nervous systems is augmented. At the 5th International Congress of Neuroimmunology held in Montreal, Canada, in August 1998, it was convincingly demonstrated that neuropathologies in the CNS result not only from defects of the immune system, but also from failure of normal CNS mechanisms. Recently, it has been pointed out that modulating the CNS might be a promising approach for immune therapy.[1] The local interaction between the autonomic nervous system and the immune system in lymphoid and non-lymphoid tissues represents one rationale for immunotherapy in MS to control immune responses.[1,33,34]

ACKNOWLEDGEMENTS

These studies have been supported by the Swedish MS Society (NHR), the Swedish Medical Research Council and Karolinska Institute Research Funds.

REFERENCES

1. Straub RH, Westermann J, Schölmerich J, Falk W. Dialogue between the CNS and the immune system in lymphoid organs. *Immunol Today* 1998; **19**: 409–413.
2. Lotan M, Schwartz M. Cross talk between the immune system and the nervous system in response to injury: implications for regeneration. *FASEB J* 1994; **8**: 1026–1033.
3. Merrill J, Jonakait GM. Interactions of the nervous and immune systems in development, normal brain homeostasis, and disease. *FASEB J* 1995; **9**: 611–618.
4. Owens T, Renno T, Taupin V, Krakowski M. Inflammatory cytokines in the brain: does the CNS shape immune responses? *Immunol Today* 1994; **15**: 566–571.
5. Xiao BG, Link H. Immune regulation within the central nervous system (review). *J Neurol Sci* 1998; **157**: 1–12.
6. Freeman GJ, Borriello F, Hodes RJ et al. Murine B7-2, an alternative CTLA-4 counter-receptor that costimulates T cell proliferation and interleukin 2 production. *J Exp Med* 1993; **178**: 2178–2192.
7. Chen H, Hendricks RL. B7 costimulatory requirements of T cells at an inflammatory site. *J Immunol* 1998; **160**: 5045–5052.
8. Griffith TS, Brunner T, Fletcher SM et al. FasL-induced apoptosis as a mechanism of immune privilege. *Science* 1995; **270**: 1189–1192.
9. White CA, McCombe PA, Pender MP. The roles of Fas, Fas ligand and Bcl-2 in T cell apoptosis in the central nervous system in experimental autoimmune encephalomyelitis. *J Neuroimmunol* 1998; **82**: 47–55.
10. Maria RO, Testi R. Fas–FasL interactions: a common pathogenetic mechanism in organ-specific autoimmunity. *Immunol Today* 1998; **19**: 121–125.
11. Sriram S, Rodriguez M. Indictment of the microglia as the villain in multiple sclerosis. *Neurology* 1997; **48**: 464–470.
12. Chabot S, Williams G, Yong VW. Microglial production of TNF-α is induced by activated T lymphocytes. Involvement of VLA-4 and inhibition by interferon beta-1b. *J Clin Invest* 1997; **100**: 604–612.
13. Dhib-Jalbut S, Gogate N, Jiang H et al. Human microglia activate lymphoproliferative responses to recall viral antigens. *J Neuroimmunol* 1996; **65**: 67–73.
14. Sun D, Coleclough C, Whitaker J. Nonactivated astrocytes downregulate T cell receptor expression and reduce antigen-specific proliferation and cytokine production of myelin basic protein-reactive T cells. *J Neuroimmunol* 1997; **78**: 69–78.
15. Hewett SJ, Misko TP, Keeling RM et al. Murine encephalitogenic lymphoid cells induce nitric oxide synthase in primary astrocytes. *J Neuroimmunol* 1996; **64**: 201–208.
16. Carson MR, Lo D, Campbell IL, Sutcliffe JG. Microglia and astrocytes as interactive regulators of adaptive immune responses in the CNS (abstract). *J Neuroimmunol* 1998; **90**: 47.
17. Xiao BG, Diab A, Zhu J, van der Meide P, Link H. Astrocytes induce hyporesponses of myelin basic protein-reactive T and B cell function. *J Neuroimmunol* 1998; **89**: 113–121.
18. Kohji T, Tanuma N, Aikawa Y et al. Interaction between apoptotic cells and reactive brain cells in the central nervous system of rats with autoimmune encephalomyelitis. *J Neuroimmunol* 1998; **82**: 168–174.
19. Aloisi F, Penna G, Cerase J et al. IL-12 production by central nervous system microglia is inhibited by astrocytes. *J Immunol* 1997; **159**: 1604–1612.
20. Aloisi F, Ria, F, Penna G, Adorini L. Microglia are more efficient than astrocytes in antigen processing and Th1 but not Th2 cell activation. *J Immunol* 1998; **160**: 4671–4680.
21. Oh LY, Yong VW. Astrocytes promote process outgrowth by adult human oligodendrocytes in vitro through interaction between bFGF and astrocyte extracellular matrix. *Glia* 1996; **17**: 237–253.
22. Ford AL, Foulcher E, Lemckert FA, Sedgwick JD. Microglia induce CD4+ T lymphocyte final effector function and death. *J Exp Med* 1996; **184**: 1737–1745.

23. Hailer NP, Heppner FL, Haas D et al. Astrocytic factors deactivate antigen presenting cells that invade the central nervous system. *Brain Pathol* 1998; **8**: 45–74.
24. Vincent VA, Tiders FJ, Van Dam AM. Inhibition of endotoxin-induced nitric oxide synthase production in microglial cells by the presence of astroglial cells: a role for transforming growth factor beta. *Glia* 1997; **19**: 190–198.
25. Xiao BG, Bai XF, Zhang GX, Link H. Transforming growth factor induces apoptosis of rat microglia without relation to bcl-2 oncoprotein expression. *Neurosci Lett* 1997; **226**: 71–74.
26. Xiao BG, Zhang GX, Ma CG, Link H. Transforming growth factor-beta 1-mediated inhibition of glial cell proliferation and down-regulation of intercellular adhesion molecule-1 are interrupted by interferon-gamma. *Clin Exp Immunol* 1996; **103**: 475–481.
27. Nikcevich KM, Gordon KB, Tan L et al. IFN-γ-activated primary murine astrocytes express B7 costimulatory molecules and prime naive antigen-specific T cells. *J Immunol* 1997; **158**: 614–621.
28. Chao CC, Lokensgard JR, Sheng WS et al. IL-1-induced iNOS expression in human astrocytes via NF-κB. *NeuroReport* 1997; **8**: 3163–3166.
29. Guo H, Jin YX, Ishikawa M et al. Regulation of β-chemokine mRNA expression in adult rat astrocytes by lipopolysaccharide, proinflammatory and immunoregulatory cytokines. *Scand J Immunol* 1998; **48**: 502–508.
30. Miyagishi R, Kikuchi S, Takayama C et al. Identification of cell types producing RANTES, MIP-1α and MIP-1β in rat experimental autoimmune encephalomyelitis by in situ hybridization. *J Neuroimmunol* 1997; **77**: 17–26.
31. Xiao BG, Zhang GX, Bai XF, Link H. IFN-γ secretion of astrocytes triggered by TNF-α. *NeuroReport* 1998; **9**: 1487–1490.
32. Xiao BG, Mousa A, Kivisäkk P et al. Induction of β-family chemokine mRNA in human embryonic astrocytes by inflammatory cytokines and measles virus. *J Neurocytol* 1998; in press.
33. Neumann H, Wekerle H. Neuronal control of the immune response in the central nervous system: linking brain immunity to neurodegeneration. *J Neuropathol Exp Neurol* 1998; **57**: 1–9.
34. Exton MS, von Horsten S, Schult M et al. Behaviorally conditioned immunesuppression using cyclosporine A: central nervous system reduces IL-2 production via spenic innervation. *J Neuroimmunol* 1998; **88**: 182–191.

7

The role of autoantibodies in the action of cytokines

Moiz Bakhiet

WHAT ARE CYTOKINES?

Cytokines are peptides that act as signals between the cells of the immune system. They are liberated during activation of immunologically relevant cells. In serum, they bind to transport proteins such as $\alpha 2$ macroglobulin or to soluble receptors[1] and act by binding to specific high-affinity cell surface receptors.[2] Most cytokines act locally but some act systemically with overlapping and potentially dangerous functions.[3] Such cytokines, namely tumour necrosis factor (TNF)-α, interleukin (IL)-1α, IL-1β and interferon (IFN)-γ, may be involved in complications of severe infections or autoimmune diseases.[4,5] In central nervous system (CNS) infections (e.g. bacterial meningitis), high levels of TNF-α, IL-1β and IL-6 have been reported and these levels correlate to the severity of the disease.[6] Furthermore, IFN-γ TGF-β and perforin messenger RNA expression has been found to be up-regulated in acute aseptic meningitis.[7] In nervous system autoimmune diseases, such as Guillian–Barré syndrome, which is a major demyelinating disease of the peripheral nervous system, TNF-α,[8] IL-2[9] and IL-6[10] are believed to play an important role in the immunopathogenesis of the disease. The triggering events and the mechanism used to control the outcome of cytokine activation are not yet fully understood. It is generally believed that natural regulation may be achieved at different stages:

(a) the cytokine gene activation stage;
(b) during secretion and in circulation; and
(c) cytokine–target cell interaction.

In the soluble phase, cytokines are controlled by binding to soluble receptors or antibodies (*Fig. 7.1*).

ANTI-CYTOKINE AUTOANTIBODIES

Several studies have demonstrated the presence of antibodies against cytokines in diseased subjects as well as healthy subjects.[11,12] Anti-cytokine autoantibodies (Aabs) are defined as naturally occurring antibodies that may interfere with the activity of a cytokine and whose Fab parts bind a cytokine in a saturable manner. They are almost exclusively of the IgG class and may function as specific carriers and systemic regulators of circulating cytokines in vivo.

The detection of cytokine Aabs is difficult. False-positive results may be obtained from the non-specific and low-affinity binding that often occurs between IgG and recombinant human cytokines attached to plastic or nitrocellulose

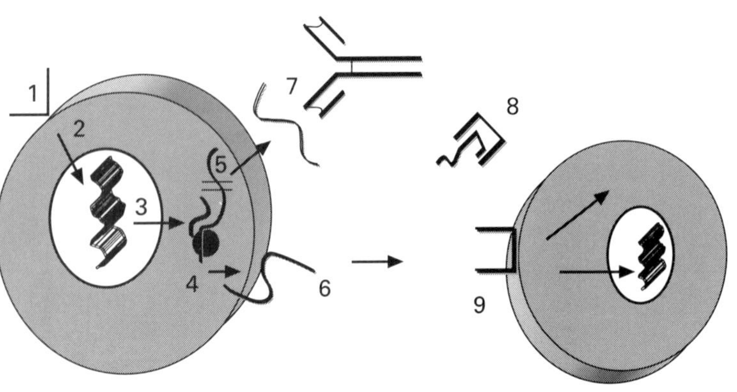

Figure 7.1 Cytokines are tightly regulated, during induction (1, 2), gene transcription (3) and translation (4), protein synthesis (5) and secretion (6). Once released, the cytokines are regulated in the circulation (7, 8) and at the receptor level on target cells (9).[13]

membranes, a procedure usually used in immunometric or immunoblotting assays for cytokines.[13] False-positive results may also arise from the use of recombinant cytokines produced, for example, in yeast cells; this is because the glycosylated molecules contain α-galactose residues that react with natural antibody to α-galactose that is present in humans and other higher primates.[14] Demonstration of binding to the Fab fragments of the immunoglobulins, combined with saturation binding analysis and demonstration of cross-binding to the native cytokines, is therefore essential to verify the presence in biological fluids of specific anti-cytokine antibodies.[15]

The biological role of specific autoantibodies to certain cytokines is not understood, although the forces by which autoantibodies bind suggest that they interfere with immune and inflammatory processes (e.g. by blocking or destroying antigen-presenting cells carrying membrane-bound cytokine or by scavenging bioactive cytokines released by cells at inflammatory sites). It has also been postulated that a maintained balance of these cytokines and anticytokine antibodies may protect from sequelae.[16] Although naturally occurring, high-avidity Aabs to IL-1α, IL-6, IL-10, IFN-α and granulocyte–macrophage colony stimulating factor (GM-CSF) are well documented, their clinical and physiological relevance is still obscure. The frequencies of healthy individuals

with these Aabs varies considerably, from up to 75% of Caucasians with Aabs to IL-1α to less than 3% with Aabs to the other cytokines.[13,17,18] Interestingly, the few people with Aabs to IFN-α and GM-CSF often possess very high titres, suggesting that high levels of Aabs to these cytokines are compatible with normal life.[19] Aabs against IL-1α, IL-6, IFN-α and GM-CSF specifically neutralize their respective recombinant and native cytokines.[20] There is an increased prevalence of IL-6 Aabs in patients with rheumatoid arthritis or systemic sclerosis,[21] and the presence of these Aabs correlates with poor survival in patients with alcoholic liver cirrhosis.[22] IL-1α Aabs are generally absent or present only at low levels in patients with Crohn's disease or atopic diseases.[13] A recent study suggested that high circulating levels of Aabs to IL-1α are associated with a better prognosis in patients with rheumatoid arthritis, making detection of these Aabs the best known predictor of less erosive disease.[23]

The occurrence of autoantibodies to proinflammatory and anti-inflammatory cytokines in cerebrospinal fluid (CSF) and plasma of patients with multiple sclerosis (MS), aseptic meningitis and stroke was recently reported. Increased levels of autoantibodies to IFN-γ, TNF-α, IL-4 and IL-10 were detected in both compartments of patients with MS and aseptic meningitis. Interestingly, in CSF of stroke patients, Aabs to IL-4 and IL-10, but not to IFN-γ or TNF-α, were detected. No significant autoantibody levels were registered in plasma of stroke patients against all four cytokines compared to healthy control subjects. Healthy controls revealed very low autoantibody levels in plasma and no detectable autoantibodies in CSF.[24]

These data showed for the first time the occurrence of cytokine autoantibodies in these diseases, but their biological significance is still unclear. However, the data should be considered in view of the evidence that MS may be mediated by autoreactive T cell exhibiting pro-inflammatory cytokine profiles such as IFN-γ and TNF-α.[25,26] As a result, the immune system may attempt to down-modulate these cytokines by inducting their natural Aabs. This was also the case for Aab responses in CSF of patients with aseptic meningitis, since the increased levels of Aab to IFN-γ and TNF-α were more conspicuous than those to IL-4 and IL-10. The relatively high anti-TNF-α Aab level in CSF of patients with aseptic meningitis is of interest because of inflammatory reactions in the subarachnoid space, which are promoted mainly by TNF-α together with IL-1.[27] The increased Aab levels to all four cytokines in plasma of patients with both MS and aseptic meningitis could be a part of a general polyclonal immune activation, resulting from mechanisms that lie behind the immunopathogenesis of MS or the symptoms of aseptic meningitis. In contrast to patients with inflammatory neurological disorders (MS and aseptic meningitis), patients with stroke as an example of a non-inflammatory neurological disorder displayed reversed patterns of anti-cytokine Aabs in CSF. Although increased Aab levels to IL-4 and IL-10 were detected in CSF of stroke patients, no Aabs to the proinflammatory cytokines IFN-γ and TNF-α were detected. Furthermore, stroke patients did not show elevated levels of Aabs to cytokines in plasma. These data may propose a role for the anti-inflammatory cytokines IL-4 and IL-10 and their Aabs, a role that should be further investigated.

In Guillain–Barré syndrome, IFN-γ is thought to be a disease-promoting cytokine. The spontaneous induction of IFN-γ and a mechanism involving the generation of neutralizing Aabs to IFN-γ that may regulate the disease has been reported. The numbers of cells spontaneously secreting IFN-γ in peripheral blood are augmented in Guillain–Barré syndrome, particularly at the peak of clinical disease, and decreased during recovery. This decrease is associated with elevated serum concentrations of IgG Aabs to IFN-γ. These Aabs specifically bind to IFN-γ and neutralize its effects. Aabs to IFN-γ are proposed to be another important regulatory mechanism in IFN-γ-driven Guillain–Barré syndrome.[28]

The basis for the beneficial effect of intravenous immunoglobulin in Guillain–Barré syndrome and certain other autoimmune diseases is not known. In line with the network theory of Jerne,[29] however, certain antibodies present in the injected immunoglobulin may down-regulate B cell populations, producing Aabs against myelin antigens in the peripheral nervous system, which in different ways contribute to the disease. Another putative mechanism for the beneficial effect of intravenous immunoglobulin is the concomitant administration of antibodies to cytokines, including IFN-γ. It can be hypothesized that the often less satisfactory effects of this treatment are due to the presence in the injected immunoglobulin preparation of insufficient amounts of antibodies to pro-inflammatory cytokines (including IFN-γ) or an over-representation of antibodies to anti-inflammatory cytokines. Such factors could possibly also result in differences in efficacy between immunoglobulin preparations from different producers and between different batches of immunoglobulin from the same producer. Defining the concentrations of antibodies to IFN-γ and other cytokines in immunoglobulin preparations might be one way of improving the usefulness of this treatment in Guillain–Barré and other autoimmune diseases. Immunoglobulin preparations are derived from the pooled serum of hundreds of donors, which may argue against the suggested magnitude of the variability. Therefore, studies to measure levels of Aabs to IFN-γ and other cytokines in such immunoglobulin preparations are currently initiated at the author's laboratories in order to resolve this question. In a recent study, naturally occurring antibodies to interferons in human IgG preparations were demonstrated. In vitro neutralization of the antiviral effect of IFN-α and IFN-β, but not of IFN-γ, was observed in 12 of 15 normal IgG preparations.[30]

CONCLUSION

In conclusion, the up-regulation of cytokines during inflammatory and autoimmune diseases is probably associated with the clinical severity. In several diseases, high serum concentrations of neutralizing Aabs to cytokines are significantly correlated with the down-regulation of cytokine levels, the down-regulation of cytokine-producing cells, and with improved clinical disability. The relationship between these three variables suggests an immunoregulatory role for the anti-cytokine Aabs as shown, for example, in Guillain–Barré syndrome. Research and clinical interest should increase when it is more widely known that Aabs interfere with the measurement of several cytokines in biological fluids, pre-existing Aabs may invalidate therapy with the corresponding cytokines and levels of certain cytokine Aabs may predict the outcome of immunoinflammatory diseases. Finally, pharmaceutically prepared normal human IgG contains high-avidity Aabs that interfere with several cytokines in vivo.

REFERENCES

1. Banchereau J. Cytokines. *Biofutur* 1993; **121**: 20–28.
2. Kishimoto T, Taga T, Akira S. Cytokine signal transduction. *Cell* 1994; **76**: 253–262.
3. Bendtzen K. Immune hormones (cytokines): pathogenic role in autoimmune rheumatic diseases and endocrine diseases. *Autoimmunity* 1989; **2**: 177–189.
4. Bernard C, Tedgui A. Cytokine network and the vessel wall: insight into septic shock pathogenesis. *Eur Cytokine Net* 1992; **3**: 19–33.
5. Panitch HS, Hirsch RL, Schindler J, Johnson KP. Treatment of multiple sclerosis with gamma interferon: exacerbations associated with activation of the immune system. *Neurology* 1987; **37**: 1097–1102.
6. Ramilo O, Saez-Liorens X, Mertsola J et al. Tumor necrosis factor-α/cachectin and interleukin-1β initiate meningeal inflammation. *J Exp Med* 1990; **172**: 497–507.
7. Navikas V, Haglund M, Link J et al. Cytokine mRNA profiles in mononuclear cells in acute aseptic meningoencephalitis. *Infect Immun* 1995; **63**: 1581–1586.
8. Sharif MK, Thompson EJ. Elevated serum levels of tumour necrosis factor-A in Guillain–Barré syndrome. *Ann Neurol* 1993; **33**: 591–596.
9. Hartung HP, Hughes RA, Taylor WA et al. T cell activation in Guillain–Barré syndrome and in MS: elevated serum levels of soluble IL-2 receptors. *Neurology* 1990; **40**: 215–218.
10. Maimone D, Annunziata P, Simon IL et al. Interleukin-6 levels in the cerebrospinal fluid and serum of patients with Guillain–Barré syndrome and chronic inflammatory demyelinating polyradiculoneuropathy. *J Neuroimmunol* 1993; **47**: 55–62.
11. Fomsgaard A, Svensen M, Benddzen K. Autoantibodies to tumour necrosis factor alpha in healthy humans and patients with inflammatory diseases and Gram-negative bacterial infection. *J Immunol* 1989; **30**: 219–223.
12. Suzuki H, Ayabe K, Kamimura J. Anti-IL-1a autoantibodies in patients with rheumatic diseases and in healthy subjects. *Clin Exp Immunol* 1991; **85**: 487–491.
13. Bendtzen K, Hansen MB, Ross C, Svenson M. Cytokine autoantibodies. In: Peter JB, Shoenfeld Y, eds. *Autoantibodies.* Amsterdam: Elsevier Science, 1996; 209–216.
14. Galili U, LaTemple DC. Natural anti-Gal antibody as a universal augmenter of autologous tumor vaccine immunogenicity. *Immunol Today* 1997; **18**: 281–285.
15. Svenson M, Hebrink P. Measurement of cytokine autoantibodies. Test development. *Biotherapy* 1997; **19**: 87–92.
16. Bakhiet M, Diab A, Mustafa M et al. Potential role of autoantibodies in the regulation of cytokine responses in bacterial infections. *Infect Immun* 1997; **65**: 3300–3303.
17. Menetrier-Caux C, Briere F, Jouvenne P et al. Identification of human IgG autoantibodies specific for IL-10. *J Clin Exp Immunol* 1996; **104**: 173–179.
18. Svenson M, Hansen MB, Ross C et al. Antibody

to granulocyte–macrophage colony-stimulating factor is a dominant anti-cytokine activity in human IgG preparations. *Blood* 1998; **91**: 2054–2061.

19. Bendtzen K, Hansen MB, Ross C, Svenson M. High avidity autoantibodies to cytokines. *Immunol Today* 1998; **19**: 209–211.

20. Ross C, Svensson M, Nielsen H et al. Increased in vivo antibody activity against interferon alpha, interleukin-1alpha, and interleukin-6 after high-dose Ig therapy. *Blood* 1997; **90**: 2376–2380.

21. Suzuki H, Takemura H, Yoshizaki K et al. IL-6–anti-IL-6 autoantibody complexes with IL-6 activity in sera from some patients with systemic sclerosis. *J Immunol* 1994; **152**: 935–942.

22. Homann C, Hansen MB, Graudal N et al. Anti-interleukin-6 autoantibodies in plasma are associated with an increased frequency of infections and increased mortality of patients with alcoholic cirrhosis. *Scand J Immunol* 1996; **44**: 623–629.

23. Jouvenne P, Fossiez F, Banchereau J, Miossec P. High levels of neutralizing autoantibodies against IL-1 alpha are associated with a better prognosis in chronic polyarthritis: a follow-up study. *Scand J Immunol* 1997; **46**: 413–418.

24. Elkarim R, Mustafa M, Link H, Bakhiet M. Cytokine autoantibodies in multiple sclerosis, aseptic meningitis and stroke. *Eur J Clinic Invest* 1998; **28**: 295–299.

25. Olsson T. Critical influences of the cytokine orchestration on the outcome of myelin antigen-specific T-cell autoimmunity in experimental autoimmune encephalomyelitis and multiple sclerosis. *Immunol Rev* 1995; **144**: 245–268.

26. Navikas V, Link H. Cytokines and the pathogenesis of multiple sclerosis. *J Neurosci Res* 1996; **45**: 322–333.

27. Ossege LM, Voss B, Wiethege T et al. Detection of transforming growth factor beta 1 mRNA in cerebrospinal fluid cells of patients with meningitis by non-radioactive in situ hybridization. *J Neurol* 1994; **242**: 14–19.

28. Elkarim R, Mustafa M, Link H, Bakhiet M. Recovery from Guillain–Barré syndrome is associated with increased levels of neutralizing autoantibodies to IFN-γ. *Clin Immunol Immunopathol* 1998; **88**: 241–248.

29. Jerne NK. Toward a network theory of the immune system. *Ann Immunol* 1974; **125C**: 373–389.

30. Ross C, Svenson M, Hansen MB et al. High avidity IFN-neutralizing antibodies in pharmaceutically prepared human IgG. *J Clin Invest* 1995; **95**: 1974–1978.

PART III

Magnetic Resonance Imaging

8

Magnetic resonance imaging and its correlation to pathology in multiple sclerosis

Marianne AA van Walderveen, Paul van der Valk and Frederik Barkhof

INTRODUCTION

The pathological hallmark of MS is the white matter plaque that is widely scattered throughout the central nervous system, with a predilection for the optic nerve, brainstem, spinal cord and periventricular white matter. Although these plaques are most commonly found in the white matter, they may also extend to involve the cortex and central grey matter nuclei. Magnetic resonance imaging (MRI) is frequently used to demonstrate dissociation in space for the diagnosis of multiple sclerosis (MS). Conventional T2-weighted spin-echo MRI is highly sensitive for the delineation of MS plaques, since all (MS-related) histopathological tissue alterations increase the T2 relaxation time of the brain tissue and therefore appear bright. Comparison with histopathology shows that the number and extent of abnormalities seen on standard proton-density and T2-weighted imaging overall correlates well with that found histologically.[1,2]

In fact, many lesions seen with MRI may be difficult to detect macroscopically, especially when they lack the characteristic gliotic retraction. In unfixed brain tissue, areas of diffuse MR abnormality, with only small corresponding areas of abnormality on pathology, have been observed; it is suggested that they represent areas of increased vascular permeability and increased extracellular water content.[3] On the other hand, small lesions detected histologically (e.g. on Klüver staining) may be difficult to detect with MRI. Especially tiny cortical lesions can go undetected with conventional imaging, owing to higher background signal in grey matter.[4]

Using high-resolution MRI, it is feasible to obtain post mortem MRI of spinal cord tissue with high image contrast and quality.[5] One preliminary post mortem study, involving 10 MS patients, showed that MS lesions have a heterogeneous appearance in the spinal cord: apart from the classical wedge-shaped focal areas of increased signal intensity, poorly demarcated increases in signal intensity could also be visualized. In two cases, the entire cord specimen was affected, with only small areas of normal spinal cord left. Interestingly, the grey matter was affected in all spinal cord specimens investigated.[6]

Although conventional T2-weighted spin-echo MRI is the most sensitive paraclinical test in diagnosing MS (even outmatching evoked potentials), its specificity is markedly lower. Any pathology from oedema and mild demyelination through completely destroyed plaques may appear bright, and there is evidence that even remyelinated lesions have

Table 8.1 Histopathologic characteristics of MS plaques with their (presumed) MR marker.

Inflammation	Gd enhancement, Cho ↑, lactate ↑, diffusion ↓
Oedema	Increased T1 and T2 relaxation times
Demyelination	Presence of neutral lipids, Cho ↑, MTR ↓, loss of short T2 component, ADC ↑
Gliosis	Increase in T1 relaxation time, Cr ↑, inositol ↑
Axonal loss	Increase in T1 relaxation time, T1 hypointensity, MTR ↓, NAA ↓, ADC ↑
Remyelination	(?) Normalization of MTR values, (?) partial recovery of ADC, (?) disappearance of hypointense lesions

Cho, NAA, Cr, lactate, inositol and neutral lipids are all visible using ^{1}H-MRS.

abnormal signals.[7] This lack of histopathological specificity accounts in part for the clinical radiological paradox in MS. Therefore, other MRI parameters have been evaluated in comparison with either histopathology or clinical parameters (or both) to improve our understanding of the histopathological developments in MS lesions (*Table 8.1*).

GADOLINIUM ENHANCEMENT

Until recently, there was only one type of MS lesion on MRI that was well defined in terms of pathology. Gadolinium (Gd)-enhancement is a marker for breakdown of the blood–brain barrier; it allows a differentiation between active inflammatory lesions and lesions with less active inflammation or chronic inactive lesions (thus demonstrating dissociation in time). Pathological studies have shown that gadolinium-enhancement correlates with the initial phase of lesion development, which consists of macrophage infiltration and astroglial response, and this relates to the presence of active demyelination.[8,9] After 2–6 weeks, enhancement subsides although myelin breakdown products may persist for up to 9 months.[9,10]

Gadolinium enhancement is therefore a sensitive indicator of the initial inflammatory phase of lesion development. Demyelination probably progresses after breakdown of the blood–brain barrier has subsided and therefore gadolinium enhancement is not a sensitive indicator of ongoing demyelination or chronic inflammation.

MAGNETIC RESONANCE SPECTROSCOPY

Magnetic resonance spectroscopy (^{1}H-MRS) provides an in vivo method for characterization of tissue metabolites, including N-acetyl aspartate (NAA), choline-containing compounds (Cho), creatine plus phosphocreatine (Cr), lactate and inositol in localized areas of the brain. Urenjak et al[11] analysed the [1]H-nuclear magnetic resonance profile of major neural cell types and identified that NAA is present in high concentration in neurones and oligodendrocyte-type 2 astrocyte (O-2A) progenitors but absent in other cells (NAA is undetectable in mature oligodendrocytes). Decreased levels of NAA may therefore be used as a marker for axonal integrity or axonal loss. Cr is present in astrocytes and oligodendrocytes and to a minor extent in neurones; increased Cr levels may therefore reflect gliosis. Increased levels of Cho (constituents of cell membranes) may reflect increased membrane turnover or increased number of cells.

Furthermore, the presence of neutral lipids or lactate in the brain can be identified using short-echo proton magnetic resonance spectroscopy. Magnetic resonance spectroscopy studies in MS patients have shown that a reduction of the NAA:Cr ratio and an increase in the Cho:Cr ratio is present in MS lesions compared to normal-appearing white matter.[12–14] In active MS lesions that show Gd-enhancement, depressed NAA levels are observed[15] which return to baseline levels after enhancement ceases. Furthermore, active lesions show increased levels of lactate (indicating the invasion of macrophages)[16,17] and increased levels of Cho (indicating increased membrane turnover, e.g. demyelination), in contrast to 'stable' lesions with reduced Cho levels. The identification of so-called marker peaks, present at 2.1–2.5 parts per million, occurs during enhancement of lesions, although the precise histopathological process that is responsible for these excitatory amino acids is unknown.[18,19] Recent studies have shown biochemical abnormalities in normal-appearing white matter of MS patients, implying that axonal dysfunction or damage not only occurs in lesions but extends beyond their borders into areas that have normal appearance on MRI.[20–22]

HYPOINTENSE LESIONS ('BLACK HOLES') ON T1-WEIGHTED MRI

Part of the MS lesions that are visible on T2-weighted MRI have low signal intensity on corresponding T1-weighted MR images. These hypointense T1 lesions ('black holes') correlate better with disability in MS patients than do lesions on T2-weighted MR images,[23,24] and therefore seem more suitable for monitoring disease progression than the overall T2 lesion load. This hypothesis was recently substantiated by histopathological findings of matrix destruction and axonal loss in hypointense lesions, which correlated with degree of hypointensity of lesions on T1-weighted images (see *Figs 8.1 and 8.2*).[7,25] In a more extensive histopathological study involving 17 MS cases, almost the same correlation between contrast

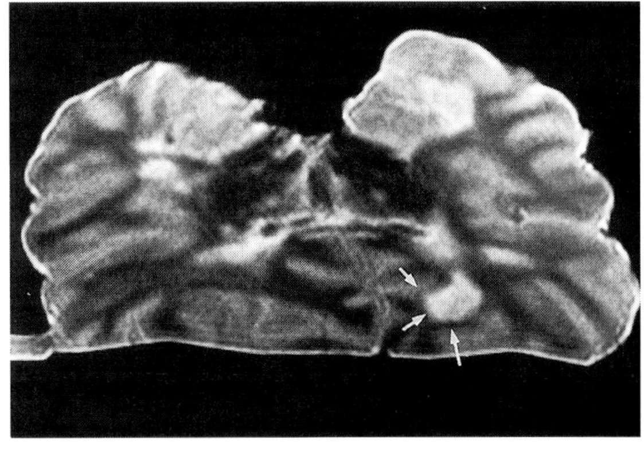

(a)

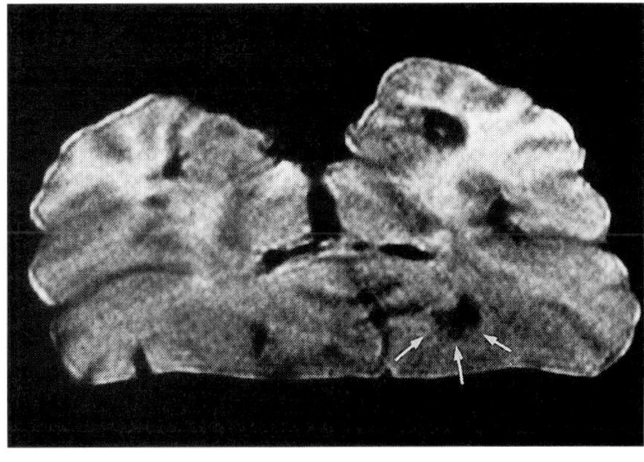

(b)

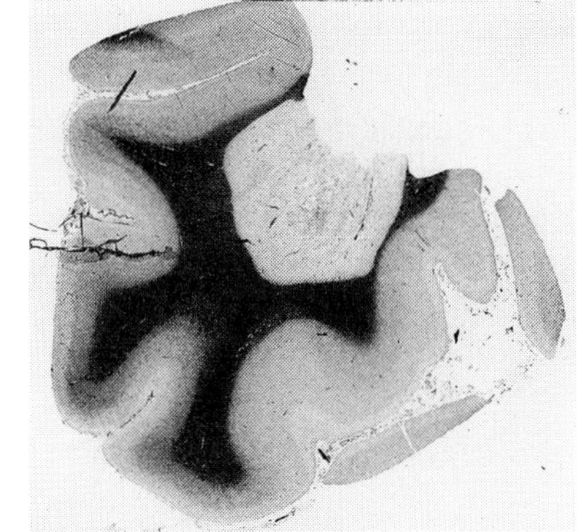

(c)

Figure 8.1 (a) A postmortem T2-weighted spin-echo MRI; (b) a T1-weighted spin-echo MR image. The lesion (arrows), which is visible on the T2-weighted spin-echo MRI appears severely hypointense on the corresponding T1-weighted spin-echo MRI. (c) The corresponding Klüver–Barrera section of this lesion.

ratio on T1-weighted images and the percentages of residual axons was found (R = 0.74).[26] Using in vivo magnetic resonance spectroscopy, one preliminary study showed that in hypointense lesions, a more pronounced reduction of NAA resonance intensity is present than in isointense lesions. Furthermore, Cr resonance intensity was shown to be more substantially reduced in hypointense lesions (see *Fig. 8.3*).[27] These in vivo spectroscopic results substantiate the assumption that hypointense lesions represent the more destructive MS lesions, which renders them suitable for monitoring disease progression, especially in the evaluation of treatment trials.[28] One should take into account that most enhancing lesions on post-contrast T1-weighted images also appear hypointense on precontrast T1-weighted images.[29] Part of these 'acute' (or 'wet') hypointense lesions are capable of returning to isointensity after 1–6 months, which probably relates to resorption of oedema and inflammatory cells, and possibly to remyelination. In line with Truyen et al,[24] who found a strong correlation between the rate of clinical progression and the accumulation of hypointense lesions in secondary progressive MS patients, temporarily hypointense lesions are less common in secondary progressive MS patients, indicating that a failure of remission probably occurs when patients enter the progressive phase of the disease.

Because part of the enhancing lesions remain hypointense at follow-up, one would intuitively expect a close correlation between enhancing activity and increase in hypointense lesion load at long term follow-up. Although such a correlation does exist it has been shown to be only moderate, and a more robust correlation has been found for initial hypointense lesion load.[30] At this moment, the development of hypointense lesions seems to be related to the base-line hypointense lesion load and the clinical course of the disease in MS patients, whereas disease activity as depicted by Gd enhancement on MRI plays a minor role. Further research on the immunogenetic factors that contribute to the development of the more destructive MS lesions is therefore mandatory.

MAGNETIZATION TRANSFER IMAGING

In contrast to conventional MRI techniques, which acquire their signal from the free water protons, magnetization transfer (MT) contrast is based on the saturation of the macromolecular protons and the subsequent exchange of magnetization into the free proton pool. The ratio of MT (MTR) provides an index of macromolecular integrity, since high MTR values are reported in myelinated white matter. From the

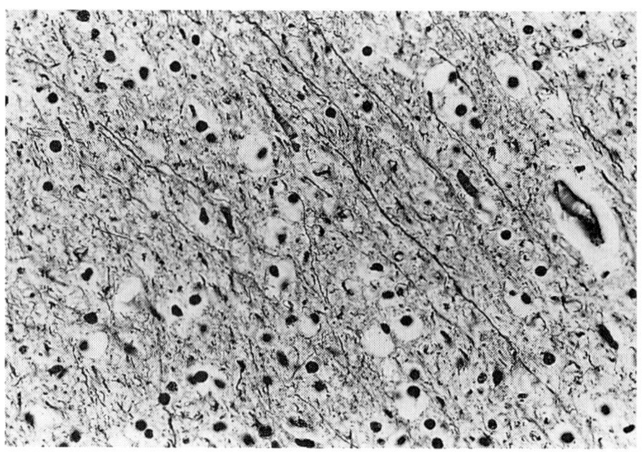

(a)

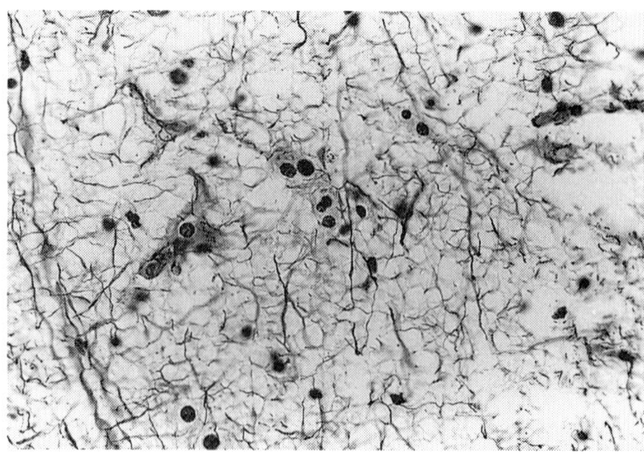

(b)

Figure 8.2 Photomicrographs taken from (a) normal-appearing white matter and (b) the severely hypointense lesions in Fig. 8.1 (Bodian stain, original magnification ×400). The percentage of residual axons was 10% in the severely hypointense lesion compared to axonal density of normal-appearing white matter.

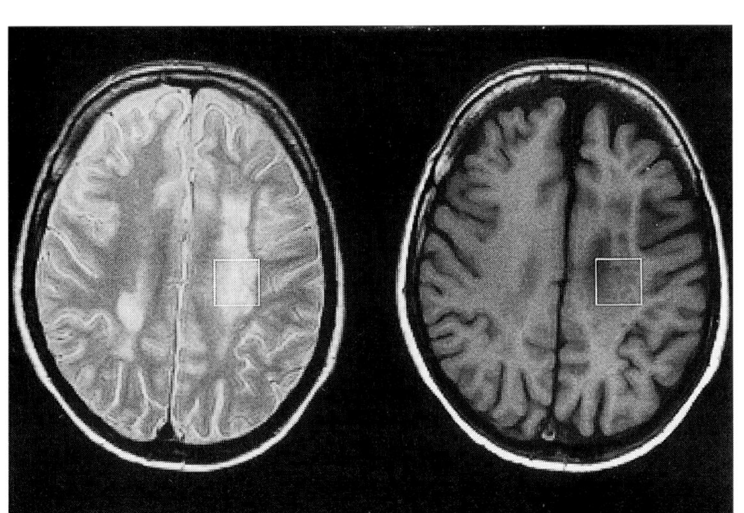

(a)

Figure 8.3 Typical magnetic resonance spectra (PRESS TR 2500/TE 135/NEX 128) from normal-appearing white matter and a hypointense T1 lesion. The T2- and T1-weighted images show the localization of the spectroscopic voxel (8 ml) of the hypointense T1 lesion. Compared with the spectrum obtained from normal-appearing white matter, the spectrum of the hypointense lesion shows a marked reduction of NAA and Cr peak integral values, indicating axonal loss (or integrity) without sufficient gliosis. (PRESS, point-resolved spectroscopy.)

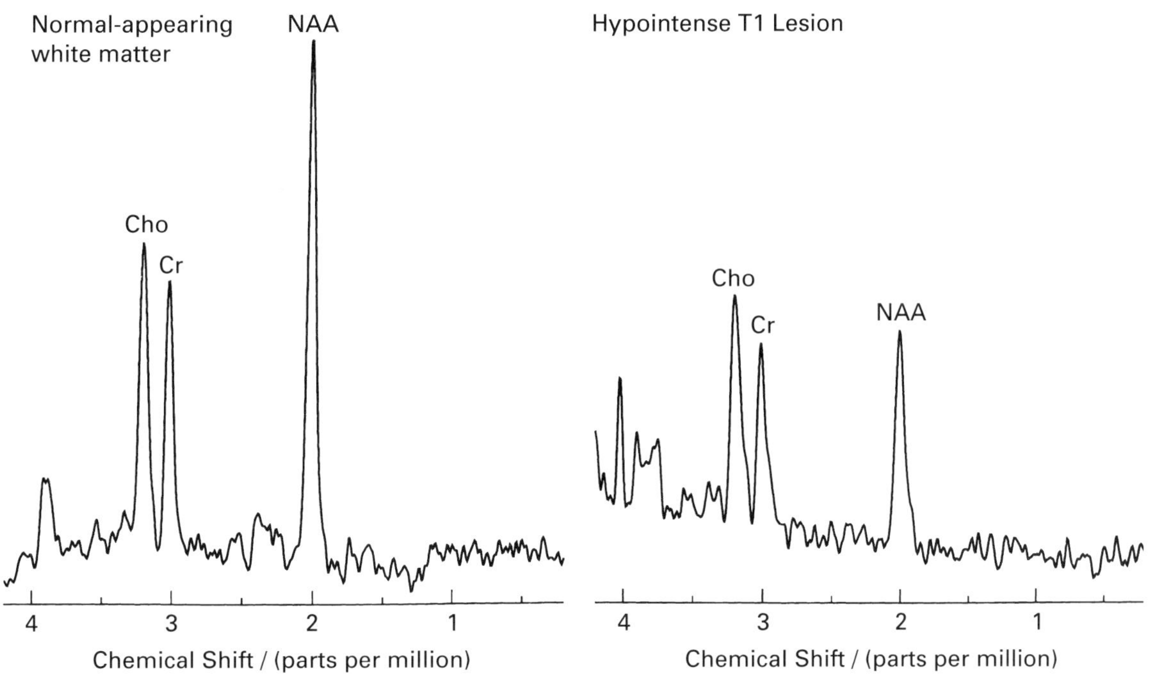

(b)

earliest studies of MT imaging in the evaluation of MS plaques, it has been suggested that MT imaging might be able to distinguish the early, oedematous stage of a lesion from the later, demyelinating or demyelinated stages. Using MT imaging, decreased MTR values have been found in severe demyelination and axonal loss, in comparison with slightly decreased values in oedema and mild demyelination.[31,32] In progressive multifocal leukoencephalopathy, a disease that essentially produces pure demyelination, marked decreases of MTR values have been observed.[33] Furthermore, reduced MTR values have been reported for the normal-appearing white matter of MS patients.[34] Preliminary results from a histopathological study[26] show that MTR values strongly correlate with the percentage of residual axons in MS lesions (in similarity with the degree of hypointensity), indicating that both MR parameters can be used as putative MR markers for persistent deficit. Furthermore, in the same histopathological study, MTR values were shown to correlate with demyelinating activity within lesions, implying that the demyelination status in MS patients may be evaluated in vivo using MT imaging.

DIFFUSION-WEIGHTED IMAGING

Diffusion weighted imaging is capable of both mapping and quantitatively assessing the in vivo diffusive motions of water protons. Randomly moving spins (in contrast to stationary spins) do not completely refocus and result in an attenuated signal. Since water protons diffuse faster along myelinated fibres than across them, the apparent diffusion coefficient (ADC) is directionally restricted (anisotropic). Diffusion-weighted imaging can therefore be used to map directional restriction (anisotropy), related to the limited freedom of mobility of water along the direction of intact myelinated fibres. Alterations in the normal patterns of diffusion anisotropy have allowed further characterization of the extracellular and intracellular barriers to diffusion that may show alterations by certain pathological conditions.

In 1992, Larsson and co-workers[35] investigated water self-diffusion in MS plaques, which were divided according to their age into acute plaques (less than 3 months of age) and chronic plaques. They found that the diffusion coefficient was higher in MS plaques than in the adjacent white matter. More recent investigations have shown that chronic MS lesions show higher ADC than contrast-enhancing lesions[36,37] and the ADC values are higher in non-enhancing hypointense lesions on T1-weighted images than in non-enhancing isointense lesions,[37] indicating that diffusion magnetic resonance may be useful in differentiating acute and chronic disease and inflammation from demyelination. Furthermore, the difference in ADC between isointense and hypointense T1 lesions may indicate that diffusion magnetic resonance could be used as an additional MR marker to monitor enlargement of the extracellular space (in similarity to hypointensity on T1-weighted images and MTR); however, pathological confirmation of this tentative assumption is so far lacking.

RELAXATION TIME MEASUREMENT

The measurement of T1 and T2 relaxation times provides indirect information about the structural composition of brain tissue. In experimental gliosis, for example, prolongation of T1 relaxation time is present, in contrast to the situation in oedema, where prolongation of T2 relaxation time is almost twice that of T1 relaxation time.[38,39] Furthermore, enlargement of the extracellular space induces a marked prolongation of T1 relaxation time and bi-exponentiality of T2 relaxation time.[40] Since both oedema and axonal loss coincides with enlargement of the extracellular space, relaxation time measurement would provide an in vivo method of monitoring inflammation or progressive axonal loss.

Previous studies have shown that there is prolongation of T1 relaxation time in both lesions and normal-appearing white matter of MS patients. However, there is a wide variability of T1 values between and within MS patients.[41,42] There is prolongation of T2 relaxation time in normal-appearing white matter of MS patients,[43] and some of these magnetization decay curves are bi-exponential.[43–45] Furthermore, most T2 decay curves in MS lesions are best fitted using a bi-exponential function. Although the precise histopathological basis for prolongation of T1 and T2 relaxation time and for the bi-exponentiality of T2 relaxation time is not known (apart from enlargement of the extracellular space), it has been suggested that there is a monoexponential decay with a long

T2 in lesions in which tissue destruction and axonal loss has occurred if the tissue destruction has been profound, whereas the short T2 component relates to the presence of myelin protons. If there remains normal white matter or sufficient amounts of gliosis to give a measurable short T2 component, T2 relaxation time will decay in a bi-exponential fashion. Furthermore, preliminary results from a study in which magnetic resonance spectroscopy of MS lesions was performed in relation to T1 relaxation time measurement showed that T1 relaxation time was highest for hypointense lesions, which is compatible with enlargement of the extracellular space caused by axonal loss. More interestingly, NAA and Cr resonance intensities of MS lesions at ^{1}H-MRS were shown to correlate with the T1 relaxation time of the lesions within the spectroscopic voxel. This indicates that T1 relaxation time measurement might be used to monitor decrease in axonal density (NAA) and decrease in glial density (Cr) in future.[28]

TISSUE-SPECIFIC MAGNETIC RESONANCE PARAMETERS: WHERE DO WE STAND?

In the past few years, novel magnetic resonance techniques have been evaluated in order to differentiate MS lesions on MRI into their various histopathological characteristics, which coincide with lesion development. Although T2-weighted spin-echo MRI remains the most sensitive modality for detecting lesions, its specificity in delineating the histopathological features of MS is inherently lower. Magnetic resonance markers, which relate more specifically to certain histopathological stages in lesion development, are therefore needed. The initial phase of lesion development, inflammation with disruption of the blood brain barrier, can be visualized by enhanced T1 weighted spin-echo MRI. On ^{1}H-MRS an increase in Cho and lactate concentrations may reflect the increase in cell density (e.g. macrophages). A temporary dysfunction of axons within the acute lesion lowers NAA resonance intensity; this returns to normal after restoration of axonal integrity. After inflammation, the subsequent demyelination leads to myelin breakdown products (e.g. neutral lipids) on short echotime ^{1}H-MRS and an increase in Cho resonance intensity (indicating increased membrane turnover) on short or long echotime ^{1}H-MRS.

Preliminary evidence indicates that demyelination or cellular activity can be monitored by MT imaging. Furthermore, diffusion-weighted imaging promises to be a valuable tool, since demyelination alters ADC values and reduce anisotropy. Increases in inositol concentrations on ^{1}H-MRS occurs when gliosis is present, a feature that is also reflected by the Cr concentration. In the end-phase of lesion development, axonal loss occurs, with a subsequent increase in the extracellular space. ^{1}H-MRS provides a direct in vivo method of monitoring axonal loss, since NAA occurs solely in neurones. Indirect MR markers of axonal loss—measuring the extracellular space—are hypointensity on T1-weighted images ('black holes'), and decreased MTR values. Using ^{1}H-MRS, T1 hypointensity and MTR, an improved correlation between MRI and disability in MS patients is possible (which will result in higher positive predictive value).

Given the visibility of shadow plaques with poorly demarcated boundaries on T2-weighted images, remyelination areas can not be distinguished from completely demyelinated lesions. Since remyelinated lesions are functionally effective, a specific magnetic resonance marker that can identify this kind of histopathology would be desirable. Apart from ^{1}H-MRS, MT imaging promises to be valuable in monitoring remyelination. In temporarily hypointense lesions, for example, MTR values strongly increase during follow-up, although they do not recover to 'normal' values. This near normalization of MTR values may be related to abnormal myelin density after remyelination has occurred.[29]

REFERENCES

1. Nagara H, Inoue T, Koga T et al. Formalin fixed brains are useful for magnetic resonance imaging (MRI) study. *J Neurol Sci* 1987; **81**: 67–77.

2. Stewart WA, Hall LD, Berry K, Paty DW. Correlation between NMR scan and brain slice: data in multiple sclerosis. *Lancet* 1984; **II**: 412.

3. Newcombe J, Hawkins CP, Henderson L et al. Histopathology of multiple sclerosis lesions detected by magnetic resonance imaging in unfixed postmortem central nervous system tissue. *Brain* 1991; **114**: 1013–1023.

4. Kidd D, Barkhof F, McConnell R et al. Cortical lesions in multiple sclerosis. *Brain*; 1999; **122**: 17–26.

5. Lycklama à Nijeholt GJ, Nicolay K, Barkhoff F et al. Postmortem MR appearance of the spinal cord in MS at 4.7 T. *J Neurol* 1997; **244**(Suppl): S65–S66.

6. Lycklama à Nijeholt GJ, Nicolay K, Barkhoff F et al. Postmortem appearance of multiple sclerosis in the spinal cord: conventional and high resolution MRI. *Proc ISMRM* 1997; **1**: 429.

7. van Walderveen MAA, Kamphorst W, Scheltens P et al. Histopathologic correlate of hypointense lesions on T1-weighted spin-echo MRI in multiple sclerosis. *Neurology* 1998; **50**: 1282–1288.

8. Katz D, Taubenberger J, Raine C et al. Gadolinium-enhancing lesions on magnetic resonance imaging: neuropathological findings. *Ann Neurol* 1990; **28**: 243.

9. Nesbit GM, Forbes GS, Scheithauer BW et al. Multiple sclerosis: histopathologic and MR and/or CT correlation in 37 cases at biopsy and 3 cases at autopsy. *Radiology* 1991; **180**: 467–474.

10. Hawkins CP, Munro PM, Mackenzie J et al. Duration and selectivity of blood–brain barrier breakdown in chronic relapsing experimental allergic encephalomyelitis studied by gadolinium-DTPA and protein markers. *Brain* 1990; **113**: 365–378.

11. Urenjak J, Williams SR, Gadian DG et al. Proton nuclear magnetic resonance spectroscopy unambiguously identifies different neural cell types. *J Neurosci* 1993; **13**: 981–989.

12. Matthews PM, Grancis G, Antel J et al. Proton magnetic resonance spectroscopy for metabolic characterization of plaques in multiple sclerosis. *Neurology* 1991; **41**: 1251–1256.

13. Arnold DL, Matthews PM, Francis G, Antel J. Proton magnetic resonance spectroscopy of human brain in vivo in the evaluation of mul-

tiple sclerosis: assessment of the load of disease. *Magn Reson Med* 1990; **14**: 154–159.

14. Arnold DL, Matthews PM, Francis GS et al. Proton magnetic resonance spectroscopic imaging for metabolic characterization of demyelinating plaques. *Ann Neurol* 1992; **31**: 235–241.

15. Narayana PA, Doyle TJ, Lai D, Wolinsky JS. Serial proton magnetic resonance spectroscopic imaging, contrast-enhanced magnetic resonance imaging, and quantitative lesion volumetry in multiple sclerosis. *Ann Neurol* 1998; **43**: 56–71.

16. Landtblom AM, Sjoqvist L, Soderfeldt B et al. Proton MR spectroscopy and MR imaging in acute and chronic multiple sclerosis—ringlike appearance in acute plaques. *Acta Radiol* 1996; **37**: 278–287.

17. De Stefano N, Matthews PM, Antel JP et al. Chemical pathology of acute demyelinating lesions and its correlation with disability. *Ann Neurol* 1995; **38**: 901–909.

18. Grossman RI, Lenkinski RE, Ramer KN et al. MR proton spectroscopy in multiple sclerosis. *AJNR* 1992; **13**: 1535–1543.

19. Hiehle JF, Lenkinski RE, Grossman RI et al. Correlation of spectroscopy and magnetization transfer imaging in the evaluation of demyelinating lesions and normal appearing white matter in multiple sclerosis. *Magn Reson Med* 1994; **32**: 285–293.

20. Fu L, Matthews PM, De Stefano N et al. Imaging axonal damage of normal-appearing white matter in multiple sclerosis. *Brain* 1998; **121**: 103–113.

21. Husted CA, Goodin DS, Hugg JW et al. Biochemical alterations in multiple sclerosis lesions and normal-appearing white matter detected by in vivo ^{31}P and ^{1}H spectroscopic imaging. *Ann Neurol* 1994; **36**: 157–165.

22. Rooney WD, Goodkin DE, Schuff N et al. MRSI of normal appearing white matter in multiple sclerosis. *Multiple Sclerosis* 1997; **3**: 231–237.

23. van Walderveen MAA, Barkhof F, Hommes OR et al. Correlating MRI and clinical disease activity in multiple sclerosis: relevance of hypointense lesions on short-TR/short-TE (T1-weighted) spin-echo images. *Neurology* 1995; **45**: 1684–1690.

24. Truyen L, van Waesberghe JHTM, van Walderveen MAA et al. Accumulation of hypointense lesions ('black holes') on T1 SE MRI in multiple sclerosis correlates with disease progression. *Neurology* 1996; **47**: 1469–1476.

25. Bruck W, Bitsch A, Kolenda H et al.

Inflammatory central nervous system demyelination: correlation of magnetic resonance imaging findings with lesion pathology. *Ann Neurol* 1997; **42**: 783–793.

26. van Waesberghe JHTM, Kamphort W, van Walderveen MAA et al. Histopathologic correlate of MTR and hypointense signal intensity on T1 SE in multiple sclerosis lesions. A direct post-mortem study. Presented at the 14th Congress of the European Committee for treatment and research in multiple sclerosis (ECTRIMS). Stockholm, Sweden, 9–12 September 1998.

27. van Walderveen MAA, Barkhof F, Pouwels PJW et al. Neuronal damage in T1-hypointense multiple sclerosis lesions demonstrated in vivo using proton magnetic spectroscopy. *Ann Neurol* 1999; in press.

28. Miller DH, Albert PS, Barkhof F et al. Guidelines for the use of magnetic resonance techniques in monitoring the treatment of multiple sclerosis. *Ann Neurol* 1996; **39**: 6–16.

29. van Waesberghe JHTM, van Walderveen MAA, Castelijns JA et al. Patterns of lesion development in multiple sclerosis: longitudinal observations with T1-weighted spin-echo and magnetization transfer MR. *AJNR* 1998; **19**: 675–683.

30. van Walderveen MAA, Truyen LLA, van Oosten BW et al. Degree of inflammatory activity only partially predicts development of hypointense lesions on T1 weighted spin-echo MRI in multiple sclerosis. *Arch of Neurol* 1999; **56**: 345–351

31. Dousset V, Grossman RI, Ramer KN et al. Experimental allergic encephalomyelitis and multiple sclerosis: lesion characterization with magnetization transfer imaging. *Radiology* 1992; **182**: 483–491.

32. Dousset V, Brochet B, Vital A et al. Lysolecithin-induced demyelination in primates: preliminary in vivo study with MR and magnetization transfer. *AJNR* 1995; **16**: 225–231.

33. Dousset V, Armand JP, Lacoste D et al. Magnetization transfer study of HIV encephalitis and progressive multifocal leukoencephalopathy. *AJNR* 1997; **18**: 895–901.

34. Loevner LA, Grossman RI, Cohen JA et al. Microscopic disease in normal-appearing white matter on conventional MR images in patients white matter on conventional MR images in patients with multiple sclerosis: assessment with magnetization–transfer measurements. *Radiology* 1995; **196**: 511–515.

35. Larsson HBW, Thomsen C, Frederiksen J et al. In vivo magnetic resonance diffusion measurement in the brain of patients with multiple sclerosis. *Magn Reson Imaging* 1992; **10**: 7–12.

36. Gass A, Gaa J, Schreiber W et al. Assessment of the apparent diffusion coefficient in contrast-enhancing and chronic MS lesions. Proceedings of the ISMRM, 6th Scientific Meeting, Sydney, Australia, 18–24 April 1998: 1328.

37. Nusbaum AO, Lu D, Atlas SW. Diffusion measurements in multiple sclerosis lesions and normal white matter. American Society of Neuroradiology, 36th Annual Meeting, 17–21 May 1998.

38. Barnes D, McDonald WI, Johnson G et al. Quantitative nuclear magnetic resonance imaging: characterization of experimental cerebral oedema. *J Neurol Neurosurg Psychiatry* 1987; **50**: 125–133.

39. Barnes D, McDonald WI, Landon DN, Johnson G. The characterisation of experimental gliosis by quantitative nuclear magnetic resonance imaging. *Brain* 1991; **114**: 1271–1280.

40. Barnes D, Munro PMG, Youl D et al. The long-standing MS lesion. A quantitative MRI and electron microscopic study. *Brain* 1991; **114**: 1271–1280.

41. Larsson HBW, Frederiksen J, Kjaer L et al. *In vivo* determination of T1 and T2 in the brain of patients with severe but stable multiple sclerosis. *Magn Reson Med* 1988; **7**: 43–55.

42. Miller DH, Johnson G, Tofts PS et al. Precise relaxation time measurements of normal-appearing white matter in inflammatory central nervous system disease. *Magn Reson Med* 1989; **11**: 331–336.

43. Armspach JP, Gounot D, Rumbach L et al. In vivo determination of multi-exponential T2 relaxation in the brain of patients with multiple sclerosis. *Magn Reson Imag* 1991; **9**: 107–113.

44. Kidd D, Barker GJ, Tofts PS et al. The transverse magnetization decay characteristics of long-standing lesions and normal-appearing white matter in multiple sclerosis. *J Neurol* 1997; **244**: 125–130.

45. Larsson HBW, Frederiksen J, Petersen J et al. Assessment of demyelination, edema, and gliosis by in vivo determination of T1 and T2 in the brain of patients with acute attack of multiple sclerosis. *Magn Reson Med* 1989; **11**: 337–348.

9

Magnetic resonance markers and disease course and activity in multiple sclerosis

Giancarlo Comi, Marco Rovaris and Massimo Filippi

INTRODUCTION

Soon after its initial use as a diagnostic tool in multiple sclerosis (MS), it was apparent that magnetic resonance imaging (MRI) had the potential to provide useful information on the pathophysiology and course of the disease, whether natural or modified by treatment.[1] In the past few years, an increasing number of papers on these topics have been published and many scientific meetings have focused on the value and limitations of MRI in the assessment of MS patients. Nevertheless, the use of MRI in MS, considering the wide amount of information that it can provide, is still limited. This is because the transfer of acquired knowledges from research centres to day-to-day clinical activity is inevitably delayed, but it might also be due to reluctance on the part of most clinicians to accepting surrogate instrumental measures of clinical parameters. The low pathological specificity of conventional MRI and the poor correlations between conventional MRI and clinical findings are usually considered the strongest arguments in favour of this conservative approach, although nowadays the combined use of several conventional and non-conventional MRI techniques may provide more complete information on MS and partially overcome the aforementioned limitations of MRI.

Central nervous system (CNS) damage in MS consists of both visible lesions and microscopic lesions in the white matter which appears normal on conventional scans.[2] The severity of this damage depends on the amount of CNS tissue affected by the lesions and on the degree of tissue disruption within the individual lesions, which can be quite variable, particularly according to their age. This review attempts to show that MRI techniques are more sensitive and accurate than clinical manifestations in describing the CNS damage in MS and, moreover, that they may provide useful information for short-term and long-term prognosis of the disease. The implications of the use of MRI for studies of natural history of MS and monitoring of clinical trials are briefly presented.

MRI AND PATHOLOGICAL FINDINGS

Several studies have analysed the correlations between histological and MRI findings in MS.[3–7] Post mortem studies[3,4,8] have clearly demonstrated the high sensitivity of T2-weighted MRI in detecting MS lesions: the number of plaques detected morphologically and radiologically is approximately the same. However, T2-weighted images have a low pathological specificity: oedema, demyelination, gliosis and axonal loss may all determine increased signal on T2-weighted MR.[8] T2-weighted MRI findings correspond to a specific pathology only for the so-called target lesions[6] (i.e. the plaques where a ring of relative hypointensity that surrounds a hyperintense core and is surrounded by another area of hyperintensity is visible on T2-weighted images). The area of relative T2 hypointensity has been attributed to the massive macrophage infiltration observed in the active demyelinating zone at the plaque border.[6]

Clinical and experimental studies have both demonstrated that areas of enhancement on T1-weighted images after administration of gadolinium-DTPA (Gd) identify MS lesions with ongoing blood–brain barrier damage and acute inflammation.[9,10] Gd enhancement in MS lesions usually lasts from 2 to 6 weeks.[10] A longitudinal study with weekly MRI scanning[11] showed that almost all newly developed lesions seen on T2-weighted scans are enhancing at their first appearance. A modest enhancement can also be observed in chronic lesions that do not show signs of inflammation or active demyelination at pathological study;[6] this phenomenon has been attributed to a persistent damage to the blood–brain barrier.[11] It is now widely known that the use of higher doses of Gd (e.g. a triple dose) significantly increases the harvest of enhancing lesions to be detected in MS patients.[12–15] Several pieces of evidence suggest that the degree of pathological changes in MS lesions that enhance only after the injection of a triple dose of Gd is less severe than in those that enhance after the standard dose,[16,17] since the former lesions are characterized by a milder and briefer increase in the permeability of the blood–brain barrier.

Newer, non-conventional magnetic resonance techniques may provide additional information on the pathological substrates of MS lesions. Both acute and chronic lesions may show a variable degree of hypointensity on unenhanced T1-weighted MR images; these hypointense areas, the so-called black holes, are mostly related to extracellular oedema and demyelination in new lesions and to axonal loss and demyelination in chronic lesions.[6,7] On MRI

scans obtained with a magnetization transfer (MT) saturation pulse, a reduction of MT ratio (MTR) values can be observed in MS lesions;[18] this indicates a reduced capacity of the brain matrix molecules to exchange energy with the surrounding water molecules, thus reflecting damage to the myelin or of the axonal membrane. Studies performed in animals affected by experimental allergic encephalomyelitis also suggest that active demyelination may cause reduction in MTR.[19–21] Decrease of MTR has also been found in the normal-appearing white matter of MS patients[22,23] and has been related to microscopic pathological changes affecting the white matter.

Another marker of demyelination in MS plaques is the appearance of peaks of mobile lipids in the spectrum of some acute lesions on magnetic resonance spectroscopy (MRS),[24,25] although it is not clear why these lipid peaks can be detected only in some acute lesions. Interestingly, in a recent MRS study,[26] lipid peaks were also found in areas of white matter without any Gd enhancement and visible lesions on T2-weighted scans; this observation suggests that demyelination might happen independently of local inflammation and breakdown in the blood–brain barrier. MRS also provides very useful information on axonal pathology: a reduction of the N-acetylaspartate (NAA) peak is observed in chronic MS lesions and has been related to neuronal or axonal damage or dysfunction.[25,27,28]

Some longitudinal MRI studies have addressed the problem of the evolution of MS lesions. Van Waesberghe et al[29] showed that, on unenhanced T1-weighted scan, about 80% of the enhancing lesions appear hypointense and 20% appear isointense. During a 6-month follow-up, most of the isointense lesions and about a half of the hypointense lesions become isointense, while a quarter of the isointense lesions and about a half of the hypointense lesions remain hypointense. A strong decrease in the MTR at the time of initial enhancement and a ring enhancement were predictive of a persistent T1 hypointensity.

Some insights about lesion evolution have also come from comparative MRI studies with standard and triple dose of Gd and with MT imaging (MTI). Lesions that enhance only after a triple dose of Gd have higher MTR values than lesions that enhance after single dose of Gd, both at the time of their enhancement and 3 months later; moreover, lesions with enhancement of longer duration tend to have a lower MTR.[17,30] About 50% of the new lesions develop in areas of normal-appearing white matter where a significant reduction of MTR can be detected before the initial enhancement.[31] These changes in MTR values may occur 1–3 months before lesions become evident on conventional MRI scans and are not seen in areas of white matter where no enhancing lesions appear in the subsequent 3 months.

All these studies provide in vivo evidence of the pathological heterogeneity of MS lesions and suggest that some immunological abnormalities might occur in the areas of future lesion development before the breakdown of the blood–brain barrier. Moreover, the severity and duration of the disruption to the blood–brain barrier seem to have a pivotal role in determining the residual persistent damage of the white matter.

MRI AND DISEASE ACTIVITY

MRI-active lesions are any new or enlarging lesion seen on serial (unenhanced) T2-weighted scans and any Gd-enhancing lesion seen on postcontrast T1-weighted images. The presence of a new or enhancing lesion indicates that the disease is active at the time the MRI is obtained. Gd enhancement may precede the onset of clinical symptoms.[32] The presence of new or enlarging T2 lesions indicates that disease activity occurred in the time elapsed between two consecutive scans. A comparison between the sensitivity of monthly unenhanced and enhanced scans of the brain in detecting active lesions showed that enhanced MRI is about twice as sensitive as unenhanced MRI,[33] whereas the combination of the two MRI techniques results in a sensitivity about five to 10 times higher than that of clinical measures.[34] Finally, the number of active lesions detected by enhanced

MRI is about 10 times higher in the brain than in the spinal cord.[35,36]

Several studies report a clear correlation between clinical and MRI activity.[32,33,37–40] The frequency of active scans and active lesions increases shortly before and during clinical relapses.[38,41] During a spinal cord attack, most patients have active lesions in the spinal cord; 78% of patients with isolated spinal cord syndromes that are suggestive of MS have spinal cord lesions consistent with clinical manifestations at the time of presentation (personal observation; unpublished data). Conversely, 30–40% of active lesions in the spinal cord are symptomatic.[35,36,42]

MRI activity is different for the different clinical courses of MS. Patients with relapsing–remitting (RR) and secondary progressive (SP) MS have higher MRI activity (on average about 20 active lesions per year), whereas patients with primary progressive (PP) and benign courses have lower MRI activity (three active lesions per year and nine active lesions per year, respectively).[37,43] Some recent serial MRI studies have showed that patients with RRMS develop more active lesions than patients with SPMS.[40,44] Longitudinal MRI studies with a follow-up duration ranging from several months to more than 5 years[36,38,40] showed that in each patient the number of enhancing lesions fluctuates widely from month to month, but the intra-subject variability is indeed lower than the inter-subject one. These studies also suggest that, in RRMS patients, MRI activity is already high in the early phases of the disease and subsequently increases when the patients begin to accumulate some clinical disability.[45] The frequency and extent of active lesions is predictive of the short-term clinical and MRI activity. Koudriavtseva et al[46] reported that, in RRMS patients, the presence of enhancing lesions is predictive of the number of relapses and MRI active lesions in the subsequent 6 months. In the same study,[46] a weak correlation between baseline volume of enhancing lesions and change of total lesion volume of T2-weighted scans in the following 6 months was also found. Filippi et al,[47] in a 1-year follow-up study with monthly MRI scans, found a significant correlation between the number of enhancing lesions and the changes in T2-weighted and magnetization transfer imaging (MTI) lesion load in SPMS patients but not in RRMS patients. However, Molyneux et al[40] found a correlation between the number of active lesions and changes in T2-weighted lesion load in both RRMS and SPMS patients. These relationships of MRI activity to MR markers of long-term disease evolution reinforce the clinical observations that in RRMS patients the frequency of relapses often correlates with the progression of disability, and this may have major implications for the interpretation of the results of clinical trials where MRI activity is a paraclinical endpoint.

The relationship of MRI activity with clinical disability is a controversial issue. Longitudinal studies of short duration (6–12 months) have failed to demonstrate a relationship between baseline MRI lesion load and its changes over time with the accumulation of disability.[40,46] Two hundred and eighty-one patients with varying MS courses underwent two unenhanced T2-weighted scans at intervals of 2–3 years; only in RRMS patients did the number of active lesions correlated significantly (albeit weakly) with the changes in disability.[48] Stone et al[45] found a moderate correlation between the degree of clinical disability and the mean frequency of enhancing lesions over 3 months in a group of RRMS patients. Losseff et al[49] found that, in patients with SPMS, the number of enhancing lesions detected with monthly MRI scans over a 6-month follow-up correlated with clinical worsening 5 years later. The results of all these correlative studies suggest that the effects of MRI activity on the accumulation of disability may be demonstrated only in studies with long enough follow-up periods, in part because only some of the active lesions will determine a persistent neurological deficit, according to their pathological characteristics and to their sites (see below).

Many factors may decrease the sensitivity of MRI in detecting MS activity, with the potential to lessen the correlations between clinical and MRI findings. More frequent scanning schedules may increase the likelihood of detecting active lesions. However, this issue has poor relevance, since it has been reported that weekly scans detect about 10% more active lesions than monthly scans,[11] at the expense of increased costs and patient discomfort. On the other hand, the use of a triple dose of Gd detects 50–70% more enhancing lesions than a standard dose,[12–15] both cross-sectionally[12–15] and longitudinally.[50] Increased sensitivity in detecting new lesions on serial unenhanced MRI scans can be obtained by using acquisition schemes with thin slices (e.g. 3 mm instead of 5 mm)[51] and also by using fast-fluid attenuated inversion recovery (FLAIR) instead of conventional T2-weighted sequences.[52] The combination of triple-dose Gd-enhanced scans with FLAIR scans maximizes the harvest of active lesions detectable on serial, monthly MRI scans in RRMS patients.[52] The application of a MT pulse in standard-dose and triple-dose Gd-enhanced MRI[15,53] also significantly increases the sensitivity of the two techniques for detecting enhancing lesions.

All these newer approaches still need to be validated in large-scale studies with longer follow-up periods. The clinical usefulness of such a high MRI sensitivity has not yet been demonstrated, although, in a preliminary study,[54] it has been reported that the use of triple-dose Gd-enhanced MRI can detect an early and significant effect of low doses of interferon-β-1a on MRI activity in RRMS patients.

MRI AND DISEASE BURDEN

The most commonly used MRI measure of disease burden in MS is the assessment of brain lesion load on unenhanced T2-weighted images. The brain lesion load on T2-weighted images is significantly higher in SPMS than in RRMS patients and is also significantly higher in SPMS than in PPMS patients matched for disease duration.[55] In another cross-sectional study,[56] it has been reported that patients with benign MS with a mean disease duration of 15 years had the same load of 12-weighted lesions as patients with RRMS with 4.4 years of disease duration.

Several cross-sectional studies found poor

correlations or none at all between brain MRI lesion load and disability in MS patients.[57–59] In the large cohort of RRMS patients included in the North American Interferon-β-1b trial, the correlation coefficient between MRI lesion load and expanded disability status scale (EDSS) score was 0.23.[60] Stronger correlations were found in more recent studies, partly because of the better quality of the MRI techniques, particularly when more homogenous groups of patients were studied.[61] Mammi et al[62] studied a large group of patients with varying disease courses and found a correlation coefficient of 0.3 between T2-weighted total lesion volume and EDSS in the whole group; the coefficient increased to 0.5 when only patients with RRMS and SPMS were considered.

The situation is similar for longitudinal studies correlating changes in disability and changes in lesion load. Van Walderveen et al[63] found only a weak correlation (R = 0.19) between increase in disability and increase in lesion load on T2-weighted images in 48 patients with clinically definite MS who were followed up for 2 years. Similar correlation coefficients were found in the North American Interferon-β-1b trial.[60]

Stronger correlations have been reported between brain MRI lesion load and global cognitive dysfunction[55,64,65] and between lesion location and specific cognitive changes.[66,67] The reason why correlation of brain MRI lesion load with cognitive dysfunction is more robust than with global disability can be explained by the disruption of the complex neural networks underlying cognitive abilities caused by the white matter lesions. Lesions located in subcortical areas seem to play a predominant role in determining the typical subcortical profile of MS dementia;[68] however, recent observations[65,69] suggest that the site of the lesions could not play a major pathogenetic role, for the frontal lobe lesion load and the total lesion load have the same strength of correlation with the impairment of executive functions. Similar results were recently obtained in a case–control study performed in the authors' MS centre with two groups of MS patients. These patients were matched for age, disease course and disability

on the basis of the presence or absence of frontal lobe dementia (unpublished data, personal observation).

Few data are available on the predictive value of brain MRI lesion load for the future development of disability. A recent study found a correlation between baseline lesion load and change of disability over 1 year in RRMS patients but not in SPMS patients.[40] More interesting observations have been made in patients with clinically isolated syndromes suggestive of MS at the onset. In patients with monosymptomatic disease, abnormal brain MRI has a high positive predictive value (40–60% after 5 years) for the development of definite MS,[61,70–72] while normal MRI is associated with a low risk (3–6% after 5 years). Patients with a high lesion load at presentation have a higher risk of early conversion;[61] in a recent study,[73] after a 10-year follow-up, 85% of the patients with more than 10 brain lesions on MRI at presentation converted to clinically definite MS, and 75% had moderate disability (i.e. an EDSS score >3).

Many factors may weaken the strength of clinical–MRI correlations. First inaccuracies in measuring lesion load may do this. Subjective, conventional scores are inaccurate and poorly reproducible,[74] while quantitative techniques are characterized by higher accuracy and reproducibility of measurements.[74,75] By using new MRI sequences such as FLAIR, which achieves a higher level of lesion visualization, higher lesion loads can be detected and measurement reproducibility can also be improved.[76] Acquisition schemes with thinner slices also increase the sensitivity of MRI for detecting MS lesions in the brain. It has been demonstrated that brain MRI scans with slices of 3 mm thickness detect lesion volumes about 9% greater than those detected with 5 mm thick slices.[51] In large-scale, multicentre studies, poor patient repositioning[77] and inter-scanner differences among centres[78] may add noise to the system, making any MRI–clinical correlation hard to find.

All the aforementioned technical and methodological factors may interfere with the possibility of correlating patient disability with the burden of brain lesions on T2-weighted

MRI, but other factors should be considered to explain the weakness of this correlation:

(a) the EDSS scale is non-linear, poorly reproducible and primarily related to locomotor disability;[79]
(b) lesions that look the same on conventional T2-weighted MRI may be pathologically heterogeneous, as discussed above;
(c) invisible pathology in the normal-appearing white matter may significantly contribute to the disability;[23,80]
(d) most of the brain lesions do not influence locomotor disability.

There have been several attempts to overcome some of these problems. Measures derived from newer magnetic resonance techniques that have a higher pathological specificity do correlate better with disability than conventional T2-weighted MRI findings. Strong correlations have been found between disability and hypointense lesion load on T1-weighted images.[63] In patients with SPMS, the rate of accumulation of hypointense lesions is strongly related to the rate of disability progression.[81] Average lesion MTR is more strictly correlated with disability than brain T2-weighted total lesion load.[18] The creation of histograms of MTR values for the whole brain or for selected brain regions provides extensive data on the burden of disease in the examined volume.[65,82,83] This technique has two advantages: it is observer-independent, since there is no preliminary identification of the lesions, and it provides a more complete picture of macroscopic and microscopic disease burden. Brain MTR histograms in normal subjects are characterized by a narrow peak; in MS patients, the height of the peak is significantly reduced and the peak is shifted to the left, indicating that fewer pixels have MTR values in the normal range.[82] Patients with benign MS and clinically isolated syndromes have brain histograms that overlap the normal ones; patients with PPMS have a reduced amplitude of the peak, but the spectrum does not shift to the left; however, RRMS and, even more, SPMS patients have a reduction of peak amplitude and a clear shift of the spectrum to the left.[84] MTR histogram parameters for selected brain regions such as the brainstem and cerebellum, which are critical sites for the development of disability, correlate with the degree of impairment of the corresponding functional systems better than the regional T2-weighted lesion loads.[85] Using MRS, a decrease in NAA has been found in the brains of patients with MS.[86,87] The relative decreases in NAA can be reversible in acute lesions over relatively short periods of time.[28,88] The ratio of NAA to Cr ratio is significantly more reduced in chronic lesions of SPMS patients than in chronic lesions of patients with benign MS.[89] The decrease in brain NAA:Cr ratio is greater in SPMS patients than in RRMS patients, and the difference is mainly dependent on changes in the normal-appearing white matter, which can be explained by diffuse axonal loss.[90] Some cross-sectional studies[91,92] have reported an inverse relation between NAA peaks and the degree of disability. In a longitudinal study, NAA decrease in the normal-appearing white matter correlated strongly with changes in disability.[90]

Atrophy is an indirect measure of axonal degeneration; several cross-sectional studies have found strong correlations between physical disability and both spinal cord[93,94] and cerebellar atrophy[95] and between measures of cerebral atrophy and cognitive impairment.[55,64] Interestingly, in patients with PPMS, disability was not significantly correlated to MRI lesion load, but it was correlated to spinal cord atrophy.[94] Longitudinal studies have found correlations between the progression of disability and the decrease in spinal cord cross-sectional area[96] and cerebral white matter volume.[97]

CONCLUSIONS

In assessing the overall damage to the CNS caused by MS, MRI provides information that cannot be derived by clinical examination. In assessing disease activity, MRI is more sensitive than clinical evaluation. Moreover, MRI activity provides unique information on the short-term disease evolution. As a consequence, MRI-derived measures are widely accepted as surrogate markers to test treatment effects in phase 2 clinical trials. In the last few years, newer MR techniques have allowed a more accurate estimate of the pathological damage, not only for the visible lesions, but also for the normal-appearing white matter. Most of the MRI techniques can now provide precise and reproducible measures, whereas clinical measures are often imprecise, inaccurate and poorly reproducible. Nevertheless, no single MRI measure is accepted as a substitute for the clinical measures of impairment and disability in phase 3 trials, since the observed correlations between clinical and MRI measures are still unsatisfactory. The weakness of these correlations is mainly dependent on the fact that MRI and clinical parameters measure different aspects of the disease, which are related to each other but do not completely overlap. MRI provides information on the disease pathology; clinical measures reflect the consequences of the pathological process.

REFERENCES

1. Filippi M, Miller DH. MRI in the differential diagnosis and monitoring the treatment of multiple sclerosis. *Curr Opin Neurol* 1996; **9**: 178–186.
2. Allen IV, McKeown SR. A historical, histochemical and biochemical study of the macroscopically normal white matter in multiple sclerosis. *J Neurol Sci* 1979; **41**: 81–91.
3. Nesbit GM, Forbes GS, Scheithauser BW et al. Multiple sclerosis: histopathologic and MR and/or CT correlation in 37 cases at biopsy and three cases at autopsy. *Radiology* 1991; **180**: 467–474.
4. Newcombe J, Hawkins CP, Henderson CL et al. Histopathology of multiple sclerosis lesions detected by magnetic resonance imaging in unfixed postmortem central nervous tissue. *Brain* 1991; **114**: 1013–1023.
5. Katz D, Taubenberger JK, Cannella B et al. Correlation between magnetic resonance imaging findings and lesion development in multiple sclerosis. *Ann Neurol* 1993; **34**: 661–669.
6. Bruck W, Bitsch A, Kolenda H et al. Inflammatory central nervous system demyelination: correlation of magnetic resonance imaging findings with lesion pathology. *Ann Neurol* 1997; **42**: 783–793.
7. van Walderveen MAA, Kamphorst W, Scheltens et al. Histopathologic correlate of hypointense lesions on T1-weighted spin-echo MRI in multiple sclerosis. *Neurology* 1998; **50**: 1282–1288.
8. Ormerod IEC, Miller DH, McDonald WI et al. The role of MRI in the assessment of MS and isolated neurological lesions: a quantitative study. *Brain* 1987; **110**: 1579–1616.
9. Hawkins CP, Munro PMG, Mackenzie F et al. Duration and selectivity of blood–brain barrier breakdown in chronic relapsing experimental allergic encephalomyelitis studied by gadolinium-DTPA and protein markers. *Brain* 1990; **113**: 365–378.
10. McDonald WI, Miller DH, Barnes D. The pathological evolution of multiple sclerosis. *Neuropathol Appl Neurobiol* 1992; **18**: 319–334.
11. Lai M, Hodgson T, Gawne-Cain ML et al. A preliminary study into the sensitivity of disease activity detection by serial weekly magnetic resonance imaging in multiple sclerosis. *J Neurol Neurosurg Psychiatry* 1996; **60**: 339–341.
11. Prineas JW, Barnard RO, Kwon EE et al. Multiple sclerosis: remyelination of nascent lesions. *Ann Neurol* 1993; **33**: 137–151.
12. Filippi M, Yousry T, Campi A et al. Comparison of triple dose versus standard dose gadolinium-DTPA for detection of MRI enhancing lesions in patients with multiple sclerosis. *Neurology* 1996; **243**: 379–384.
13. Filippi M, Campi A, Martinelli V et al. Comparison of triple dose versus standard dose gadolinium-DTPA for detection of MRI enhancing lesions in patients with primary progressive multiple sclerosis. *J Neurol Neurosurg Psychiatry* 1995; **59**: 540–544.
14. Filippi M, Capra R, Campi A et al. Triple dose of gadolinium-DTPA and delayed MRI in patients with benign multiple sclerosis. *J Neurol Neurosurg Psychiatry* 1996; **60**: 526–530.
15. Silver NC, Good CD, Barker GJ et al. Sensitivity of contrast enhanced MRI in multiple sclerosis. Effects of gadolinium dose, magnetization transfer contrast and delayed imaging. *Brain* 1997; **120**: 1149–1161.
16. Rovaris M, Mastronardo G, Gasperini C et al. MRI evolution of new MS lesions enhancing after different doses of gadolinium. *Acta Neurol Scand* 1998; **98**: 90–93.
17. Filippi M, Rocca MA, Rizzo G et al. Magnetization transfer ratios in MS lesions enhancing after different doses of gadolinium. *Neurology* 1998; **50**: 1289–1293.

18. Gass A, Barker GJ, Kidd D et al. Correlation of magnetization transfer ratio with disability in multiple sclerosis. *Ann Neurol* 1994; **36**: 62–67.

19. Dousset V, Brochet B, Vital A et al. Lysolecithin-induced demyelination in primates: preliminary in vivo study with MR and magnetisation transfer. *AJNR* 1995; **16**: 225–231.

20. Dousset V, Brochet B, Vital A et al. MR Imaging including diffusion and magnetisation transfer of chronic relapsing experimental encephalomyelitis-correlation with immunological and pathological datas. *Proc Int Soc Magn Reson Med* 1994; **2**: 1401.

21. Dousset V, Grossman RI, Ramer KN et al. Experimental allergic encephalomyelitis and multiple sclerosis: lesion characterization with magnetization transfer imaging. *Radiology* 1992; **182**: 483–491.

22. Loevener LA, Grossman RI, Cohen JA et al. Microscopic disease in normal-appearing white matter on conventional images in patients with multiple sclerosis: assessment with magnetization–transfer measurements. *Radiology* 1995; **196**: 511–515.

23. Filippi M, Campi A, Dousset V et al. A magnetisation transfer imaging study of normal-appearing white matter in multiple sclerosis. *Neurology* 1995; **45**: 478–482.

24. Wolinsky JS, Narayana PA, Ferstenmacher MJ. Proton magnetic resonance spectroscopy in multiple sclerosis. *Neurology* 1990; **40**: 1764–1769.

25. Larsson HBW, Christianson P, Jenson M et al. Localized in vivo proton spectroscopy in the brain of patients with multiple sclerosis. *Magn Reson Med* 1991; **22**: 23–31.

26. Narayana PA, Doyle TJ, Lai D et al. Serial proton magnetic resonance spectroscopic imaging, contrast-enhanced magnetic resonance imaging, and quantitative lesion volumetry in multiple sclerosis. *Ann Neurol* 1998; **43**: 56–71.

27. Matthews PM, Francis G, Antel J et al. Proton magnetic resonance spectroscopy for metabolic characterization of plaques in multiple sclerosis. *Neurology* 1991; **41**: 1251–1256.

28. Davie CA, Hawkins CP, Barker GJ et al. Serial proton magnetic resonance spectroscopy in acute multiple sclerosis lesions. *Brain* 1994; **117**: 49–58.

29. van Waesberghe JHTM, van Walderveen MAA, Castelijns JA et al. Patterns of lesion development in multiple sclerosis: longitudinal observations with T1-weighted spin-echo and magnetization transfer MR. *AJNR* 1998; **19**: 675–683.

30. Filippi M, Rocca MA, Comi G. Magnetization transfer ratio of multiple sclerosis lesions with variable durations of enhancement. *J Neurol Sci* 1998; **159**: 162–165.

31. Filippi M, Rocca MA, Martino G et al. Magnetization transfer changes in the normal-appearing white matter precede the appearance of enhancing lesions in patients with multiple sclerosis. *Ann Neurol* 1998; **43**: 809–814.

32. Kermode AG, Tofts PS, Thompson AJ et al. Heterogeneity of blood–brain barrier changes in multiple sclerosis: an MRI study with gadolinium-DTPA enhancement. *Neurology* 1990; **40**: 229–235.

33. Miller DH, Barkhof F, Nauta JJP. Gadolinium enhancement increased the sensitivity of MRI in detecting disease activity in MS. *Brain* 1993; **116**: 1077–1094.

34. Miller DH, Rudge P, Johnson G et al. Serial gadolinium enhanced magnetic resonance imaging in multiple sclerosis. *Brain* 1988; **111**: 927–939.

35. Capra R, Marcianò N, Vignolo LA et al. Gadolinium-pentetic acid magnetic resonance imaging in patients with relapsing remitting multiple sclerosis. *Arch Neurol* 1992; **49**: 687–689.

36. Thorpe JW, Kidd D, Moseley IF et al. Serial gadolinium-enhanced MRI of the brain and spinal cord in early relapsing–remitting multiple sclerosis. *Neurology* 1996; **46**: 373–378.

37. Thompson AJ, Kermode AG, Wicks D et al. Major differences in the dynamics of primary and secondary progressive multiple sclerosis. *Ann Neurol* 1991; **29**: 53–62.

38. Smith ME, Stone LA, Albert PS et al. Clinical worsening in multiple sclerosis is associated with increased frequency and area of gadopentetate dimeglumine-enhancing magnetic resonance imaging lesions. *Ann Neurol* 1993; **33**: 480–489.

39. Bastianello S, Pozzilli C, Bernardi S et al. Serial study of gadolinium-DTPA MRI enhancement in multiple sclerosis. *Neurology* 1990; **40**: 591–595.

40. Molyneux PD, Filippi M, Barkhof F et al. Correlations between monthly enhanced MRI lesion rate and changes in T2 lesion volume in multiple sclerosis. *Ann Neurol* 1998; **43**: 332–339.

41. Willoughby EW, Grochowski E, Li DKB et al. Serial magnetic resonance scanning in multiple sclerosis: a second prospective study in relapsing patients. *Ann Neurol* 1989; **25**: 43–49.

42. Wiebe S, Lee DH, Karlik SJ et al. Serial cranial and spinal cord magnetic resonance imaging in multiple sclerosis. *Ann Neurol* 1992; **32**: 643–650.

43. Thompson AJ, Miller DH, Youl BD et al. Serial gadolinium-enhanced MRI in relapsing/remitting multiple sclerosis of varying disease duration. *Neurology* 1992; **42**: 60–63.

44. Filippi M, Rossi P, Colombo B et al. Serial contrast-enhanced MR in patients with multiple sclerosis and varying levels of disability. *AJNR* 1997; **18**: 1549–1556.

45. Stone LA, Smith ME, Albert PS et al. Blood–brain barrier disruption on contrast-enhanced MRI in patients with mild relapsing–remitting multiple sclerosis: relationship to course, gender, and age. *Neurology* 1995; **45**: 1122–1126.

46. Koudriavtseva T, Thompson AJ, Fiorelli M et al. Gadolinium enhanced MRI disease activity in relapsing–remitting multiple sclerosis. *J Neurol Neurosurg Psychiatry* 1997; **62**: 285–287.

47. Filippi M, Rocca MA, Horsfield MA, Comi G. A one year study of new lesions in multiple sclerosis using monthly gadolinium enhanced MRI: correlations with changes of T2 and magnetization transfer lesion loads. *J Neurol Sci* 1998; **158**: 203–208.

48. Filippi M, Paty DW, Kappos L et al. Correlations between changes in disability and T_2-weighted brain MRI activity in multiple sclerosis: a follow up study. *Neurology* 1995; **45**: 255–260.

49. Losseff N, Kingsley D, McDonald WI et al. Clinical and magnetic resonance imaging predictors in primary and secondary progressive MS. *Multiple Sclerosis* 1996; **1**: 218–222.

50. Filippi M, Rovaris M, Capra R et al. A multicentre, longitudinal study comparing the sensitivity of enhanced brain MRI after the injection of standard and triple dose gadolinium-DTPA for detecting active lesions in multiple sclerosis (abstract). *Neurology* 1997; **48**(Suppl 3): A362.

51. Filippi M, Horsfield MA, Campi A et al. Resolution-dependent estimates of lesion volumes in magnetic resonance imaging studies of the brain in multiple sclerosis. *Ann Neurol* 1995; **38**: 749–754.

52. Filippi M, Mastronardo G, Bastianello S et al. A longitudinal brain MRI study comparing the sensitivities of the conventional and a newer approach for detecting active lesions in multiple sclerosis. *J Neurol Sci* 1998; **159**: 94–101.

53. Metha RC, Pike GB, Enzmann DR. Improved detection of enhancing and non-enhancing lesions of multiple sclerosis with magnetization transfer. *AJNR* 1995; **16**: 1771–1778.

54. Filippi M, Rovaris M, Capra R et al. Serial standard- and triple-dose MRI to monitor the effect of interferon β-1a on multiple sclerosis activity (abstract). *Neurology* 1998; **50**: A323.

55. Comi G, Filippi M, Martinelli V et al. Brain MRI correlates of cognitive impairment in primary and secondary multiple sclerosis. *J Neurol Sci* 1995; **132**: 222–227.

56. Filippi M, Barker GJ, Horsfield MA et al. Benign and secondary progressive multiple sclerosis: a preliminary quantitative MRI study. *J Neurol* 1994; **241**: 246–251.

57. Baumhefner RW, Tourtellotte WW, Syndulko K et al. Quantitative multiple sclerosis plaque assessment with magnetic resonance imaging. Its correlation with clinical parameters, evoked potentials and intra-blood–brain barrier IgG synthesis. *Arch Neurol* 1990; **47**: 19–26.

58. Koopmans RA, Li DK, Grochowski E et al. Benign versus chronic progressive multiple sclerosis: magnetic resonance imaging features. *Ann Neurol* 1989; **25**: 74–81.

59. Thompson AJ, Kermode AG, MacManus DG et al. Patterns of disease activity in multiple sclerosis: clinical and magnetic resonance imaging study. *Br Med J* 1990; **300**: 631–634.

60. Paty DW, Li DKB, UBC MS/MRI Study Group, IFNB Multiple Sclerosis Study Group. Interferon beta-1b is effective in relapsing–remitting multiple sclerosis. II. MRI analysis results of a multicenter, randomized, double-blind, placebo-controlled trial. *Neurology* 1993; **43**: 662–667.

61. Filippi M, Horsfield MA, Morrissey SP et al. Quantitative brain MRI lesion load predicts the course of clinically isolated syndromes suggestive of MS. *Neurology* 1994; **44**: 635–641.

62. Mammi S, Filippi M, Martinelli V et al. Correlation between brain MRI lesion volume and disability in patients with multiple sclerosis. *Acta Neurol Scand* 1995; **94**: 93–96.

63. van Walderveen MAA, Barkhof F, Hommes OR et al. Correlating MRI and clinical disease activity in multiple sclerosis: relevance of hypointense lesions on short TR/short TE (T_1-weighted) spin-echo images. *Neurology* 1995; **45**: 1684–1690.

64. Rao SM, Leo GJ, Haughton VM et al. Correlation of magnetic resonance imaging with neuropsychological testing in multiple sclerosis. *Neurology* 1989; **39**: 161–166.

65. Rovaris M, Filippi M, Falautano M et al. Relation between MR abnormalities and patterns of cognitive impairment in multiple sclerosis. *Neurology* 1998; **50**: 1601–1608.

66. Arnett PA, Rao SM, Bernardin L et al.

Relationship between frontal lobe lesions and Wisconsin Card Sorting Test performance in patients with multiple sclerosis. *Neurology* 1994; 420–425.

67. Swirsky-Sacchetti T, Mitchell DR, Seward J et al. Neuropsychological and structural brain lesions in multiple sclerosis: a regional analysis. *Neurology* 1992; **42**: 1291–1295.

68. Damian MS, Schilling C, Bachmann G et al. White matter lesions and cognitive deficits: relevance of lesions pattern? *Acta Neurol Scand* 1994; **90**: 430–436.

69. Foong J, Rozewicz L, Quaghebeur G et al. Executive functions in multiple sclerosis. The role of frontal lobe pathology. *Brain* 1997; **120**: 15–26.

70. Beck RW, Cleary PA, Trobe JD et al. The effect of corticosteroids for acute optic neuritis on the subsequent development of multiple sclerosis. *N Engl J Med* 1993; **329**: 1764–1769.

71. Martinelli V, Comi G, Filippi M et al. Paraclinical tests in acute-onset optic neuritis: basal data and results of a short-follow-up. *Acta Neurol Scand* 1991; **84**: 231–236.

72. Morrissey SP, Miller DH, Kendall BE et al. The significance of brain magnetic resonance imaging abnormalities at presentation with clinically isolated syndromes suggestive of multiple sclerosis. *Brain* 1993; **116**: 135–146.

73. O'Riordan JI, Thompson AJ, Kingsley DPE et al. The prognostic value of brain MRI in clinically isolated syndromes of the CNS. A 10-year follow-up. *Brain* 1998; **121**: 495–503.

74. Filippi M, Horsfield MA, Bressi S et al. Intra- and inter-observer agreement of brain MRI lesion volume measurements in multiple sclerosis: a comparison of techniques. *Brain* 1995; **118**: 1583–1592.

75. Filippi M, Horsfield MA, Tofts PS et al. Quantitative assessment of MRI lesion load in monitoring the evolution of multiple sclerosis. *Brain* 1995; **118**: 1601–1612.

76. Rovaris M, Yousry T, Calori G et al. Sensitivity and reproducibility of fast-FLAIR, FSE and TGSE sequences for the assessment of brain MRI lesion load in multiple sclerosis: a preliminary study. *J Neuroimaging* 1997; **7**: 98–102.

77. Filippi M, Marcianò N, Capra R et al. The effect of imprecise repositioning on lesion volume measurements in patients with multiple sclerosis. *Neurology* 1997; **49**: 274–276.

78. Filippi M, van Waesberghe JH, Horsfield MA et al. Interscanner variation in brain MRI lesion load measurements in multiple sclerosis. *Neurology* 1997; **49**: 371–377.

79. Noseworthy JH, Vandervoort MK, Wong CJ et al. Interrater variability with the Expanded Disability Status Scale (EDSS) and Functional Systems (FS) in a multiple sclerosis clinical trial. *Neurology* 1990; **40**: 971–975.

80. Barbosa S, Blumhardt LD, Roberts N et al. Magnetic resonance relaxation time mapping in multiple sclerosis: normal appearing white matter and the 'invisible' lesion load. *Magn Reson Imaging* 1994; **12**: 33–42.

81. Truyen L, van Waesberghe JHTM, van Walderveen MAA et al. Accumulation of hypointense lesions ('black holes') on T1 spin-echo MRI correlates with disease progression in multiple sclerosis. *Neurology* 1997; **47**: 1469–1476.

82. van Buchem MA, McGowan JC, Kolson DL et al. Quantitative volumetric magnetization transfer analysis in multiple sclerosis: estimation of macroscopic and microscopic disease burden. *Magn Reson Med* 1996; **36**: 632–636.

83. van Buchem MA, Grossman RI, Armstrong C et al. Correlation of volumetric magnetization transfer imaging with clinical data in MS. *Neurology* 1998; **50**: 1609–1617.

84. Rovaris M, Iannucci G, Minicucci L et al. Assessment of disease severity in multiple sclerosis patients with magnetization transfer histograms (abstract). *J Neurol* 1998; **245**: 444.

85. Filippi M, Iannucci G, Rocca MA et al. Correlations between clinical and MRI involvement in multiple sclerosis: assessment with T2, T1 and MT histograms (abstract). *J Neurol* 1998; **245**: 383–384.

86. Arnold DL, Matthews PM, Francis G, Antel J. Proton magnetic resonance spectroscopy of human brain in vivo in the evaluation of multiple sclerosis: assessment of the load of disease. *Magn Reson Med* 1990; **14**: 154–159.

87. van Hecke P, Marchal G, Johannik K et al. Human brain proton localized NMR spectroscopy in multiple sclerosis. *Magn Reson Med* 1991; **18**: 199–206.

88. Arnold DL, Matthews PM, Francis G et al. Proton magnetic resonance spectroscopic imaging for metabolic characterisation of demyelinating plaques. *Ann Neurol* 1992; **31**: 235–241.

89. Falini A, Calabrese G, Filippi M et al. Benign versus secondary progressive multiple sclerosis: the potential role of ^{1}H MR spectroscopy in defining the nature of disability. *AJNR* 1998; **19**: 223–229.

90. Fu L, Matthews PM, De Stefano N et al. Imaging

axonal damage of normal-appearing white matter in multiple sclerosis. *Brain* 1998; **121**: 103–113.

91. De Stefano N, Matthews PM, Antel JP et al. Chemical pathology of acute demyelinating lesions and its correlation with disability. *Ann Neurol* 1995; **38**: 901–909.

92. Matthews PM, Pioro E, Narayana S et al. Assessment of lesion pathology in multiple sclerosis using quantitative MRI morphometry and magnetic resonance spectroscopy. *Brain* 1996; **119**: 715–722.

93. Filippi M, Campi A, Colombo B et al. A spinal cord MRI study of benign and secondary progressive multiple sclerosis. *J Neurol* 1996; **243**: 502–505.

94. Losseff NA, Webb SL, O'Riordan JI et al. Spinal cord atrophy and disability in multiple sclerosis: a new reproducible and sensitive MRI method with potential to monitor disease progression. *Brain* 1996; **119**: 701–708.

95. Davie CA, Barker GJ, Webb S et al. Persistent functional deficit in multiple sclerosis and autosomal dominant cerebellar ataxia is associated with axon loss. *Brain* 1995; **118**: 1583–1592.

96. Filippi M, Colombo B, Rovaris M et al. A longitudinal magnetic resonance imaging study of the cervical cord in multiple sclerosis. *J Neuroimaging* 1997; **7**: 78–80.

97. Losseff NA, Wang L, Lai HM et al. Progressive cerebral atrophy in multiple sclerosis. A serial MRI study. *Brain* 1996; **119**: 2009–2019.

10

Is the normal-appearing white matter so normal?

Paul M Matthews, Martin Lee and Nikos Evangelou

INTRODUCTION

Magnetic resonance imaging (MRI) has become the primary technique with which neurologists monitor the pathological evolution of multiple sclerosis (MS). Patients with MS characteristically show multifocal areas of hyperintense signal on T2-weighted MRI sequences. Clinical–radiological correlations have established that these areas of hyperintense signal correspond to the oedematous, demyelinated or gliotic plaques found on post mortem examination.[1] In consequence, MRI has become an important laboratory test to support the diagnosis of MS. More recently, analysis of changes in volumes of T2 hyperintense lesion load or of gadolinium-enhancement associated with breakdown of the blood–brain barrier in the acute inflammatory stage of lesions have been used as surrogate markers of biological activity for treatment trials.[2]

After segmentation of hyperintense lesions on T2-weighted images, 'normal-appearing white matter' (NAWM) is defined conventionally as the white matter volume outside areas of abnormally high white matter signal intensity. However, 'normal-appearing' volumes are curiously evanescent, as the volume of brain defined may be substantially different (or may even disappear!) if a different magnetic reso-

nance pulse sequence (or other method) is used for its definition. As is reviewed below, the authors believe that all white matter volumes show some evidence of pathological change in patients with established MS if imaging techniques with appropriate sensitivity are used.

Why should researchers concern themselves with NAWM? A primary goal of MRI and other laboratory tests in MS is to understand the pathological basis of functional impairment and disability. Logically, if one is interested in defining the brain pathology that is responsible for functional impairment and disability, one should focus on analysis of functional systems. This demands an understanding of the ways in which neurones interact via axonal projections in the white matter. Such functionally defined white matter tracts in general include both volumes of lesions and NAWM. Secondly, with the recognition of the extent of axonal injury and transection that occurs even in acute lesions,[3,4] it has become clear that pathological changes secondary to axonal damage from Wallerian degeneration must extend well beyond the borders of focal lesions identified by T2-weighted MRI. Finally, while the conventionally obvious pathology lies in the plaques on post mortem examination or the lesions on T2-weighted images taken in vivo, this macroscopic lesion load in a typical MS brain constitutes at most a few percent of the total white matter volume. Thus, the bulk of changes (considered in terms of volume) must occur in the NAWM.

It is as if MS is adopting a well-known principle of animal camouflage: distraction by presentation of an arresting detail. Like the leopard's prey in the jungle, our eyes are drawn to the spots, potentially missing the beast!

MAGNETIC RESONANCE MEASURES OF PATHOLOGICAL CHANGE SHOW ABNORMALITIES IN THE NAWM

Progressive loss of volume of the NAWM in MS

Late stages of chronic MS have long been recognized to be associated with brain atrophy. More recent quantitative MRI studies have demonstrated that white matter volume loss occurs even early in the progression of the disease. Losseff and coworkers[5] have shown that relative atrophy of the spinal cord at the third cervical level (C3) is correlated with the degree of disability. In addition, they have described a measurable progressive change in cross-sectional area of the spinal cord at C3 with time. In a later study,[6] they used a measure of cerebral atrophy based on analysis of segmented white matter volumes in axial slices from the central brain. Just as for the spinal cord, it was found that MS patients show measurable atrophy of white matter with time. Because lesion volumes constitute only a small proportion of the total white matter volume in the brain, it is clear that atrophy must occur in white matter outside lesion volumes. Lossef et al,[6] for example, found an average 3% reduction in brain volume (equivalent to an approximate 15 cm^3 white matter volume loss) over 18 months in patients who demonstrated significant atrophy, despite measuring only a 3.3 cm^3 increase in T2 lesion burden over the same period.

Relaxation time measurements show diffuse changes in NAWM

Free water has a relatively long proton MR T2 ('spin–spin') relaxation time of approximately 2500 msec. As water becomes less mobile (e.g. by association with protein-rich myelin), the relaxation time of water is markedly reduced by energy exchange with macromolecules. Thus, the water in normal white matter has a T2 of about 85 msec.[7,8] Detailed analysis of the white matter T2 decay demonstrates that the water signal originates from distinct tissue compartments, each with a characteristic T2. The compartment with the shortest T2 relaxation time (10–55 msec) is thought to represent myelin-associated water, whereas that with a longer T2 relaxation time (70–95 msec) is thought to represent cytoplasmic and extracellular water.[9] Following demyelination there is a decrease in the relative volume of the myelin-associated water compartment and an increase in extracellular water, leading to an increase in the overall T2 relaxation time.

Early studies consistently reported longer relaxation times within NAWM in MS patients than in healthy controls.[10–12] More recent demonstration of bi-exponential T2 decays within NAWM provides more direct evidence of an expansion of the extracellular water compartment in MS.[8,13,14] Prolonged T1 relaxation times have also been reported within NAWM in MS, which also suggests an increase of mobile, extracellular water.[12]

Magnetization transfer is abnormally low in NAWM

Magnetization transfer (MT) imaging generates contrast that also varies with the extent and nature of interactions between tissue water and macromolecules. This technique involves applying an off-resonance radio frequency pulse to saturate spins of the relatively immobile protons of water associated with the macromolecules (of which those of myelin are quantitatively the largest). With exchange of macromolecular bound and free water, there is a reduction in signal intensity. The extent of this so called 'magnetization transfer' decreases with loss of these macromolecular structures.

MT appears to be particularly sensitive to demyelination. MT changes are found in hyperintense lesions on T2-weighted MRI, although the heterogeneity of changes is high, which is consistent with the expected heterogeneity of pathology of the lesions.[15] Several studies also demonstrated a significantly reduced MT for NAWM of patients with MS.[16,17] This diffuse quantitative change in water–macromolecular interactions suggests diffuse demyelination and extracellular matrix loss.

Diffusion anisotropy is abnormally increased in NAWM

With the use of high-gradient field strengths, MRI can be made sensitive to the diffusivity of water in tissue. Consistent with evidence cited above for diffuse demyelination, magnetic resonance diffusion contrast studies suggest diffuse expansion of the extracellular space within the NAWM in MS. Recent work has demonstrated an increase in the apparent diffusion coefficient, both in lesions and (to a lesser extent) in the NAWM of MS patients.[18] The diffusion coefficient of water depends on cell type, size and shape and on the proportion of intercellular to extracellular water. An increased diffusion coefficient is believed to reflect, in part, increased extracellular water.

Magnetic resonance spectroscopy shows evidence for diffuse axonal injury in NAWM

Proton magnetic resonance spectroscopy (MRS) provides a unique tool for in vivo evaluation of biochemical changes associated with brain pathology. The technique is similar to that of MRI, differing in that information on the resonance frequencies of protons observed in the tissue are preserved. This allows analysis of the relative spatial distributions and concentrations of small molecules. As intracellular metabolites are much less abundant than water, the spatial resolution is much lower than with conventional MRI (of the order of just under 1 cm^3) with current instrumentation. However, loss of sensitivity is compensated for by a gain in pathological specificity compared to conventional MR imaging. Water-suppressed localized ^{1}H spectroscopy yields spectra dominated by resonances of N-acetyl aspartate (NAA), creatine (Cr) and phosphocreatine, and choline. NAA is exclusively localized within neurones in the mature brain[19] and is therefore used as a marker of axonal density and integrity. NAA measured using brain MRS spectroscopy has often been expressed relative to Cr, the concentration of which is believed to vary little.

Brain proton MRS in patients with MS has demonstrated substantially reduced NAA:Cr ratios in both chronic[20–22] and acute[23,24] lesions. Irreversible decreases in the relative NAA concentrations in lesions must reflect axonal volume loss (i.e. either a decrease in the number of axons or in their aggregate cross-sectional area). Reversible changes must be a marker of axonal dysfunction rather than loss.[25] The possibility that significant biochemical changes occur outside areas of focal inflammation (i.e. within NAWM) was highlighted by the finding that reductions in the NAA:Cr ratio from a large volume of interest within the brain were relatively independent of T2 hyperintense lesion volumes and could be found with even very large voxels that included relatively small lesion volumes.[21,22] Later studies directly demonstrated a reduced NAA:Cr ratio adjacent to[23] or even distant from lesions in areas of the brain containing only NAWM.[26] Using more sophisticated methodology, the reduction in the NAA:Cr ratio within NAWM has been confirmed and has been shown to be more marked in patients with secondary progressive MS than in those with relapsing–remitting MS.[27,28] A trend to reduction in the absolute NAA concentration within the NAWM has been reported in relapsing MS patients[26] and shown in a subgroup of patients with primary progressive MS,[29] confirming that decreases in the relative NAA concentration (i.e. NAA:Cr) in NAWM do not occur primarily because of increases in Cr.

The reduced NAA:Cr ratio or reduction in absolute NAA signal within NAWM could arise from reduced axonal density (owing to net axon loss or relative volume decrease), reduction in axonal NAA concentration within axons[30] or altered relaxation times. Early studies suggested that relaxation time changes are unlikely to be great enough to have a large effect on the NAA:Cr ratio.[21] Decreases in neuronal NAA concentration occur in response to an acute inflammatory insult and can be reversible.[31,32] However a reduction in the NAA signal within large areas of macroscopically NAWM in patients who have not suffered a recent relapse most likely reflects chronic changes in axonal morphology or density.

Although the greatest effect on the NAA:Cr ratio comes from decreases in NAA, more modest increases in Cr may occur. Increased absolute Cr signal has been shown by proton MRS, and an increased phosphocreatine signal in the NAWM has been measured by phosphorus MRS.[26] Rooney and co-workers[33] have suggested that in some early relapsing–remitting MS patients who show only small reductions in the NAA:Cr ratio in NAWM, the ratio changes may primarily reflect an increased Cr signal. However, studies on post mortem tissue have not shown increased Cr concentrations within NAWM in MS,[34] suggesting that any increase in Cr must be relatively small. Creatine is found in all brain cells but is thought to be particularly high in astrocytes, oligodendrocytes and microglia.[35] Astrocyte and microglial proliferation within NAWM therefore could lead to small increases in Cr signal with MRS.

RECENT PATHOLOGICAL STUDIES CONFIRM THAT THERE IS SUBSTANTIAL DAMAGE IN THE NAWM

Just as the MRI definition of NAWM can vary with the pulse sequence, the pathological definition of 'normal' varies according to the histopathological technique used. For example, immunoreactivity for myelin-associated glycoprotein is decreased in white matter that appears normal for myelin basic protein immunohistochemistry or with luxol fast blue.[36] Since the early observations of Charcot,[37] and Greenfield and King,[38] transection of axons in chronic MS lesions has been recognized. Transection must be associated with rarefaction of axons in the surrounding NAWM after secondary Wallerian degeneration of transected axonal projections extending from the lesions.

Diffuse gliosis is another characteristic finding in MS. Gliosis is most obvious in plaques but it is also found in NAWM, where it is probably secondary to axonal damage and degeneration. Such diffuse axonal loss and gliosis is a plausible correlate of atrophy of the white matter in MS. Until very recently, quantitative estimates of axonal density had been made only for lesions. Ferguson and co-workers[3] studied the distribution of amyloid precursor protein (APP), a relatively sensitive marker of axonal injury. They found abnormal accumulations of APP at the borders of active chronic lesions. These APP accumulations were presumed to be associated with active inflammation in chronic active plaques, since similar changes also were found inside acute plaques. Trapp et al[4] reported abnormal hypophosphorylated neurofilaments in white matter distant from lesions.

Esiri and co-workers[39] recently reported measurements of the density of axons in the spinal cord at the third cervical and second thoracic levels. A novel aspect of their study was that they focused on assessment of axonal density in volumes that did not include lesions. They found a reduction of up to 45% in axonal density compared to controls. There was an intriguing sex-related difference, with greater reduction of axonal density in males. The analysis of the histogram distribution of axonal changes showed a preferential loss of smaller fibres.

Further work reported by Evangelou[40] has focused on analysis of the corpus callosum. This volume of the cerebral white matter is ideal for quantitative axonal counting, since fibres are arranged in an orderly fashion. The density of axons was measured, as well as the total cross-sectional area of the corpus callosum in areas distant from macroscopic lesions. There was no evidence of 'microscopic' lesions in the tissue examined. A mean decrease of axonal density of approximately 35% was measured, although it varied across the length of the corpus callosum from 16% to 56%. This occurred in addition to relative atrophy of the corpus callosum by a mean of approximately 35%. This work therefore confirms that in cerebral white matter there is substantial loss of axons. In addition, the study emphasizes that the degree of total axonal loss is underestimated by measures of atrophy alone. Combined morphological and axonal density measures are needed to appreciate the full extent of axonal loss in NAWM, which (at least for the chronic MS brains studied by Evangelou) can be estimated to be about 45%.

PATHOLOGICAL CHANGES IN NAWM CORRELATE WITH DISABILITY AND PROGRESSION OF DISABILITY

As described above, measurements of atrophy of the cervical cord or of the brain correlate better with clinical disability than do the T2 lesion volumes. These MRI measures may be considered to reflect the cumulative damage from MS lesions, which appears to occur early in the disease, as well as in the later, secondary progressive phase.

Supporting this concept has been work based on analysis of the T1 hypointense lesion load. Following observations that demonstrated a strong correlation between the T1 hypointense load within T2 hyperintense lesion volumes ('black holes') with pathological matrix destruction and axonal loss and clinical disability,[41,42] recent work has used quantitative measures of signal change on T1-weighted images in order to explore the relationship between changes in NAWM and disability.[43] Evangelou and co-workers[43] were able to demonstrate that the 'microscopic' T1-hypointense lesion load in the NAWM correlated as significantly with disability, as the macroscopic 'black hole' lesion volume did.

MT changes in the white matter (which, as described above, is largely NAWM) also correlate with disease state and disability in cross sectional studies.[44]

MRS studies provide a more specific index of axonal injury. The earliest MRS studies reported that large voxel MRS measurements of brain NAA were lower in patients with higher disability scores than in those with lower disability scores.[20] Fu and co-workers[45] later co-registered MRS imaging with conventional images in which the lesions had been segmented in order to produce an independent definition of the relationship between axonal injury in lesions or NAWM and progression of disability. They found a correlation between decreases in NAA in NAWM and progression of disability. It is notable that a similar correlation was not found between NAA decreases in lesions and disability. In contrast, Davie et al[29] noted the correlation between overall axonal injury in lesions and disability in a cross-sectional study. Perhaps measurement of NAA in the aggregate lesion load is difficult and not as sensitive to change over time as are changes in NAWM. The potential utility of NAA measurements in NAWM was further emphasized in a recent large voxel study.[31] Longitudinal follow-up of the same relapsing–remitting and secondary progressive MS patient cohort followed by Fu et al[45] demonstrated a strong correlation between progression of disability and decreases in relative NAA concentrations in a large central volume of white matter.

Lee and co-workers[46] have recently taken a 'functional systems'-focused approach to analysis of the relationship between axonal injury and disability. A group of patients with asymmetric upper limb weakness was identified. The corticospinal tract was defined anatomically and MRS voxels were placed in the corticospinal tract at the level of the internal capsule in both hemispheres. The relative decrease in the concentrations of NAA in the volumes were then compared with the relative motor impairments in the contralateral limb. A strong correlation between the extent of the relative decreases in NAA in the corticospinal tract measured in this way and the relative functional impairment of the appropriate side was found. Since the voxels were located in NAWM, they reflected injury through the tract rather than changes in specific lesions impinging on the tract. This suggests that in specific functionally defined systems there is a relationship between the extent of axonal injury in NAWM (including projecting axons of that functional system) and the degree of functional deficit.

PATHOLOGICAL CHANGES IN NAWM: WHAT IS NOT KNOWN

It is clear that MRI is highly sensitive to the inflammatory lesions of MS. However, there are limits to the sensitivity. Very small lesions (particularly those under the dimension of a pixel) will be difficult to detect because of partial volume effects on signal intensity. Cortical lesions are poorly detected because of poor contrast changes between lesions and surrounding grey matter. In a similar way, it is possible that there may be more diffuse disease throughout NAWM than is apparent from segmentation of the macroscopic hyperintense lesions on the T2-weighted image. This is one possible explanation for the diffuse nature of changes identified in NAWM with other techniques. However, although plaques located in the cortical grey matter are usually only a few millimetres in diameter and are difficult to detect by either MRI or gross inspection, this is not typical for lesions in the central white matter in most patients. For example, in the corpus callosum of eight patients with MS, no 'microscopic' lesions occult to careful gross inspection were identified, even in patients with a short duration of disease (Evangelou N, Esiri M, unpublished data).

Remyelination is prominent in some MS patients, especially early in the disease. So-called shadow plaques seen at post mortem are defined by myelin that is abnormally thin and similar in appearance to the remyelinating plaques observed in experimental demyelinating diseases. The extent of remyelination and the number of shadow plaques probably varies substantially between individual patients. Prineas found evidence of remyelination in 38 out of 105 plaques in five patients who died 3–10 months after the onset of the disease.[47] The extent to which shadow plaques are visible on

conventional MR imaging is not certain. What is the degree of remyelination required for a previously demyelinated plaque that is visible on MRI to become invisible on a T2-weighted MRI, for example?

Diffusible factors, such as proteolytic enzymes, cytokines or nitric oxide and other free radicals, are generated in foci of inflammatory activity, but they may damage axons and glial cells more diffusely.[48,49] Immunoglobulins directed against axonal membrane channels may cause damage or dysfunction. The potential significance of widespread changes was suggested by recent work that describes reversible axonal changes in diffuse areas of white matter that are associated with acute relapse. The extent to which such mechanisms might contribute to diffuse irreversible axonal injury needs to be defined.

There are few data on the spatial relationship between changes in NAWM and the focal lesions of MS. Narayanan and co-workers[50] used a probabilistic mapping technique to define the relationship between T2 hyperintense lesions and decreases in NAA in the white matter. They showed that, although decreases in NAA occur most prominently in areas where there is a high probability of lesions (i.e. in the immediate periventricular area), there also is more widespread distribution of relative NAA decreases extended well beyond the borders of high lesion probability volumes, which is consistent with secondary degeneration of axons around areas of convergence of fibre tracts through lesions. It is clear from MRS imaging studies of large demyelinating lesions that areas adjacent to acute lesions can show at least transient injury patterns.[23] This suggests that the axonal damage occurring in NAWM has a major component from the secondary damage extending from focal lesions of MS. Defining this in greater detail will be critical to testing the hypotheses that most or all of the damage in the NAWM arises secondary to the macroscopic lesions measured by conventional MRI.

THE SIGNIFICANCE OF CHANGES IN NAWM

Although their genesis is not fully appreciated, changes in NAWM are widespread and are correlated with disability and its progression. Lesions of MS identified on T2-weighted images are clearly heterogeneous in size, shape and underlying pathology. However, in an effort to relate pathological change to functional disability, it may be more relevant to identify damage in functional systems traversing the entire white matter tract, focusing necessarily largely on changes that occur in NAWM. This may offer a more robust approach to quantitative evaluation of pathology in patients, since anatomical landmarks can be used for clear definition of functional systems, particularly with use of image registration methods to represent data in a common brain space. Assessment of the load of disease in terms of NAWM using pathologically more specific MRI criteria, such as changes in MT imaging, diffusion anisotropy or NAA, may offer improved ways of defining both sensitivity and specificity of the progression of pathology relevant to disability. Global measures of disease (e.g. from large, single voxels in critical areas of white matter such as the corpus callosum) may provide efficient approaches to assessment of change.

Alternatively, analysis of clinically eloquent functional systems such as the corticospinal tract may provide a relatively direct surrogate for assessment of the functional significance of pathological change in individual patients, particularly if the pathology of lesions within an individual patient is relatively homogeneous throughout the brain.

It is important in our enthusiasm for analysis of MRI that we do not become transfixed by the most obvious qualitative changes. Quantitative MRI methods are essential for sensitive detection of change. Consideration of the brain from a systems point of view may offer important advantages for understanding the clinical relevance of MRI findings and for making them clinically predictive as a surrogate. In doing this, we must learn to see the leopard, not just his spots.

REFERENCES

1. McDonald WI, Miller DH, Barnes D. The pathological evolution of multiple sclerosis. *Neuropathol Appl Neurobiol* 1992; **18**: 319–334.
2. Miller DH, Albert PS, Barkhof F et al. Guidelines for the use of magnetic resonance techniques in monitoring the treatment of multiple sclerosis. US National MS Society Task Force. *Ann Neurol* 1996; **39**: 6–16.
3. Ferguson B, Matyszak MK, Esiri MM, Perry VH. Axonal damage in acute multiple sclerosis lesions. *Brain* 1997; **120**: 393–399.
4. Trapp BD, Peterson J, Ransohoff RM et al. Axonal transection in the lesions of multiple sclerosis [see comments]. *N Engl J Med* 1998; **338**: 278–285.
5. Losseff NA, Webb SL, O'Riordan JI et al. Spinal cord atrophy and disability in multiple sclerosis. A new reproducible and sensitive MRI method with potential to monitor disease progression. *Brain* 1996; **119**: 701–708.
6. Losseff NA, Wang L, Lai HM et al. Progressive cerebral atrophy in multiple sclerosis. A serial MRI study. *Brain* 1996; **119**: 2009–2019.
7. Barbosa S, Blumhardt LD, Roberts N et al. Magnetic resonance relaxation time mapping in multiple sclerosis: normal appearing white matter and the 'invisible' lesion load. *Magn Reson Imaging* 1994; **12**: 33–42.
8. Kidd D, Barker GJ, Tofts PS et al. The transverse magnetisation decay characteristics of long-standing lesions and normal-appearing white matter in multiple sclerosis. *J Neurol* 1997; **244**: 125–130.
9. MacKay A, Whittall K, Adler J et al. In vivo visualization of myelin water in brain by magnetic resonance. *Magn Reson Med* 1994; **31**: 673–677.
10. Lacomis D, Osbakken M, Gross G. Spin-lattice relaxation (T1) times of cerebral white matter in multiple sclerosis. *Magn Reson Med* 1986; **3**: 194–202.
11. Larsson HB. In vivo characterization of the multiple sclerosis plaque by magnetic resonance imaging and spectroscopy. *Acta Neurol Scand Suppl* 1995; **159**: 1–44.
12. Miller DH, Johnson, G, Tofts PS et al. Precise relaxation time measurements of normal-appearing white matter in inflammatory central nervous system disease. *Magn Reson Med* 1989; **11**: 331–336.
13. Barnes D, McDonald WI, Johnson G et al. Quantitative nuclear magnetic resonance imag-

ing: characterisation of experimental cerebral oedema. *J Neurol Neurosurg Psychiatry* 1987; **50**: 125–133.

14. Naruse S, Horikawa Y, Tanaka C et al. Proton nuclear magnetic resonance studies on brain edema. *J Neurosurg* 1982; **56**: 747–752.

15. Dousset V, Grossman RI, Ramer KN et al. Experimental allergic encephalomyelitis and multiple sclerosis: lesion characterization with magnetization transfer imaging [published erratum appears in *Radiology* 1992; **183**: 878]. *Radiology* 1992; **182**: 483–491.

16. Filippi M, Campi A, Dousset V et al. A magnetization transfer imaging study of normal-appearing white matter in multiple sclerosis. *Neurology* 1995; **45**: 478–482.

17. Loevner LA, Grossman RI, Cohen JA et al. Microscopic disease in normal-appearing white matter on conventional MR images in patients with multiple sclerosis: assessment with magnetization-transfer measurements. *Radiology* 1995; **196**: 511–515.

18. Horsfield MA, Lai M, Webb SL et al. Apparent diffusion coefficients in benign and secondary progressive multiple sclerosis by nuclear magnetic resonance. *Magn Reson Med* 1996; **36**: 393–400.

19. Simmons ML, Frondoza CG, Coyle JT. Immunocytochemical localization of N-acetyl-aspartate with monoclonal antibodies. *Neuroscience* 1991; **45**: 37–45.

20. Arnold DL, Matthews PM, Francis G, Antel J. Proton magnetic resonance spectroscopy of human brain in vivo in the evaluation of multiple sclerosis: assessment of the load of disease. *Magn Reson Med* 1990; **14**: 154–159.

21. Matthews PM, Francis G, Antel J, Arnold DL. Proton magnetic resonance spectroscopy for metabolic characterization of plaques in multiple sclerosis [published erratum appears in *Neurology* 1991; **41**: 1828]. *Neurology* 1991; **41**: 1251–1256.

22. Van HP, Marchal G, Johannik K et al. Human brain proton localized NMR spectroscopy in multiple sclerosis. *Magn Reson Med* 1991; **18**: 199–206.

23. Arnold DL, Matthews PM, Francis GS. Proton magnetic resonance spectroscopic imaging for metabolic characterization of demyelinating plaques. *Ann Neurol* 1992; **31**: 235–241.

24. Davie CA, Hawkins CP, Barker GJ. Serial proton magnetic resonance spectroscopy in acute multiple sclerosis lesions. *Brain* 1994; **117**: 49–58.

25. De Stefano N, Matthews PM, Antel JP et al. Chemical pathology of acute demyelinating lesions and its correlation with disability. *Ann Neurol* 1995; **38**: 901–909.

26. Husted CA, Goodin DS, Hugg JW et al. Biochemical alterations in multiple sclerosis lesions and normal-appearing white matter detected by in vivo 31P and 1H spectroscopic imaging. *Ann Neurol* 1994; **36**: 157–165.

27. Matthews PM, Pioro E, Narayanan S et al. Assessment of lesion pathology in multiple sclerosis using quantitative MRI morphometry and magnetic resonance spectroscopy. *Brain* 1996; **119**: 715–722.

28. Fu L, Wolfson C, Worsley KJ et al. Statistics for investigation of multimodal MR imaging data and an application to multiple sclerosis patients. *NMR Biomed* 1996; **9**: 339–346.

29. Davie CA, Barker GJ, Thompson AJ et al. 1H magnetic resonance spectroscopy of chronic cerebral white matter lesions and normal appearing white matter in multiple sclerosis. *J Neurol Neurosurg Psychiatry* 1997; **63**: 736–742.

30. Matthews PM, Cianfaglia L, McLaurin J et al. Demonstration of reversible decreases in N-acetylaspartate (NAA) in a neuronal cell line: NAA decreases as a marker of sublethal neuronal dysfunction. *Proc Soc Magn Reson Med* 1995; **1**: 147.

31. De Stefano N, Matthews PM, Fu L. Axonal damage correlates with disability in patients with relapsing–remitting multiple sclerosis. Results of a longitudinal magnetic resonance spectroscopy study. *Brain* 1998; **121**: 1469–1477.

32. De Stefano N, Matthews PM, Arnold DL. Reversible decreases in N-acetyl aspartate after acute brain injury. *Magn Reson Med* 1995; **34**: 721–727.

33. Rooney WD, Goodkin DE, Schuff N et al. 1H MRSI of normal appearing white matter in multiple sclerosis. *Multiple Sclerosis* 1997; **3**: 231–237.

34. Davies SE, Newcombe J, Williams SR et al. High resolution proton NMR spectroscopy of multiple sclerosis lesions. *J Neurochem* 1995; **64**: 742–748.

35. Urenjak J, Williams SR, Gadian DG, Noble M. Proton nuclear magnetic resonance spectroscopy unambiguously identifies different neural cell types. *J Neurosci* 1993; **13**: 981–989.

36. Itoyama Y, Sternberger NH, Webster HD et al. Immunocytochemical observations on the distribution of myelin-associated glycoprotein and myelin basic protein in multiple sclerosis lesions. *Ann Neurol* 1980; **7**: 167–177.

37. Charcot J. Histologie de la sclerose en plaques. *Gaz Hop (Paris)* 1868; **41**: 554–566.

38. Greenfield J, King L. Observations on the histopathology of the cerebral lesions in disseminated sclerosis. *Brain* 1936; **59**: 445–459.

39. Ganter P, Prince C, Esiri MM. Spinal cord axonal loss in multiple sclerosis: a post mortem study. *Multiple Sclerosis* 1998; **4**: 272.

40. Evangelou N, Esiri MM, Palace J, Matthews PM. A quantitative pathological study of axonal loss in the corpus callosum in multiple sclerosis. *Multiple Sclerosis* 1998; **4**: 287.

41. van Walderveen MA, Kamphorst W, Scheltens P et al. Histopathologic correlate of hypointense lesions on T1-weighted spin-echo MRI in multiple sclerosis. *Neurology* 1998; **50**: 1282–1288.

42. Truyen L, van Waesberghe JH, van Walderveen MA et al. Accumulation of hypointense lesions ('black holes') on T1 spin-echo MRI correlates with disease progression in multiple sclerosis. *Neurology* 1996; **47**: 1469–1476.

43. Evangelou N, Lee M, Palace J, Matthews PM. Correlation between volume of T1 hypointense white matter signal and disability in relapsing remitting MS. *Multiple Sclerosis* 1997; **3**: 299.

44. Gass A, Barker GJ, Kidd D et al. Correlation of magnetization transfer ratio with clinical disability in multiple sclerosis. *Ann Neurol* 1994; **36**: 62–67.

45. Fu L, Matthews PM, De SN et al. Imaging axonal damage of normal-appearing white matter in multiple sclerosis. *Brain* 1998; **121**: 103–113.

46. Lee MA, Blamire AM, Ho KH et al. Asymmetry of NAA in the internal capsule of patients with MS correlates with lateralisation of motor impairment: a spectroscopic, clinical and electrophysiological study. *J Neurol* 1998; **245**: 384.

47. Prineas JW, Barnard RO, Kwon EE et al. Multiple sclerosis: remyelination of nascent lesions. *Ann Neurol* 1993; **33**: 137–151.

48. Bo L, Dawson TM, Wesselingh S et al. Induction of nitric oxide synthase in demyelinating regions of multiple sclerosis brains. *Ann Neurol* 1994; **36**: 778–786.

49. Hohlfeld R. Biotechnological agents for the immunotherapy of multiple sclerosis. Principles, problems and perspectives. *Brain* 1997; **120**: 865–916.

50. Narayanan S, Fu L, Pioro E et al. Imaging of axonal damage in multiple sclerosis: spatial distribution of magnetic resonance imaging lesions. *Ann Neurol* 1997; **41**: 385–391.

11

Diffusion magnetic resonance imaging in multiple sclerosis

David J Werring, Chris A Clark and David H Miller

IMAGING DIFFUSION USING MAGNETIC RESONANCE

Diffusion is the random translational motion of molecules in a fluid system. A large proportion of the living brain is in a fluid state owing to its high water content, and diffusion plays a vital role in the transport of metabolites and the regulation of the tissue environment. Diffusion is influenced by the microstructural components of tissue, including cell membranes and organelles, and measurement of diffusion in the brain (in particular of water molecules) thus gives unique information about its structure. Diffusion may be understood by conceptually following a molecule of water in a glass beaker, whose direction is altered every time it interacts with another water molecule. The longer we observe the molecule, the further it has travelled, on average, from its original position when the observation began. The diffusion coefficient relates the observation time and the average distance travelled, and is a characteristic of the fluid under consideration. Diffusion is a three-dimensional process and when (as in a glass of water) it is the same in any direction in space, it is termed isotropic or free diffusion. Because the diffusion coefficient reflects the kinetic or motional energy of the molecules, its value is approximately proportional to temperature.

Magnetic resonance imaging (MRI) can be used to measure diffusion coefficients non-invasively. The technique is based on the application of large pulsed field gradients, which sensitize the nuclear magnetic resonance (NMR) signal to diffusive motion.[1] This sensitization results in an irreversible dephasing of the transverse magnetization, which causes signal attenuation. The degree of signal attenuation is related to the diffusion coefficient of the sample and to the properties (including the magnitude, separation and duration) of the diffusion sensitizing gradients, described by the gradient b factor. By collecting a series of signals with different b factors, it is possible to calculate the diffusion coefficient of the sample. Diffusion MRI can therefore provide a new type of tissue contrast and produce maps of diffusion coefficients throughout the brain.[2–4]

In biological tissues, the value of the diffusion coefficient is less than in free water at the same temperature. This is because the structural components of tissue, including cell membranes and organelles, present obstacles to water diffusion. Thus, if we observe water molecules for a sufficiently long time they will eventually reach an element of the cellular structure. If a cell membrane is completely impermeable to water molecules, the molecules will be reflected back so that their progress across the membrane is impeded: this is termed restricted diffusion. If the membrane is semipermeable then only a proportion of the diffusing water molecules proceed across the membrane, causing a more modest reduction in the diffusion coefficient, termed hindered diffusion. Measuring diffusion in a biological system such as the brain therefore results in an apparent diffusion coefficient (ADC), so named in order to distinguish it from true free diffusion.[5]

In a diffusion-weighted image (DWI) of the brain, regions in which there is high diffusion, such as the cerebrospinal fluid, show marked signal attenuation, whereas areas with lower diffusion, such as grey or white matter, have less signal attenuation. (In addition to these effects, blood flow in capillaries may cause subtle changes in the signal attenuation.) This approach can yield useful information, for example by revealing reduced diffusion in acute cerebral infarction,[6] which is probably due to a shift of water into cells from the extracellular space ('cytotoxic oedema'). However, this approach is qualitative, and the interpretation of DWIs is often complicated by a T2 relaxation component observed in addition to the effects of diffusion.

Quantitation of diffusion (i.e. measurement of the ADC) is possible by obtaining two or more images with different degrees of sensitization to diffusion (b factors) and fitting the data to the exponential function:

$$\frac{S}{S_0} = \exp(-bADC)$$

where S is the attenuated NMR signal in the presence of diffusion gradients, S_0 is the signal in their absence, and b is the gradient b factor.

In some biological tissues, the degree of restriction or hindrance of diffusion may change with direction owing to oriented structural barriers to diffusion such as axonal membranes, myelin and the neurofilamentary cytoskeleton. In this situation, where the diffusion coefficient is directionally dependent, diffusion is said to be anisotropic. This phenomenon has been observed in the white matter tracts of the brain by applying the diffusion sensitizing gradients in two or more directions.[7,8] A higher ADC is seen parallel to the fibre direction than is the case perpendicular to the fibres. Anisotropy in the brain depends on the structural coherence of fibre tracts, and it is therefore of potential interest in assessing the impact of pathology on tract integrity, but accurate quantification presents a considerable challenge.

Diffusion imaging has recently been revolutionized by the recognition that the diffusion tensor, D (a mathematical matrix quantity), is required to describe anisotropic diffusion adequately and that it may be characterized using MRI.[9] The magnitude of diffusion as measured by the diffusion tensor (known as the mean diffusivity) has the special property of rotational invariance. This means that, unlike the ADC calculated with only one axis of sensitization, mean diffusivity has the same value regardless of the orientation of the brain in the magnet. This property is particularly desirable for longitudinal patient studies and for studies involving different laboratories. Furthermore, Basser and Pierpaoli[10,11] have demonstrated that true quantification of diffusion anisotropy is possible using measurements derived from the diffusion tensor; proposed anisotropy indices include fractional anisotropy and the volume ratio.

Unfortunately sensitization of the imaging sequence to diffusion also results in greatly increased sensitivity to patient motion. Early diffusion imaging studies were limited by severe motion artefacts resulting in an inaccurate assessment of the ADC. A number of strategies have been employed to circumvent this problem, including the use of cardiac gating and navigator echoes that correct for the effects of bulk subject motion.[12] Perhaps the most notable development, however, has been the use of echo–planar imaging (EPI).[13] EPI acquires images in a fraction of a second, thus freezing physiological motion. This method effectively avoids the motion problem and is sufficiently rapid to enable the collection of DWIs with the multiple b factors and axes of sensitization required for imaging the diffusion tensor. EPI is now becoming more widely used on many commercial MRI systems for diffusion imaging.

Thus, diffusion imaging has benefited from a

Table 11.1 Hypothetical effects of pathological changes in multiple sclerosis lesions on diffusion (mean diffusivity) and diffusion anisotropy (fractional anisotropy).

Pathological element	Acute lesions		Chronic lesions	
	Change in mean diffusivity	Change in fractional anisotropy	Change in mean diffusivity	Change in fractional anisotropy
Vasogenic oedema	↑	↓	—	—
Cellular infiltration (macrophages etc)	↓	↓	—	—
Inflammation (oedema and cellular infiltration)	↑	↓	—	—
Demyelination (loss of myelin)	↑	↓	↑	↓
Axonal loss	↑	↓	↑	↓
Myelin breakdown products	↓	↓	↓	↓
Remyelination	—	—	↓	↑
Gliosis	—	—	↓	↓

number of methodological improvements, which today make DWI and diffusion tensor imaging (DTI) realistic tools for clinical investigation. The following section demonstrates that these developments have been reflected in the application of diffusion imaging to study multiple sclerosis (MS).

DIFFUSION MRI IN MS

Rationale for using diffusion MRI in MS

Conventional MRI is able to detect the white matter lesions of MS with excellent sensitivity,[14] and it has an established role in diagnosis. However, both cross-sectional and longitudinal studies show only a modest relationship between T2-weighted cranial MRI abnormalities and the severity and progression of disability. An important contributory factor is the lack of pathological specificity of T2 signal change:

all of the pathological hallmarks of MS (inflammation, oedema, demyelination, gliosis and axonal loss) alter tissue water content and thus T2 signal, but they may have very different effects on neuronal function and clinical deficit. It has been suggested that a number of newer MRI techniques have greater pathological specificity: these include magnetization transfer imaging (a putative marker for demyelination or axonal loss),[15] spectroscopy of N-acetyl aspartate (a measure of axonal loss or dysfunction),[16] T1-weighted imaging (in which hypointensity of lesions appears to relate to the degree of axonal loss)[17] and quantitation of brain or cord atrophy.[18] These techniques have all shown significant correlations with disability, suggesting that axonal loss and persistent demyelination are contributory factors. There remains, however, a need for new magnetic resonance techniques that can detect more specifically the structural changes that underpin clinical deficit, in order to gain a better understanding of the mechanisms of disability and to monitor the effects of therapeutic interventions.

Diffusion MRI, as discussed above, is able to probe structural properties of tissue (including the size, shape, integrity and orientation of water spaces) that are inaccessible to other imaging methods. The pathological elements of multiple sclerosis alter the permeability or geometry of structural barriers to water diffusion in the brain, which may allow diffusion MRI to provide a quantitative estimate of the degree of tissue disruption and to increase understanding of the mechanisms underlying reversible and persistent disability. *Table 11.1* provides a hypothetical framework of the changes in diffusion properties anticipated to result from each pathological element in MS.

Diffusion imaging in clinical studies of multiple sclerosis

Diffusion MRI has been extensively used to investigate acute stroke, but it has not been widely applied to the study of MS. The first report of water diffusion in MS was published by Larsson et al in 1992.[19] Although limited by motion artefact, this study demonstrated higher diffusion in MS plaques than in normal-appearing white matter (NAWM). Plaques judged to be less than 3 months old showed the highest diffusion values. A subsequent paper[20] used strategies to reduce motion artefact (bi-polar gradients and cardiac gating), which resulted in more stable measurements and con-firmed the previous observations. In this study it was also noted that NAWM in MS patients showed higher diffusion than NAWM in healthy control subjects. These early studies suffered from technical limitations, particularly of motion artefact, limited brain coverage and an ability to examine only large lesions with diffusion gradients applied in a single direction. A study by Horsfield et al[21] used a volume selective technique that permitted three-axis diffusion measurement in a reasonable time frame without major motion artefact, although only large lesions could be studied. No signifi-cant differences in ADC were detected between

benign and secondary progressive phenotypes of MS. The finding of increased ADC in lesions was again confirmed, and a single acute lesion had the highest value with subsequent normal-ization almost to the NAWM value. NAWM in MS patients was found to exhibit higher water diffusion than NAWM in normal controls, in keeping with earlier work. The method used in this study did not, however, allow lesion mor-phology and the surrounding structure to be visualized on ADC maps.

A more recent study[22] used a navigator echo strategy to correct for motion artefact in a spin-echo diffusion sequence; this study obtained high-quality ADC maps, albeit of a limited por-tion of the brain. Here too an increase in diffu-sion in lesions compared to NAWM was observed, with the highest diffusion values found in T1 hypointense lesions ('T1 black holes'). There is evidence that T1 black holes represent lesions containing substantial axonal loss.[17] The reason for T1 hypointense lesions showing high water diffusion may therefore be an extensive loss of axons and a consequent expansion in the extracellular space. Acute (enhancing) lesions had higher diffusion than chronic (non-enhancing) lesions in this study, which could be accounted for by acute vaso-genic (extracellular) oedema in contrast-enhancing lesions.[23] Some large enhancing lesions were observed to have a rim of tissue with relatively hindered water diffusion, which may represent an accumulation of inflamma-tory cells, including macrophages, at the edge of the lesion (*Fig. 11.1*).[23]

The studies discussed so far, although encouraging, were subject to technical limita-tions, most notably of motion artefact and of a limited volume of sampled tissue. Both of these problems are addressed by the use of EPI, which is less susceptible to motion and permits greater brain coverage, with more diffusion-sensitized gradient directions, in a given time. Some recent studies have used EPI diffusion in MS, although there are few pub-lished data. All studies show that diffusion is higher in lesions than in NAWM, in keeping with the findings from other techniques.[24,25] One study estimated a (non-rotationally invari-

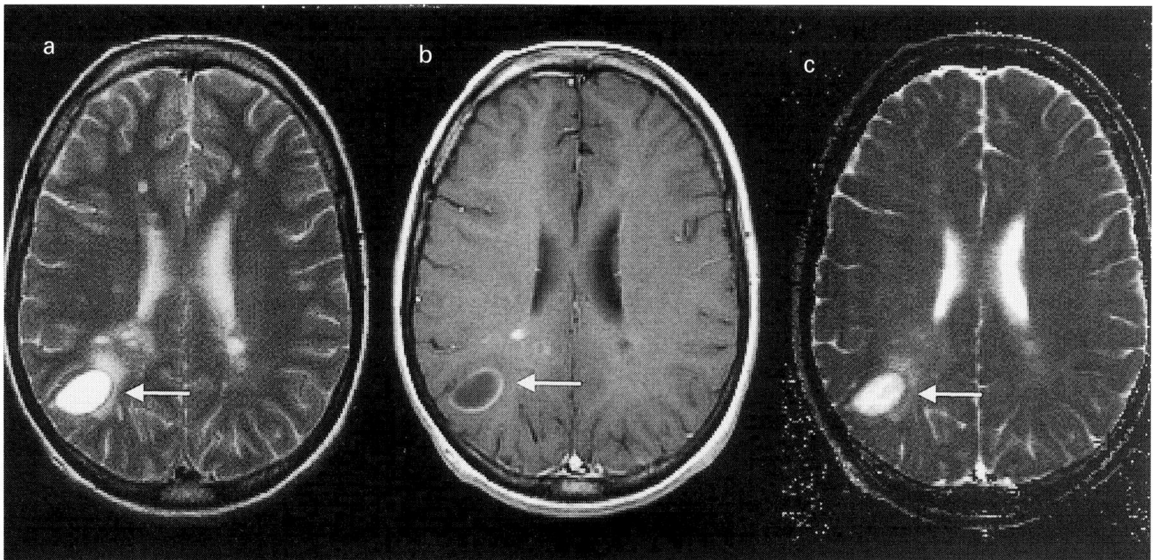

Figure 11.1 Axial MRI scans in a patient with relapsing–remitting sclerosis. (a) T2-weighted scan showing large lesion posteriorly in the right hemisphere (arrow). (b) T1-weighted scan following administration of gadolinium-DTPA contrast. The lesion enhances in a 'ring' pattern, showing that there is active inflammatory activity. (c) ADC map calculated from diffusion-weighted images acquired using a navigator-corrected spin echo diffusion sequence. The lesion shows a heterogeneous pattern of ADC measurements; diffusion is high centrally with an area of restricted diffusion curving around its left side. This area may represent the accumulation of inflammatory cells at the rim of the acute lesion.

ant) index of anisotropy, which was found to reduced within lesions.[24] In common with previous data, areas of restricted diffusion have been observed in EPI diffusion studies of both acute and chronic lesions, and these areas may represent inflammatory cell accumulation.[23]

There are few data examining the relationship between diffusion changes in the brain in MS and clinical phenotype or disability. A navigator-corrected spin-echo study in 40 patients with a range of disabilities found no significant correlation of mean lesion ADC with disability as measured by Kurtzkes's expanded disability status scale (EDSS).[22] Studies to date suggest that there are not large differences in the ADC of lesions or white matter between the clinical MS phenotypes,[21,22] although more work is required to establish this conclusively.

Diffusion tensor imaging in multiple sclerosis

DTI offers the prospect of a fuller exploration of the structural changes in the lesions and NAWM of patients with MS. It is the only method that allows the accurate quantitation of diffusion anisotropy, a property that is likely to be closely linked to the structural integrity of tissue. It provides exquisite delineation of white matter tracts in the living brain (*Fig. 11.2*). A preliminary study has demonstrated the feasibility of using the technique in MS;[26] findings suggest that there is a reduction in anisotropy in lesions. A recent DTI study demonstrated lower anisotropy and higher mean diffusivity in acute (enhancing) lesions than in chronic (non-enhancing) lesions.[27] These changes probably relate to acute vasogenic oedema and

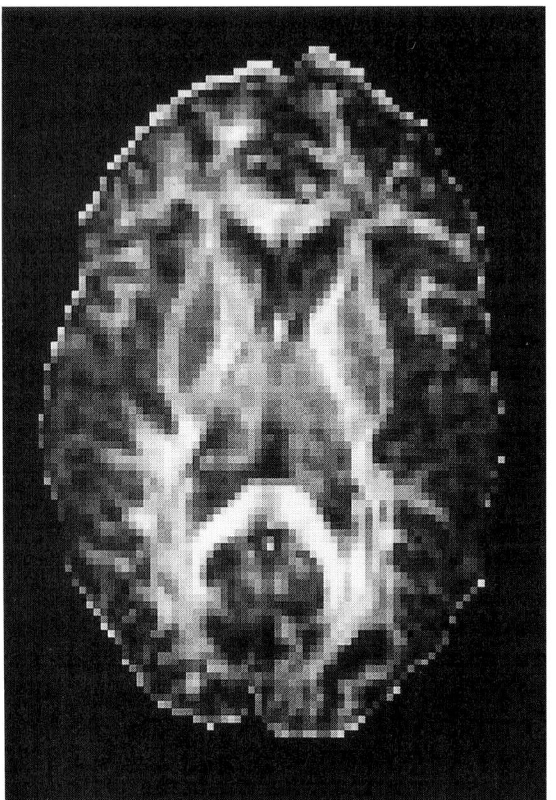

Figure 11.2 Map of fractional anisotropy, derived from DTI data. Bright voxels are those in which anisotropy is high, implying a high degree of fibre tract coherence. The white matter tracts including the internal capsule, corpus callosum and optic radiation are well demonstrated.

axonal loss, and it will be interesting to determine how much structural disruption is permanent as the lesions evolve. Anisotropy maps derived from DTI reveal tract anatomy, and the effects of lesions upon them, in a way that is not possible with other MRI methods. An example of how the DTI findings correlate with the clinical symptoms in a patient during an acute relapse is shown in *Fig. 11.3*. DTI may also reveal changes in anisotropy distinct from the plaque itself (*Fig. 11.3d*). The mechanism underlying these changes is not yet understood, but one possibility could be Wallerian degeneration of axons traversing the lesion.[28] DTI may thus

be a way of investigating the role of Wallerian degeneration in the pathophysiology of MS. Such effects on tracts may have important functional consequences on connected cerebral areas.

Diffusion imaging in experimental models of multiple sclerosis

A study of water diffusion in an animal model of MS (experimental allergic encephalomyelitis) reported that in evolving lesions, DWI signal intensity increased before any detectable change in conventional T2-weighted images,[29] an observation that is yet to be investigated in MS in human subjects. Increased ADC values were seen in lesions. Another study provided evidence of a relative preservation of diffusion anisotropy in chronic compared to acute lesions of experimental allergic encephalomyelitis.

Diffusion MRI of the optic nerve and spinal cord

Diffusion imaging of the optic nerve presents a considerable technical challenge. The optic nerve is a small structure that is prone to movement during imaging sequences; it is also subject to geometric distortions in EPI sequences owing to the proximity of air–bone interfaces. For these reasons there have been few studies of diffusion in the human optic nerve. One study has successfully obtained diffusion magnetic resonance measurements in patients with optic neuritis.[31] It showed increased diffusion in the affected nerve, despite problems caused by head motion. The optic nerve is an attractive region in which to study pathophysiological mechanisms in demyelinating diseases. It is clinically eloquent, and conduction along the nerve may be investigated using electrophysiological methods. There are also simple clinical measures of function (visual acuity, colour appreciation). Thus, if the technical challenges of diffusion imaging in the optic nerve are overcome, it may increase our understanding of mechanisms of impairment and recovery in MS.

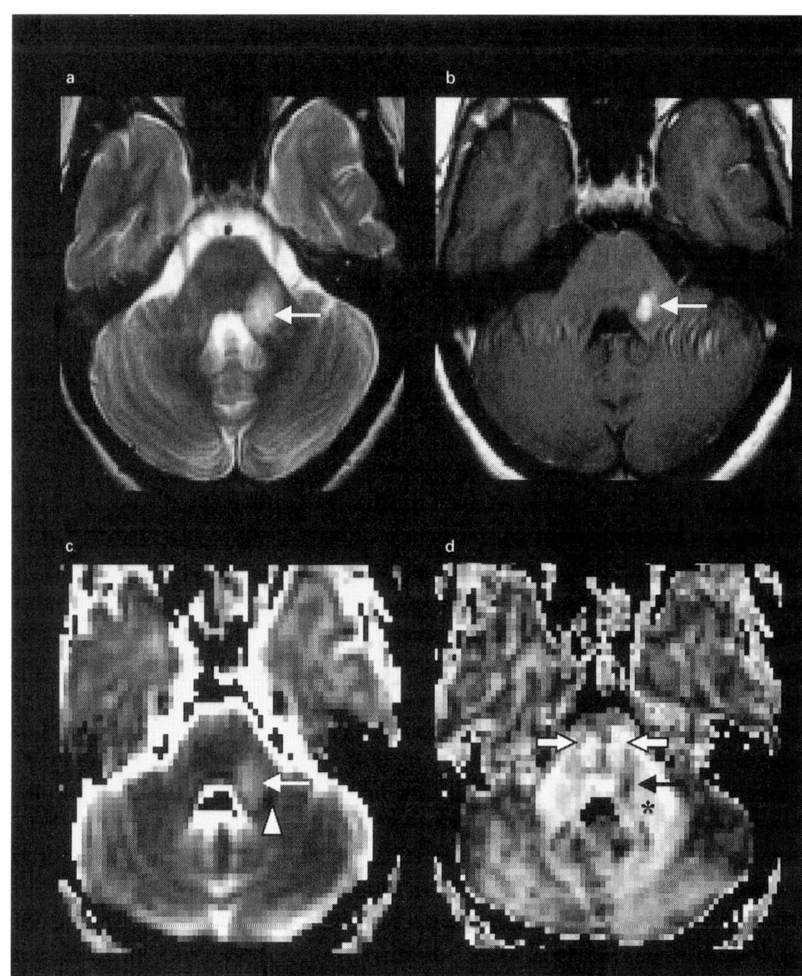

Figure 11.3 Axial MRI scans from a 26-year-old woman with relapsing–remitting MS, taken during an acute relapse. The patient had symptoms of left facial weakness and numbness and left sided ataxia (upper and lower limb), but no pyramidal deficit. (a) T2-weighted scan showing a lesion in the left middle cerebellar peduncle (white arrow). (b) T1-weighted scan showing central contrast enhancement (white arrow). (c) Mean diffusivity map showing the lesion clearly (white arrow), but revealing abnormally low diffusion posteriorly and to the left of the lesion (white arrowhead). (d) Fractional anisotropy map showing low anisotropy within the lesion (black arrow) but also reduced anisotropy distal to the lesion in the white matter tract (asterisk). Note that the corticospinal tracts (white arrows) show preserved anisotropy, in keeping with the clinical findings.

Diffusion in the spinal cord also presents technical difficulties because of its small size, its tendency to move during imaging and its location deep to substantial bony and soft tissue structures. This last problem makes EPI particularly difficult owing to susceptibility artefacts. The first successful diffusion-weighted images of the human cervical cord have recently been obtained, however (*Fig. 11.4*).[32] In this study, the ADC was observed to be greater along the spinal cord than across it, in keeping with the rostrocaudal orientation of the majority of fibre tracts. Spinal cord disease is likely to be a major determinant of locomotor disability in MS; the quantification of water diffusion in the spinal cord of MS patients is therefore of considerable interest.

CONCLUSION

This chapter has described the basic principles of diffusion MRI and has given an overview of recent methodological developments. Some data from clinical studies in MS have been presented. Diffusion imaging appears to give

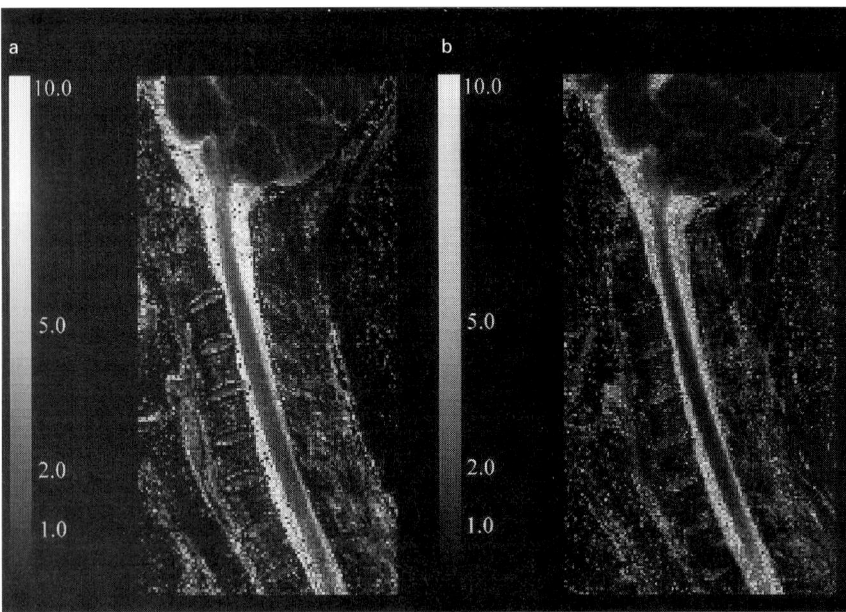

Figure 11.4 ADC maps of the healthy human cervical cord (a) with diffusion sensitized gradients applied in the superoinferior direction; and (b) in the anteroposterior direction. Note that diffusion is greater in the superoinferior direction than the anteroposterior direction, indicating that diffusion in the spinal cord is anisotropic.

complementary information to conventional MRI methods: it can detect structural abnormalities in NAWM and can quantitatively distinguish between lesions of different pathological severity (as evidenced by T1-weighted imaging hypointensity) or stages of evolution (as evidenced by the presence of contrast enhancement). Diffusion imaging also reveals new information about the morphology of MS plaques, which may relate to pathophysiological changes. The recent development of DTI allows the precise quantification of anisotropy in patients with MS, which promises to shed further light on mechanisms of disability by showing the effects of lesions on white matter tract integrity and orientation. The application of diffusion imaging to clinically eloquent structures, including the spinal cord and optic nerves, presents technical difficulties but may be rewarding in providing a better understanding of mechanisms of deficit and recovery in demyelinating disease.

REFERENCES

1. Stejskal EO, Tanner JE. Spin diffusion measurements: spin echoes in the presence of a time-dependent field gradient. *J Chem Phys* 1965; **42**: 288–292.
2. Le Bihan D, Breton E. Imagerie de diffusion in vivo par resonance magnétique nucléaire. *C R Acad Sci (Paris)* 1985; **301**: 1109–1112.
3. Taylor DG, Bushell MC. The spatial mapping of translational diffusion coefficients by the NMR imaging technique. *Phys Med Biol* 1985; **30**: 345–349.
4. Merboldt KD, Hanicke W, Frahm J. Self-diffusion NMR imaging using stimulated echoes. *J Magn Reson* 1985; **64**: 479–486.
5. Le Bihan D, Breton E, Lallemand D et al. MR imaging of intravoxel incoherent motions: applications to diffusion and perfusion in neurologic disorders. *Radiology* 1986; **161**: 401–407.
6. Warach S, Chien D, Li W et al. Fast magnetic resonance diffusion-weighted imaging of acute human stroke. *Neurology* 1992; **42**: 1717–1723.
7. Chien D, Buxton RB, Kwong KK et al. MR diffusion imaging of the human brain. *J Comput Assist Tomogr* 1990; **14**: 514–520.

8. Chenevert TL, Brunberg JA, Pipe JG. Anisotropic diffusion in human white matter: demonstration with MR techniques in vivo. *Radiology* 1990; **177**: 401–405.

9. Basser PJ, Le Bihan D, Mattiello J. Estimation of the effective self-diffusion tensor from the NMR spin echo. *J Magn Reson (B)* 1994; **103**: 247–254.

10. Basser PJ, Pierpaoli C. Microstructural and physiological features of tissues elucidated by quantiative diffusion tensor MRI. *J Magn Reson (B)* 1996; **111**: 209–219.

11. Pierpaoli C, Basser PJ. Toward a quantitative assessment of diffusion anisotropy. *Magn Reson Med* 1996; **36**: 893–906.

12. Ordidge RJ, Helpern JA, Qing ZQ et al. Correction of motional artifacts in diffusion-weighted MR images using navigator echoes. *Magn Reson Imaging* 1994; **12**: 455–460.

13. Turner R, Le Bihan D. Single-shot diffusion imaging at 2.0 Tesla. *J Magn Reson* 1990; **86**: 445–452.

14. Young IR, Hall AS, Pallis CA et al. Nuclear magnetic resonance imaging of the brain in multiple sclerosis. *Lancet* 1981; **ii**: 1063–1066.

15. Gass A, Barker GJ, Kidd D et al. Correlation of magnetisation transfer ratio with clinical disability in multiple sclerosis. *Ann Neurol* 1994; **36**: 62–67.

16. Davie CA, Barker GJ, Webb S et al. Persistent functional deficit in multiple sclerosis and autosomal dominant cerebellar ataxia is associated with axonal loss. *Brain* 1995; **118**: 1583–1592.

17. van Walderveen MAA, Barkhof F, Hommes R et al. Histopathologic correlate of hypointense lesions on T1-weighted spin-echo MRI in multiple sclerosis. *Neurology* 1998; **50**: 1282–1288.

18. Lossef NA, Webb SL, O'Riordan JL et al. Spinal cord atrophy and disability in multiple sclerosis: a new reproducible and sensitive MRI method with potential to monitor disease progression. *Brain* 1996; **119**: 2009–2019.

19. Larsson HBW, Thomsen C, Frederiksen J et al. In vivo magnetic resonance diffusion measurement in the brain of patients with multiple sclerosis. *Magn Reson Imaging* 1992; **10**: 7–12.

20. Christiansen P, Gideon P, Thomsen M et al. Increased water self-diffusion in chronic plaques and in apparently normal white matter in patients with multiple sclerosis. *Acta Neurol Scand* 1993; **87**: 195–199.

21. Horsfield MA, Lai M, Webb SL et al. Apparent diffusion coefficients in benign and progressive multiple sclerosis by nuclear magnetic resonance. *Magn Reson Med* 1996; **36**: 393–400.

22. Droogan AG, Clark CA, Werring DJ et al. Comparison of multiple sclerosis clinical subgroups using navigated spin echo diffusion-weighted imaging. *Magn Reson Imaging* 1999; in press.

23. Katz D, Taubenberger JK, Cannella B et al. Correlation between magnetic resonance imaging findings and lesion development in chronic, active multiple sclerosis. *Ann Neurol* 1993; **34**: 661–669.

24. Graham GD, Zhong J, Guarnaccia JB. Echo-planar imaging of water diffusion and diffusion anistropy within multiple sclerosis plaques (abstract). *Proc ISMRM* 1995; **1**: 278.

25. Gass A, Gaa J, Schreiber W et al. Assessment of the apparent diffusion coefficient in contrast-enhancing and chronic lesions (abstract). *Proc ISMRM* 1998; **2**: 1328.

26. Tievsky AL, Ptak T, Wu O et al. Evaluation of MS lesions with full tensor diffusion weighted imaging and anisotropy mapping (abstract). *Proc ISMRM* 1997; **2**: 666.

27. Werring DJ, Clark CA, Barker GJ et al. Diffusion tensor imaging of lesions and normal appearing white matter in multiple sclerosis. *Neurology* 1999; in press.

28. Trapp BD, Peterson J, Ransohof RM et al. Axonal transection in the lesions of multiple sclerosis. *N Engl J Med* 1998; **388**: 278–285.

29. Heide AC, Richards TL, Alvord EC et al. Diffusion imaging of experimental allergic encephalomyelitis. *Magn Reson Med* 1993; **4**: 478–484.

30. Verhoye MR, 's-Gravenmade EJ, Raman ER et al. In vivo noninvasive determination of abnormal water diffusion in the rat brain studied in an animal model for multiple sclerosis by diffusion-weighted NMR imaging. *Magn Reson Imaging* 1996; **14**: 521–532.

31. Iwasawa T, Matoba H, Ogi A et al. Diffusion-weighted imaging of the human optic nerve: a new approach to evaluate optic neuritis in multiple sclerosis. *Magn Reson Med* 1997; **38**: 484–491.

32. Clark CA, Barker GJ, Tofts P. Magnetic resonance diffusion imaging of the human cervical spinal cord *in vivo* (abstract). *Proc ISMRM* 1998; **1**: 529.

PART IV
Therapy

12

Emerging therapeutic options in multiple sclerosis

John H Noseworthy

BACKGROUND

With the emergence of three[1–7] or possibly four[8] partially effective therapies for patients with relapsing multiple sclerosis (MS), there are new challenges to those designing and conducting randomized controlled trials.[9] These partially effective therapies dictate that the sample size in future trials in relapsing MS will need to be increased by at least 30% to demonstrate efficacy. We may now have reached the end of the 'placebo era' for patients with relapsing–remitting MS. Trials comparing new agents against these established treatments will be significantly more complex in that the 'accepted standard treatments' are costly, parenterally administered and, to a greater or lesser degree, have recognizable adverse side effects, which makes blinding difficult. MS investigators have now entered into a new relationship with sponsors (largely industry) and to a large extent have assumed a more passive role with regard to clinical trial design and data analysis. There are a limited and diminishing number of 'treatment-naïve' patients. In addition, one must repeatedly determine whether there is 'equipoise' when designing randomized controlled trials to test new agents against these proven, albeit only partially effective, agents.[10,11]

Serial gadolinium-enhanced MRI studies are a sensitive but expensive screening tool for determining whether putative candidate agents alter blood–brain barrier permeability.[12] There remains, however, a limited ability to screen new agents for clinical efficacy, especially in the case of agents that may not affect the early inflammatory phase of the illness. MS investigators struggle with a limited ability to detect clinical evidence of efficacy in small phase 1 and 2 trials. There is limited validity to the current rules that are used to 'stop for efficacy and futility'. Phase 2 trials are long and costly and perhaps of limited value in moving the field towards the recognition of effective agents. As this burgeoning field is surveyed, it is prudent to ponder a few of the key questions facing the MS clinical trial community. What are the important mechanisms of tissue injury and recovery in MS? How important are the following components: resolution of inflammatory and edema, remyelination, sodium-channel rearrangements, axonal sprouting? What is the role of the immune response in determining the degree of recovery? Can axonal injury be recognized early in the course of the illness, and will currently available treatments slow or reduce the development of further axonal injury? Is an anti-immune strategy the correct approach? Are there alternatives to identifying candidate agents for future phase 3 randomized controlled trials?

CONVENTIONAL IMMUNOSUPPRESSIVE THERAPIES

Each of the following 'conventional' approaches to immunosuppressive therapy has its proponents worldwide: total lymphoid irradiation,[13,14] cladribine,[15,16] mitoxantrone,[17] lymphocytapheresis (P Bloom, personal communication), azathioprine,[18,19] interferon-α,[20] and intravenous immunoglobulin.[8,21,22] A number of trials with these agents are currently in progress, including the Erazimus trial in France (interferon β-1a ± azathioprine) and ongoing European studies of mitoxantrone.

PARTIALLY EFFECTIVE AGENTS

There is now consensus that interferon β-1b (Betaseron®; Berlex; Betaferon, Schering),[1–3] interferon β-1a (Avonex®, Biogen; Rebif®,[4,5] Ares-Serono)[23] and glatrimer acetate (Copaxone®. Teva-Marion)[6,7] each reduce relapse rate in patients with active relapsing–remitting disease. The advantages and disadvantages of these agents, their relative effectiveness in reducing relapse rate and altering progression of disability as measured by the Expanded Disability Status Scale, their impact on MRI behavior, and the likelihood and relevance of the development of neutralizing antibodies to these agents are beyond the scope of this review.

Investigators worldwide are building on these early successes in a large number of ongoing trials in patients with relapsing–remitting and secondary progressive disease. Recently released reports from an interim analysis suggest that interferon (IFN)β-1b may significantly alter disability progression over a period of 2–3 years.[24] This finding led to early termination of a large European study of this agent. The field anxiously awaits the publication of this peer-reviewed report. It is anticipated that this find-

ing may have a significant impact on the integrity of several ongoing trials and may influence the design of future trials in patients with secondary progressive disease. Phase 3 trials are nearing completion to determine whether interferon β-1a delays the onset of the second event in patients presenting with mono-symptomatic, isolated episodes of presumed inflammatory–demyelinating disease (e.g. does INFβ-1a delay the development of clinically definite MS?).

Have these agents been administered at the optimal dose? Is it possible that alternate routes of administration (whether intravenous, subcutaneous or oral)[25–27] might provide more efficacy and improved patient tolerance? Might these agents work synergistically in combination either with each other (e.g. IFN-β with glatiramer acetate)[28] or with other immuno-modulatory therapies (e.g. azathioprine or corticosteroids)?

The research community is now exploring the complexity of combination trials using partially effective agents. In designing a trial in which one agent is tested alone and in combination with a second 'partially effective' agent (e.g. agent A versus agent A + agent B), one agent is clearly the dominant drug. A design of this type requires co-operation from at least one pharmaceutical company, perhaps more. Safety issues are paramount in such trials, as demonstrated by the apparent worsening of the course of experimental allergic encephalomyelitis when glatiramer acetate and interferon-α are given together (J Wolinsky, personal communication).

ANTI-VIRAL DRUGS

The studies designed to determine whether anti-viral drugs may have a role in the treatment of MS patients are reviewed in Chapter 14. Recent attention has focused on the herpes virus group of pathogens (including human herpes virus 6) with studies of valacyclovir and acyclovir.[29] The possibility that other infectious agents (e.g. chlamydia) may be important either primarily or secondarily in this disease are being considered by others.[30]

EMERGING IMMUNOMODULATORY STRATEGIES

It is currently widely held that the immune system may be involved primarily (e.g. antigen-specific assault on oligodendroglial or myelin antigens) or secondarily (e.g. non-specific immune activation) in mediating the tissue injury in MS. Many clinicians are familiar with the major principles of immunology but admit difficulty in understanding the complexities of the immune response and are challenged to remain up to date with this rapidly changing field (see the superb reviews by Hohlfield[31] and Xiao and Link[32]).

Stated simply, it is likely that either a unique antigen or a common antigen (or group of antigens) somehow triggers an initial phase of immune activation within or adjacent to the central nervous system (CNS). Thereafter, a series of events leads to amplification of this primary immune response, and, over time, reactivation with recurrent or continuous immune-mediated damage to oligodendrocytes, myelin, and ultimately, axons and neurons. At the center of this immune response is the tri-molecular complex comprising the antigen-presenting cell (macrophage, monocyte, astrocyte, dendritic cell and others), antigen, and the T cell. Conceptually, there are important similarities in the recognition of antigen by T cells of differing classes (e.g. $CD4^+$ and $CD8^+$ T cells). Antigen is recognized in the context of major histocompatibility complex (MHC) antigens (class I for $CD8^+$ T cells and class II for $CD4^+$ T cells) that are expressed on the surface of antigen-presenting cells using either the CD4 or CD8 molecule on the T cell. Immediately after the antigen is bound by the T-cell receptor and the MHC molecules on the antigen-presenting cell, signal transduction is mediated by the CD3 molecule complexed to the T-cell receptor, and a series of co-stimulatory events occur.

CTLA, cytotoxic T lymphocyte-associated antigen

LFA, leucocyte function-associated antigen

VLA, very late antigen

ICAM, intercellular adhesion molecule

VCAM, vascular cell adhesion molecule

These events include molecular–ligand interactions (e.g. CD40–ligand on the T cell with the CD40 molecule on the antigen-presenting cell, CD28–CTLA-4 molecule on the T cell with the B7-1,2 molecule on the antigen-presenting cell) and interactions cytokines between cytokine receptors (e.g. involving interleukin (IL)-2). Cytokines are pleotropic, redundant, inducible peptides that are secreted by multiple cell types and that act through signal proteins. These peptides bind to high-affinity receptors on cell surfaces, which, on binding, activate secondary intracellular signaling and ultimately lead to T cell activation and differentiation. Co-stimulatory signals enhance the expression of adhesion molecules on T cells and antigen-presenting cells. There is then binding of adhesion molecules between the T cell and antigen-presenting cell (e.g., CD2, LFA-2, VLA-4 on the T cell with LFA-3, ICAM-1, -2, and VCAM on the antigen-presenting cell). These steps in T-cell activation are followed by a series of local immune amplification steps, which include intracellular signaling, cytokine production, T-cell and B-cell differentiation, and the initiation of a complex interaction of T cells, B cells, complement, antigen-presenting cells, and supporting glia.

There are enormous complexities in each stage of the immune response. One area that has drawn particular attention is the concept of 'immune deviation'. $CD4^+$ T-helper (Th) cells produce different cytokines depending on a number of factors that occur during the development of the Th cell. Th_0 cells may be induced to the Th_1 ('pro-inflammatory') lineage if the cytokines IL-12 and IFN-γ are present locally. Similarly, Th_0 cells may develop along the Th_2 ('anti-inflammatory') lineage in the presence of IL-4 and IL-10. In addition, the concentration of the relevant antigen adjacent to the Th_0 cell determines whether a Th_0 cell develops into a Th_1 cell or a Th_2 cell. High and low local concentrations of antigen promote the Th_2 lineage whereas an intermediate concentration leads to the preferential development of Th_1 cells. As indicated, Th_1 cells secrete 'pro-inflammatory' cytokines, including IFN-γ, tumor necrosis factor (TNF)-α, TNF-β, and IL-2. Th_2 cells secrete 'anti-inflammatory' cytokines, including interferon-β, transforming growth factor (TGF)-β, and IL-5, IL-6, IL-9, IL-10, and IL-13. This concept of 'pro-inflammatory' and 'anti-inflammatory' cytokines requires additional explanation, however. Although pro-inflammatory and anti-inflammatory cytokines may primarily up-regulate or down-regulate the immune response, these peptides may have entirely opposing effects depending on the doses and timing of their administration.[33,34]

A number of competing mechanisms may be involved in mediating the damage to myelin and oligodendrocytes. The pro-inflammatory cytokine products of Th_1 cells and macrophages (tumor necrosis factor-α, oxygen radicals, nitric oxide, proteases and others) may all damage myelin membranes. Antibodies secreted locally by B cells may activate complement, resulting in the formation of membrane-attack complexes that may injure oligodendrocytes and myelin membranes. The Fc component of IgG may non-specifically activate lymphocytes and antigen-presenting cells by binding with Fc cell surface receptors. Once activated, T cells migrate across the blood–brain barrier into the brain parenchyma. Adhesion molecules are instrumental in mediating the interaction of lymphocytes with other cells, including endothelial cells, facilitating migration.[35,36] White blood cells, macrophages, and eosinophils secrete endoproteinases (gelatinases, stromelysins, and collagenases), loosely termed matrix metalloproteinases (MMPs). MMPs facilitate inflammation and the formation of edema by digesting extracellular matrix and cleaving peptides from cell surfaces, leading to further immune activation and immune-mediated injury. Chemokines are chromo- attractant cytokines that enhance inflammatory cell migration by promoting a conformational change in endothelial adhesion molecules (e.g. integrins).

In the course of this inflammatory–demyelinating injury, parallel processes are initiated to facilitate repair and remyelination. The factors that determine the degree of remyelination in the adult CNS are now only partially understood.[37] Whereas inflammatory cytokines inhibit nerve condition,[38] resolution of edema is following by the restoration of conduction along central axons. Rearrangements of sodium channels have been demonstrated along demyelinated axons[39,40] and there is now abundant evidence for extensive, although incomplete, remyelination (seen in 40% of MS plaques in patients who have suffered from MS for less than 5 years).[41,42] Paradoxically, remyelination may be partly assisted by the degree of the local inflammatory response. This needs to be kept in mind in the planning of trials designed to reduce the degree of inflammation within the MS lesion.

The adult CNS has immature oligodendrocyte lineage cells, which have the capacity to divide, migrate, and differentiate. Conversely, mature postmitotic oligodendrocytes are unable to divide, differentiate, or remyelinate significantly. An increasingly long list of growth factors probably contributes significantly to the survival of CNS glia and the potential for the immature oligodendrocyte to undergo mitosis, migration, and differentiation. Platelet-derived growth factor (PDGF), neutrophin (NT)-3, insulin-like growth factor (IGF)-1,2 and glial growth factor (GGF)-2 are mitogenic for oligodendrocytes whereas basic fibroblast growth factor (bFGF), especially in the presence of PDGF, blocks differentiation and enhances migration of these immature oligodendrocytes. IGF-1, IL-6, leukemia inhibitory factor, NT-3, PDGF, and ciliary neurotrophic factor enhance oligodendroglial cell survival, permitting differentiation into the adult state. This, too, probably represents a gross over-simplification of the interaction of growth factors on the ontogeny of the immature oligodendrocyte lineage cell in the adult CNS. These growth factors may have opposing effects on CNS glial cells (e.g. they may induce oligodendroglial apoptosis) depending on the state of expression of cell surface receptors, the signals that are transduced by binding with these receptors, and the ability of these cells to enter the cell cycle.

Cytokines and anti-cytokine strategies

The opportunities for influencing the immune response in a favorable manner may be predicted from the simplified summary outlined above. The agents currently being considered for 'anti-cytokine' therapies in MS include the type 1 interferons (IFN-α and IFN-β), antagonists of TNF, 'anti-inflammatory' cytokines (e.g. IL-4, IL-10, and IL-13), inhibitors of 'pro-inflammatory' cytokines (IL-1 inhibitors and transforming growth factor-β), and chemokine antagonists.

Considerable attention has been focused on inhibiting the effects of TNF in patients with MS for several reasons. TNF-α stimulates IL-1 release, enhances the expression of adhesion molecules on endothelial cells (leading to further accumulation of antigen-presenting cells and lymphocytes in the CNS), enhances the production of reactive oxygen species and nitric oxide derivatives, and leads to activation and proliferation of T cells. TNF-α has been shown to mediate damage to oligodendrocytes and myelin membranes in vitro,[43] and it is expressed along with other 'pro-inflammatory' cytokines (IL-1, IFN-γ) in MS plaques.[44] Spontaneous CNS demyelination is seen in a transgenic mouse model in which TNF is over-expressed.[45] Currently available TNF-α antagonists are incompletely selective, however. TNF-α may be needed to fight infection and inhibit tumor growth. TNF-α antagonists may induce the formation of neutralizing antibodies and may prolong the half-life of TNF-α in vitro. Paradoxically, however, TNF is protective in TNF knock-out mice and may limit the extent and duration of clinical and pathological hallmarks of experimental allergic encephalomyelitis in mice that are deficient in TNF.[46] To date, TNF-α strategies have been largely unrewarding. The following human MS trials were either negative or, indeed, suggested possible worsening of the MS disease process: TNF-α receptor–IgG soluble dimer (Lenercept, Hoffman LaRoche: increased clinical relapse rate and MRI activity),[47] IgG1K neutralizing antibodies to TNF (cA2, Centocor), and pentoxifylline.

Immune deviation

Would it be advantageous to enhance Th$_2$ ('anti-inflammatory') cell predominance? Pentoxifylline[48] has been shown to reduce Th$_1$

and to increase Th$_2$ cytokine production and is being tested further. TGF-β, IL-10, and IL-4 (alone and combined with glucocorticoids) are all being considered for pilot studies in MS.

MMP inhibitors

Preliminary data suggests that D-penicillamine and hydroxamate may inhibit MMP activity and suppress experimental allergic encephalomyelitis. In experiments, IFN-β inhibits the secretion of gelatinase[49] and reduces white blood cell migration. MMP inhibitors are somewhat non-selective and have pleotrophic actions, however. Whether they may be used acutely or in the long term in MS is currently under investigation.

Trimolecular complex, co-stimulation, and adhesion molecule strategies

There is an ever-increasing list of therapeutic strategies to modulate each of these fundamentally important steps the early immune response. Some of the earliest approaches focused on monoclonal antibodies that bound MHC peptides on antigen-presenting cells. The MHC molecule, however, is much less variable than the other contributors to the trimolecular complex, and it is perhaps less attractive for further study. An MHC class II hypervariable peptide vaccine is currently being pioneered, however.

It has been demonstrated that it is possible to produce long-lasting depletion of CD4$^+$ T cell in relapsing–remitting MS by the administration of a chimeric monoclonal antibody (cM-T412) without, unfortunately, significantly influencing clinical or MRI indicators of MS disease activity.[51] Prolonged lymphopenia followed treatment with a humanized monoclonal antibody (CAMPATH-1H) against the CD52 cell surface antigen (pan-lymphocyte marker) with short-term clinical worsening (attributed to the physiological effects of released pro-inflammatory cytokines on central conduction).[38,52] This treatment approach resulted in an apparent 18-month reduction in clinical relapses and MRI activity, yet patients continued to deteriorate clinically. It is expected that there will be other trials using monoclonal antibodies directed against differentiation molecules expressed on the T cell, perhaps following work in other putative autoimmune diseases.[53]

The finding that the oral administration of antigen is followed by immune tolerance,[54] immune cell deletion, or immune deviation to a Th_2 'anti-inflammatory' profile led to the oral administration of myelin basic protein.[55] However, this study was recently reported as being negative in MS,[56,57] despite early successes administering cartilage-derived type 2 collagen to patients with active rheumatoid arthritis.[58]

There is considerable interest in the administration of peptides that differ from the parent molecule by as few as one or two amino acids. These altered peptide ligands bind to the trimolecular complex with a varying degree of affinity and they down-regulate the immune response, resulting in T-cell anergy and an anti-inflammatory cytokine profile (Th_2). Preliminary evidence in experimental allergic encephalomyelitis has led to the initiation of at least seven industry-funded trials in MS using altered peptide ligands.

The finding that a minority of MS patients use a restricted number of T-cell receptors to bind putative myelin antigens has led to a number of T cell vaccination strategies. In each of these, the goal is to target the putative antigen-specific, autoreactive T cell through the induction of anti-idiotypic T cells or neutralizing antibodies. Whole T cells[59] and T-cell receptor peptides have been used as the immunogen in these early T-cell vaccination trials. One approach has been to attempt to induce immune tolerance by the injection of T-cell receptor antigens (e.g. complementarity determining regions of the T-cell receptors $V\beta5.2$ and 6.1). These studies have shown some immunological evidence of immunosuppressive activity[60] but there have been no reports of definitive clinical benefit. Three T-cell receptor peptide trials are underway. Another trial is in progress using T-cell receptor antibodies, and three additional trials are investigating myelin basic protein-reactive T cell vaccination studies. In the future, it may be possible to administer

'naked' T-cell receptor deoxyribonucleic acid (DNA) in vectors ('naked DNA vaccine').

Each of the steps in T-cell co-stimulation and subsequent adhesion molecule binding are being targeted for immune manipulation in patients with presumed autoimmune disease, including MS. It has been shown that one can induce antigen-specific non-responsiveness (T cell anergy) by interfering with co-stimualtory signaling. Preliminary studies have shown that anti-B 7-1 reduces the pathology in experimental allergic encephalomyelitis, and administering a CTLA-4 immunoglobulin fusion protein may reduce the clinical severity of the encephalomyelitis and down-regulate Th_1 expression. CTLA-4 immunoglobulin administration enhances allograft tolerance when this is given with an anti-CD4 monoclonal antibody. Another potential target for immunomodulatory therapy would be the CD40–CD40 ligand interaction.[61] However, targeting each of the co-stimulatory sites has the potential to either suppress or enhance the immune response, since the balance between T-cell activation and down-regulation depends on the timing, local concentration, receptor binding, cytokine concentration and type of antigen-presenting cell (e.g. microglia, astrocytes) at the tissue level. The cell surface adhesion molecules involved in the circulation, homing and transendothelial migration of lymphocytes are generally up-regulated in MS. Monoclonal antibodies against VLA-4, ICAM-1, and LFA-1 have each shown some positive effect in the experimental allergic encephalomyelitis model. Trials are nearing completion in acutely relapsing MS patients using the antibodies that block the VLA-4 receptors on T cells and anti-α-4 integrin antibodies.[62] Chemokine-receptor blocking agents are being considered for testing in patients with relapsing MS.

BONE MARROW TRANSPLANTATION

A number of centers are exploring using allogeneic or autologous $CD34^+$ hematopoietic (progenitor) stem cell infusion following myeloablative therapy.[63–65] Hematopoietic stem cells proliferate and differentiate into red blood cells, platelets, neutrophils, lymphocytes, and macrophages but may not fully reconstitute the immune spectrum of T-cell reactivity. Recent work suggests that complete myeloablative therapy ('supralethal conditioning') may not be necessary for the success of bone marrow transplantation. Rather, the adequacy of T-cell replacement may be the major determining factor for the success of the graft, with transplanted T cells playing a role in removing any surviving immune reactive or malignant cells. Peripheral expansion of T cells that follows hematopoietic stem cell infusion does not completely reconstitute the total $CD4^+$ T cell number in adult patients, presumably due to incomplete thymopoiesis. Evidence suggests that thymic-independent pathways do not allow for complete reconstitution of immunocompetence following bone marrow transplantation. Autologous bone marrow transplantation is preferred, when possible, since this is not associated with graft-versus-host response, and the 100-day mortality is significantly less than that experienced after allogeneic transplantation (1–3% against 20%).

GENE THERAPY

Gene therapy is discussed in detail in Chapter 13. Simplistically, one could imagine a gene therapy strategy that targeted the target tissue (e.g. to induce the expression of immunoregulatory cytokines through gene therapy), a gene therapy that used T cells to deliver therapeutic transgene products such as IL-4 and -10, and a gene therapy that induced regeneration (e.g. progenitor oligodendrocytes and growth factors).[66]

REMYELINATION STRATEGIES

The approaches currently being considered to enhance CNS remyelination can be predicted from what is known about remyelination in the adult CNS (see above).[37] Clearly, it may be important to arrest CNS inflammation. It may be possible to implant oligodendrocyte precur-

sors using either cells or transformed cell lines. It may be possible to harvest oligodendrocyte precursors from the patients ('autotransplantation'), which could then be expanded in vitro with growth factors[67,68] and later implanted. Growth factors could be given either alone to enhance oligodendrocyte precursor migration or transplanted in conjunction with oligodendrocyte precursors.[69]

OTHER STRATEGIES

Investigators are considering dendritic cell vaccines,[70] therapies that would induce apoptosis in activated T cells,[71] and strategies that block the Fc receptor on immune cells to reduce the immune-activating effect of non-specific IgG binding to immune cells.[72] In addition, cathepsin B inhibitors may be used to block antigen presentation; vitamins A and D may induce suppressor cell activity;[73–76] and scavengers of oxygen radicals and peroxynitrite (such as uric acid[77]) may be worth pursuing.

MATHEMATICAL MODELING: POSSIBLE ALTERNATIVES TO RANDOMIZED CLINICAL TRIALS

MS remains a largely unpredictable disease. One wonders whether it might be possible to use readily identifiable clinical and MRI variables to predict clinical and MRI behavior in certain patient groups within acceptable confidence intervals. One approach would be to access the currently available natural history and randomized clinical trial databases worldwide to define 'expected' clinical and MRI behaviors. Once accomplished, it might be possible to model patient profiles mathematically within defined confidence intervals to calculate the sample size and duration of open-label, phase 1 clinical trials that would be needed to identify potentially promising (or futile) putative agents. Patients 'observed' behavior in the setting of these phase 1 trials would then be compared in these models to determine any potential 'hint of efficacy'.

The primary purpose of this approach would be to see whether such models could help recognize more efficiently which agents should be selected for phase 3 clinical trials. If successful, this approach could essentially eliminate the need for phase 2 trials in MS patients and thereby speed the time to ultimate drug approval and license. If this approach were successful, there would then be significantly increased options for the development of multiple, simultaneous, adequately powered, unblinded, phase 1 trials, which would lead to more rapid screening of potentially effective therapies for study in definitive phase 3 studies. Inherent in this approach is the need for each of these studies to be carefully monitored by unblinded safety committees empowered to stop such trials for safety or futility.

This 'radical' and currently purely theoretical approach has evolved from the multiple and ever-increasing complexities of designing randomized clinical trials in the era of partially effective therapies in a disease that remains largely unpredictable and chronic in its evolution. The incentive behind this effort is to initiate a paradigm shift towards more rapid recognition of candidate therapies that are of potential interest while eliminating as quickly as possible those that have little likelihood of success.

The recent successes in defining agents that favorably alter the natural history of MS has enhanced the sense of urgency in applying the knowledge that has evolved from immunology and neurobiology to the care of patients. However, this success has paradoxically complicated the design of future randomized clinical trials. There are now 'too many' potentially interesting treatment approaches to permit methodical study of each agent using conventional phase 1, 2, and 3 randomized clinical trial design. The challenge remains to define more reliable and efficient methods to choose which agent to test. These concerns need to be addressed while awaiting further unraveling of the essential mystery of the etiology of this illness—a step that presumably may pave the way for a more efficient search for a cure for MS.

REFERENCES

1. The IFNB Multiple Sclerosis Study Group. Interferon beta-1b is effective in relapsing–remitting multiple sclerosis. I. Clincial results of a multicenter, randomized, double-blind, placebo-controlled trial. *Neurology* 1993; **43**: 655–661.
2. Paty DW, Li DKB, The UBC MS/MRI Study Group, The IFNB Multiple Sclerosis Study Group. Interferon beta-1b is effective in relapsing–remitting sclerosis. II. MRI analysis results of a multicenter, randomized, double-blind, placebo-controlled trial. *Neurology* 1993; **43**: 662–667.
3. The IFNB Multiple Sclerosis Study Group, The University of British Columbia MS/MRI Analysis Group. Interferon β-1b in the treatment of MS: final outcome of the randomized controlled trial. *Neurology* 1995; **45**: 1277–1285.
4. Jacobs LD, Cookfair DL, Rudick RA et al. Intramuscular interferon beta-1a for disease progression in relapsing multiple sclerosis. The Multiple Sclerosis Collaborative Research Group (MSCRG). *Ann Neurol* 1996; **39**: 285–294.
5. Rudick R, Goodkin D, Jacobs L et al. Impact of interferon beta-1a on neurologic disability in relapsing multiple sclerosis. *Neurology* 1997; **49**: 358–363.
6. Johnson KP, Brooks BR, Cohen JA et al. Copolymer 1 reduces relapse rate and improves disability in relapsing–remitting multiple sclerosis: results of a phase III multicenter, double-blind placebo-controlled trial. The Copolymer 1 Multiple Sclerosis Study Group (see comments). *Neurology* 1995; **45**: 1268–1276.
7. Johnson K, Brooks B, Cohen J et al. Extended use of glatriamer acetate (Copaxone) is well tolerated and maintains its clinical effect on multiple sclerosis relapse rate and degree of disability. *Neurology* 1998; **50**: 701–708.
8. Fazekas F, Deisenhammer F, Strasser-Fuchs S et al. Randomised placebo-controlled trial of monthly intravenous immunoglobulin therapy in relapsing–remitting sclerosis. *Lancet* 1997; **349**: 589–593.
9. Noseworthy J. MS clinical trials: old and new challenges. *Semin Neurol* 1998; **18**: 377–388.
10. Freedman B. Equipoise and the ethics of clinical research. *N Engl J Med* 1987; **317**: 141–145.
11. Johnson N, Lilford RJ, Brazier W. At what level of collective equipoise does a clinical trial become ethical? *J Med Ethics* 1991; **17**: 30–34.
12. Miller DH, Albert PS, Barkhof F et al. Guidelines

for the use of magnetic resonance techniques in monitoring the treatment of multiple sclerosis. *Ann Neurol* 1996; **39**: 6–16.

13. Cook SD, Devereux C, Troiano R et al. Combination total lymphoid irradiation and low-dose corticosteroid therapy for progressive multiple sclerosis. *Acta Neurol Scand* 1995; **91**: 22–27.

14. Cook S, Devereux C, Troiano R et al. Modified total lymphoid irradiation and low dose corticosteroids in progressive multiple sclerosis. *J Neurol Sci* 1997; **152**: 172–181.

15. Sipe JC, Romine JS, Kozoil JA, McMillan R. Cladribine in treatment of chronic progressive multiple sclerosis. *Lancet* 1994; **344**: 9–13.

16. Sipe JC, Romine JS, Kozoil J et al. Cladribine improves relapsing-remitting MS: a double-blind, placebo-controlled study (abstract). *Neurology* 1997; **48**: A340.

17. Edan G, Miller D, Clanet M et al. Therapeutic effect of mitoxantrone combined with methylprednisolone in multiple sclerosis: a randomised multicenter study of active disease using MRI and clinical criteria. *J Neurol* 1997; **62**: 112–118.

18. Cavazzuti M, Merelli E, Tassone G et al. Lesion lead quantification in serial MR of early relapsing multiple sclerosis patients in azathioprine treatment. A retrospective study. *Eur Neurol* 1997; **38**: 284–290.

19. Palace J, Rothwell P. New treatments and azathioprine in mulitple sclerosis. *Lancet* 1997; **350**: 261.

20. Durelli L, Bongioanni MR, Cavallo R et al. Chronic systemic high-dose recombinant interferon alfa-2a reduces exacerbation rate, MRI signs of disease activity, and lymphocyte interferon gamma production in relapsing–remitting multiple sclerosis. *Neurology* 1994; **44**: 406–413.

21. Achiron A, Gabbay U, Gilad R et al. Intravenous immunoglobulin treatment in multiple sclerosis: effect on relapses. *Neurology* 1998; **50**: 398–402.

22. Sorensen P, Wanscher B, Jensen C et al. Intravenous immunoglobulin G reduces MRI activity in relapsing multiple sclerosis. *Neurology* 1998; **50**: 1273–1281.

23. Ebers G, Oger J, Li D et al. The multiple sclerosis PRISMS study: prevention of relapses and disability by interferon beta-1a subcutaneously in multiple sclerosis. *Neurology* 1997; **42**: A986.

24. Kappos L, Polman C, Pozzilli C et al. Interferon beta-1b delays progression of disability in secondary progressive multiple sclerosis: results of the European multicenter study. *J Neurol* 1998; **245**: A357.

25. Brod S. Gut response: therapy with ingested immunomodultory proteins. *Arch Neurol* 1997; **54**: 1300–1302.

26. Brod S, Herman R, Nelson L et al. Ingested IFN-alpha has biological effects in humans with relapsing–remitting multiple sclerosis. *Multiple Sclerosis* 1997; **3**: 1–7.

27. Soos J, Muftabe M, Subramaniam P et al. Oral feeding of interferon tau can prevent the acute and chronic relapsing forms of experimental allergic encephalomyelitis. *J Neuroimmunol* 1997; **75**: 43–50.

28. Lublin F, Reingold S. Combination therapy for treatment of multiple sclerosis. *Ann Neurology* 1998; **44**: 7–9.

29. Lycke J, Svennerholm B, Hjelmquist E et al. Acyclovir treatment of relapsing–remitting multiple sclerosis: a randomized, placebo-controlled, double-blind study. *J Neurol* 1996; **243**: 214–224.

30. Yao S, Sriram S, Mitchell W et al. CNS infection with *C. pneumoniae* in MS. *Neurology* 1998; **50**: A423.

31. Hohlfeld R. Biotechnological agents for the immunotherapy of multiple sclerosis, principles, problems and perspectives. *Brain* 1997; **120**: 865–916.

32. Xiao B, Link H. Immune regulation within the central nervous system. *J Neurol Sci* 1998; **157**: 1–12.

33. Romagnani S. The Th 1/Th 2 paradigm. *Immunol Today* 1997; **6**: 263–266.

34. Allen J, Maizels R. Th 1–Th 2: reliable paradigm or dangerous dogma? *Immunol Today* 1997; **8**: 387–391.

35. Springer T. Traffic signals for lymphocyte recirculation and leukocyte emigration: the multistep paradigm. *Cell* 1994; **76**: 301–314.

36. Butcher E, Picker L. Lymphocytes homing and homeostasis. *Science* 1996; **272**: 60–66.

37. Compston A. Remyelination in multiple sclerosis: a challenge for therapy. The 1996 European Charcot Foundation Lecture. *Multiple Sclerosis* 1997; **3**: 51–70.

38. Moreau T, Coles A, Wing M et al. transient increase in symptoms associated with cytokine release in patients with multiple sclerosis. *Brain* 1996; **119**: 225–237.

39. Foster R, Whalen C, Waxman S. Reorganization of the axon membrane in demyelinated peripheral nerve fibers: morphological evidence. *Science* 1980; **210**: 661–663.

40. Felts P, Baker T, Smith K. Conduction in segmentally demyelinated mamalian central axons. *J Neurosci* 1997; **17**: 7267–7277.

41. Prineas JW, Connell F. Remyelination in multiple sclerosis. *Ann Neurol* 1979; **5**: 22–31.

42. Prineas JW, Kwon EE, Goldenberg PZ et al. Multiple sclerosis. Oligodendrocyte proliferation and differentiation in fresh lesions. *Lab Invest* 1989; **61**: 489–503.

43. Selmaj KW, Raine CS. Tumor necrosis factor mediates myelin and oligodendrocyte damage in vitro. *Ann Neurol* 1988; **23**: 339–346.

44. Renno T, Krakowski M, Piccirillo C et al. TNF-alpha expression by resident microglia and infiltrating leukocytes in the central nervous system of mice with experimental allergic encephalomyelitis. Regulation by Th 1 cytokines. *J Immunol* 1995; **154**: 944–953.

45. Probert L, Akassoglou K, Pasparakis M et al. Spontaneous inflammatory demyelinating disease in transgenic mice showing central nervous system-specific expression of tumor necrosis factor alpha. *Proc Natl Acad Sci USA* 1995; **92**: 11294–11298.

46. Liu J, Marino M, Wong G et al. TNF is a potent anti-inflammatory cytokine in autoimmune-mediated demyelination. *Nat Med* 1998; **4**: 78–83.

47. Paty D, The Lenercept Multiple Sclerosis Group, The UBC MS/MRI Analysis Group. TNF neutralization induces an increase in relapses in patients with multiple sclerosis. *Can J Neurol Sci* 1998; **25** (Suppl 2): S31–S32.

48. Friedman J, Zabriskie J, Bourganskaia E. A pilot study of pentoxifylline in multple sclerosis. *Arch Neurol* 1996; **53**: 956–957.

49. Leppert D, Waubant E, Burk M et al. Interferon beta-1b inhibits gelatinase secretion and in vitro migration of human T cells: a possible mechanism for treatment efficacy in multiple sclerosis. *Ann Neurol* 1996; **40**: 846–852.

50. Steinman L, Rosenbaum J, Sriram S, McDevitt H. In vivo effects of antibodies to immune response gene products: prevention of experimental allergic encephalitis. *Proc Natl Acad Sci USA* 1981; **78**: 7111–7114.

51. van Oosten B, Lai M, Hodgkinson S et al. Treatment of multiple sclerosis with monoclonal anti-CD4 antibody cM-T412: results of a randomized, double-blind, placebo-controlled, MR-monitored phase II trial. *Neurology* 1997; **49**: 351–357.

52. Moreau T, Coles A, Wing M et al. CAMPATH-IH in multiple sclerosis. *Multiple Sclerosis* 1996; **1**: 357–365.

53. Lorenz HM, Kalden J. Biological agents in rheumatoid arthritis. Which ones could be used in combination? *Biopharmaceuticals* 1998; **9**: 303–324.

54. Liblau T, Tisch R, Bercovici N et al. Systemic antigen in the treatment of T-cell-mediated autoimmune diseases. *Immunol Today* 1997; **18**: 599–604.

55. Weiner HL, Friedman A, Miller A et al. Oral tolerance: immunologic mechanisms and treatment of animal and human organ-specific autoimmune disease by oral administration of autoantigens (review). *Annu Rev Immunol* 1994; **12**: 809–837.

56. Francis G, Evans A, Panitch H. Results of a phase III trial of oral myelin in relapsing–remitting multiple sclerosis. *Ann Neurol* 1997; **42**: A467.

57. Panitch H, Francis G, Toms G. Clinical results of a phase III trial of oral myelin in relapsing–remitting multiple sclerosis (abstract). *Ann Neurol* 1997; **42**: S459.

58. Barnett M, Kremer J, St Clair EW et al. Treatment of rheumatoid arthritis with oral type II collagen. Results of a multicenter, double-blind, placebo-controlled trial. *Arthritis Rheum* 1998; **41**: 290–297.

59. Medaer R, Stinissen P, Truyen L et al. Depletion of myelin-basic protein autoreactive T cells by T-cell vaccination: pilot trial in multiple sclerosis. *Lancet* 1995; **346**: 807–808.

60. Vandenbark A, Chou Y, Whitham R et al. Treatment of multiple sclerosis with T-cell receptor peptides: results of a double-blind pilot trial. *Nat Med* 1996; **2**: 1109–1115.

61. Gerritse K, Laman J, Noelle R et al. CD40–CD40 ligand interactions in experimental allergic encephalomyelitis and multiple sclerosis. *Proc Natl Acad Sci USA* 1996; **93**: 2499–2504.

62. Keszthelyi E, Karlik S, Hyduk S et al. Evidence for a prolonged role of alpha 4 integrin throughout active experimental allergic encephalomyelitis. *Neurology* 1996; **47**: 1053–1059.

63. Burt R, Burns W, Hess A. Bone marrow transplantation for multiple sclerosis. *Bone Marrow Transplant* 1995; **16**: 1–6.

64. Burt R. BMT for severe autoimmune diseases: an idea whose time has come. *Oncology* 1997; **11**: 1001–1017.

65. Burt R, Traynor A, Cohen B et al. T cell-depleted autologous hematopoietic stem cell transplantation for multiple sclerosis: report on the first three patients. *Bone Marrow Transplant* 1998; **21**: 537–541.

66. Mathisen P, Tuohy V. Gene therapy in the treatment of autoimmune disease. *Immunol Today* 1998; **19**: 103–105.

67. Yao DL, Liu X, Hudson LD, Webster HD. Insulin-like growth factor I treatment reduces demyelination and up-regulates gene expression of myelin-related proteins in experimental autoimmune encephalomyelitis. *Proc Natl Acad Sci USA* 1995; **92**: 6190–6194.

68. Liu X, Linnington C, Webster H et al. Insulin-like growth factor-1 treatment reduces immune cell responses in acute non-demyelinating experimental autoimmune encephalomyelitis. *J Neurosci Res* 1997; **47**: 531–538.

69. McMorris F, McKinnon R. Regulation of oligodendrocyte development and CNS myelination by growth factors: prospects for therapy of demyelinating disease. *Brain Pathol* 1996; **6**: 313–329.

70. Girolomoni G, Ricciardi-Castagnoli P. Dendritic cells hold promise for immunotherapy. *Immunol Today* 1996; **18**: 102–104.

71. Weishaupt A, Gold R, Gaupp S et al. Antigen therapy eliminates T cell inflammation by apoptosis: effective treatment of experimental autoimmune neuritis with recombinant myelin protein P2. *Proc Natl Acad Sci USA* 1997; **94**: 1338–1343.

72. Deo Y, Graxiano R, Repp R, Van de Winkel J. Clinical significance of IgG Fc receptors and FcyR-directed immunotherapies. *Immunol Today* 1997; **18**: 127–135.

73. Qu Z, Dayal A, Jensen M et al. All-trans retinoic acid potentiated the ability of interferon beta-1b to augment suppressor cell function in multiple sclerosis. *Arch Neurol* 1998; **55**: 315–321.

74. Branisteanu D, Mathieu C, Casteels K et al. combination of vitamin D analogues and immunosuppressants. *Clin Immunother* 1996; **6**: 465–478.

75. Cantorna M, Hayes C, De Luca H. 1,25-Dihydroxyvitamin D3 reversibly blocks the progression of relapsing encephalomyelitis, a model of multiple sclerosis. *Proc Natl Acad Sci USA* 1996; **93**: 7861–7864.

76. Hayes C, Cantorna M, De Luca H. Vitamin D and multiple sclerosis. *Proc Soc Exp Biol Med* 1997; **216**: 21–27.

77. Hooper D, Spitsin S, Kean R et al. Uric acid, a natural scavenger of peroxynitrite, in experimental allergic encephalomyelitis and multiple sclerosis. *Proc Natl Acad Sci USA* 1998; **95**: 675–690.

13

Gene therapy: a possible future option for multiple sclerosis

Gianvito Martino, Roberto Furlan, Pietro L Poliani, Alessandra Bergami, Gaetano Desina, Giancarlo Comi and Peggy Marconi

INTRODUCTION

Multiple sclerosis (MS) is an immune-mediated demyelinating disease of the central nervous system (CNS) of unknown etiology.[1] The pathological hallmark of the disease is the presence within the CNS of inflammatory infiltrates containing few autoreactive T cells and a multitude of pathogenic non-specific lymphocytes[2] determining the typical patchy CNS demyelination, ranging from demyelination with preservation of oligodendrocytes to complete oligodendrocyte loss and severe glial scarring. In most instances, however, oligodendrocytes or their precursors are morphologically preserved in demyelinating plaques and remain capable of differentiating and remyelinating.[3] It is currently believed that CNS antigen-specific T cells provide the organ specificity of the pathogenic process and regulate the recirculation within the CNS of non-antigen-specific lymphomononuclear cells, which in turn act as effector cells by directly destroying oligodendrocytes, by releasing myelinotoxic substances, or both.

Studies performed on transgenic animals affected by experimental autoimmune encephalomyelitis (EAE), the animal model for MS, have confirmed that peripheral polyclonal expansion of lymphocytes driven by non-specific stimuli along with T cells specific for myelin antigens is actually required to attain CNS perivascular infiltration and demyelination.[4,5] A successful therapeutic approach to immune-mediated demyelinating disorders should be therefore based on the inhibition of activation of antigen-specific and non-antigen-specific immune cells or on the rescue of surviving oligodendrocytes within demyelinating plaques. However, the mechanisms underlying antigen-specific and non-antigen-specific T-cell activation as well as those underlying demyelinating and remyelinating events in the CNS of MS patients are still partially unknown. Thus, current therapies aimed at inhibiting the pathogenic process in MS are mainly based on non-specific immunomodulating treatments (e.g. immunosuppressive drugs, corticosteroids, high-dose gammaglobulins, total lymphoid irradiation), which are hampered by heavy side effects and poor clinical efficacy.[6]

GENE THERAPY IN THE CNS

Gene therapy, originally considered only as a strategy for replacing non-functioning genes in patients with inherited monozygotic recessive disorders,[7] now has a wider range of potentially useful therapeutic applications, from in situ

Table 13.1 Methodologies for delivering genes into somatic cells.

Experimental system	Methodology
Naked DNA	Plasmids
	Oligonucleotides
Physical methods	Microinjection
	Electroporation
	Gene gun
Viral vectors	Retrovirus
	Adenovirus
	Adeno-associated virus
	Herpes simplex virus
	Lentivirus
	Vaccinia virus
Lipofection	Liposomes
	Cationic lipids
	Liposome and protein specific complexes
Protein–DNA complexes	DNA–lactoferrin
	DNA–transferrin
	DNA–polylysine
	DNA–asialoglycoprotein
	DNA–viral capsid
New 'organs'	Microcapsules, macrocapsules

replacing of non-functioning genes to delivery of immunomodulatory genes.

Several gene delivery approaches are currently available (*Table 13.1*):

(a) physicochemical techniques, including deoxyribonucleic acid (DNA) transfection with current methods of calcium phosphate, cationic lipids or direct injection of naked DNA,[8] microinjection, ballistic guns delivering gold-coated DNA particles, complexed DNA as liposomes[9] or polylisine complexes;[10]

(b) implantation of non-autologous tissues: the recombinant gene products are derived from genetically modified cell lines using microcapsule or macrocapsule technology;[11] this technology has targeted neurological diseases mainly by direct implantation of encapsulated transformed cells into the brain where is necessary to deliver the therapeutic products;[12]

(c) biological vectors, an approach that is based on the development of viral vectors and that takes advantage of the properties of viruses as evolutionary gene transfer agents (viruses are essentially parasites that survive using functions of the host cell; they employ either DNA or ribonucleic acid (RNA) as genetic material encoding virus-specific components).

VIRAL VECTORS FOR GENE TRANSFER

Given the complexity of the CNS, the limitations imposed by the blood–brain barrier and the need of methods to generate reagents rapidly in order to deliver gene products in situ have led to the development and use of viral vectors that, at present, are the vehicles of choice for genetic manipulation of the adult CNS.[13] The characteristics of the viral vectors used so far for gene therapy protocols are briefly summarized here.

Retroviral vectors are the most extensively used viral vectors in gene therapy approaches[14] because of their capacity to integrate in the host chromosomal DNA and to sustain expression of the transgene.[15] Retroviruses are single-stranded RNA viruses encoding a RNA-dependent DNA polymerase (reverse transcriptase). The genome is 9 kb long and contains two long terminal repeats. Prototype retroviral vectors derived from oncoretroviruses, such as the Moloney leukaemia virus, are limited in their potential targets since they are able to integrate their genome only into replicating cells.[16,17] Ex vivo protocols for gene therapy applications using retroviruses are therefore necessary.

Recently, viral vectors obtained from human lentiviruses, such as human immunodeficiency virus (HIV), have been obtained and used. Lentiviral vectors have been deleted of env, vif, vpr, vpu and nef genes, which are involved in the virulence of the virus.[18] These vectors are able to infect non-dividing cells and they offer some hope for overcoming the limitation of the traditional retroviral vectors.[18] The actual limitation of HIV-derived vectors is the remote possibility of it recombining in vivo into a virulent form and causing the acquired immunodeficiency syndrome. Recently, retroviral vectors have been encased into heterologous vesicular stomatitis virus envelope. This new approach allows high titres of these pseudotype particles to be obtained and heterologous genes to be introduced into a broad range of tissues.[19]

Adenoviral vectors are derived from a subclass of adenovirus that is not associated with human malignancies. The genome of adenoviruses is a double-stranded DNA of approximately 36 kb with two short inverted terminal repeats.[20] The advantages of adenoviral-based vectors are their ability to infect a wide variety of cell types, including postmitotic cells[21] and

the high titres that can be obtained.[22] The major limitations of adenoviral vectors are the inability to sustain long-term expression of the transgene, the high immunogenicity of viral proteins and the virus toxicity at high doses.

Adeno-associated virus (AAV) vectors are based on a small non-pathogenic, helper-dependent human parvovirus. The AAV genome is a single-stranded DNA of approximately 5 kb with two inverted terminal repeats; it requires co-infection with helper virus (adenovirus or herpes simplex virus) to be able to replicate. AAV in helper-free conditions most frequently establishes a latent infection in vivo and in vitro by integration into the chromosomal cellular DNA.[13,23] AAV can infect various types of mammalian cells and can integrate in non-dividing cells. The advantage of this type of vector is that it can be easily manipulated; however, the amount of foreign DNA that can be inserted in AAV is limited.

Vaccinia virus (VV) vectors are derived from a member of the poxvirus family.[24] The VV genome is a double-stranded DNA of 185 kb; the virus replicates in the cytoplasm of mammalian cells. The large VV genome allows the virus to be used as a vector that contains multiple genes. It is able to infect replicating and non-replicating cells. Recombinant vectors are obtained by homologous recombination from the plasmid construct transfected into the VV-infected cells.[25] The major disadvantages of VV vectors are their high immunogenicity and cytotoxicity. The toxicity of these vectors can be reduced by using the canarypox strain or the fowlpox strain instead of the smallpox strain.

Vectors based on herpes simplex virus (HSV) have biological features allowing gene transfer into non-dividing cells. HSV, which has a double-stranded DNA genome of 152 kb, is a neurotropic human pathogen that persists in neurones in a latent state and carries a large number of viral genes, which can be replaced by foreign genes to create vectors for gene therapy.[26] Vectors based on HSV type 1 are currently:

(a) helper free amplicon;[27]
(b) replication defective viruses;[28]

(c) genetically engineered replication competent viruses with restricted host range.[29]

Plasmid-derived vector, named amplicon, consists in a plasmid that is capable of propagation and selection in bacteria and that contains an HSV origin of replication and a packaging signal that allows replication in eukaryotic cells. Concatamers of plasmids are packaged into viral particles using HSV helper virus.[30] The advantage of amplicons is that they can be easily engineered; however, the amount of foreign DNA that can be introduced in this vector is limited, as with AAV vectors.

Replication-defective or replication-restricted vectors derive from recombinants using herpesvirus as a backbone; alterations of the HSV-type 1 genome can be achieved in several ways.[31,32] Less pathogenic vectors have been created by disrupting and deleting genes that are involved in viral replication and genes that play an important role in viral cytotoxicity.[33,34] The replicative HSV-based vectors are attenuated viruses in which non-essential genes for viral replication in cultured cells are mutated or deleted. These viral mutants can only grow on genetically engineered cell lines that are able to complement their defects. These genes, which are considered 'accessory' genes for in vitro viral replication, may play an important role in the vital cycle of the virus in the natural host, and their removal may reduce neuropathogenicity.

In replication-defective HSV viral vectors, 'essential' genes for in vitro replication are mutated or deleted. The new generation of replication-defective vectors are deleted for all immediate early genes to reduce cytotoxicity,[35,36] to prevent early and late viral gene expression and to create space to introduce distinct and independently regulated expression cassettes for different transgenes.[37] The advantage of these vectors is that they can produce a therapeutic effect in some gene therapy applications requiring simultaneous and synergistic expression of multiple gene products. At present, the main limitation of HSV vectors is their inability to sustain long-term expression of the transgenes.

GENE THERAPY IN MS

Immunomodulatory cytokine-based approaches

The recent findings that non-antigen-specific priming can be induced in vitro in $CD4^+$ T cells by pro-inflammatory cytokines including tumour necrosis factor (TNF)-α, interleukin (IL)-2 and IL-6[38] and in $CD8^+$ T cells by interferons (IFNs)[39] and the in vivo evidence that these cytokines are crucial in the development of MS[40,41] suggest that pro-inflammatory cytokines not only participate in the process of myelin antigen-specific T-cell activation but may also represent the main mediators of the non-specific activation of T cells in the periphery (*Fig. 13.1*). Therefore, it is possible to consider pro-inflammatory cytokines as a possible therapeutic target in MS.

The rationale for deciding which cytokine to target when developing new therapies for MS derives from our understanding of the complex interplay between different cytokines during the immune-mediated processes that lead to demyelination. It is well documented that mouse and human $CD4^+$ (and $CD8^+$) T cells comprise three cell subsets that differ in their cytokine secretion profile. T helper 1 (Th$_1$) cells secrete IL-2, IFN-γ and TNF-β whereas T helper 2 (Th$_2$) produce IL-4, IL-5 and IL-10. Their precursor cells, named Th$_0$ cells, can produce IL-2, IFN-γ and IL-4 simultaneously.[42] The cytokines produced by each Th-cell subset are inhibitory for the opposite subset. Th$_2$ cytokines play a predominant role in immediate-type hypersensitivity; IL-4 is, in fact, the critical stimulus inducing a switch to IgE antibody production. Conversely, Th$_1$ cytokines play a role in the activation of macrophages (a pro-inflammatory function) to kill intracellular parasites, in delayed-type hypersensitivity and in IgG1 (human) or IgG2a (mouse) synthesis, but not IgE synthesis. Th$_1$ cytokines are also considered to be involved in the induction of experimental autoimmune diseases, as well as human organ-specific autoimmune diseases such as MS.[43]

Considering the central role played by Th$_1$ cytokines in experimental and human

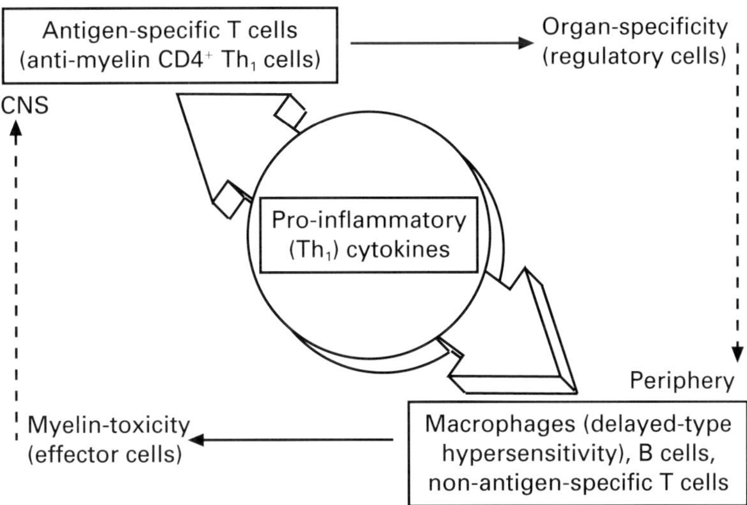

Figure 13.1 Pro-inflammatory cytokines (mainly TNF-α, TNF-β and IFN-γ) play a central role in the pathogenesis of MS. They are produced by non-antigen-specific mononuclear cells resident in the periphery, which act as myelinotoxic cells when recruited in the CNS by T cells that are specific for myelin components. These T cells in turn orchestrate this recruitment via up-regulation of the production of the same pro-inflammatory cytokines. Gene therapies aimed at turning off the pathogenic process occurring in MS should take into consideration that non-antigen-specific immune cells might be more successfully inhibited by anti-inflammatory agents, while CNS-resident myelin-specific T cells might be more susceptible to antigen-specific T-cell therapies (e.g. T-cell receptor vaccination, Th₁ versus Th₂ shift, oral tolerization).

demyelination and the close balance between Th₁ and Th₂ cytokines, cytokine-based therapies aimed at interfering with the pathogenic process leading to demyelination should encompass administration of Th₂ cytokines or cytokines able to down-regulate activity of Th₁ cytokines. This is supported by the recently reported clinical efficacy of systemic IFN-β in patients with relapsing–remitting MS,[44] which has been in part attributed to its anti-inflammatory effect.[45] However, although IFN-β improves the disease course in MS, it is only partly clinical effective. The route of administration of IFN-β in MS patients can in part explain the incomplete efficacy of this cytokine. Systemic administration of IFN-β causes the formation of anti-cytokine antibodies in 10–40% of patients after 1 year of treatment.[46] Moreover, IFN-β does not efficiently cross the blood–brain barrier and therefore does not accumulate within the CNS when administered systematically.[47]

Gene therapy in MS patients has never been attempted so far. However, some experiments, mainly based on cytokine gene delivery, have been performed in animals affected by EAE. Two different approaches have been followed so far:

(a) cytokine genes incorporated into viral vectors or plasmids have been injected into the peripheral circulation of the mice or directly into the circulating encephalitogenic T cells;

(b) cytokine genes have been directly transferred into the CNS.

When IL-4[48] or IL-10[49] genes have been transferred into autoreactive encephalitogenic T cells, EAE was ameliorated, while direct CNS injection of DNA-liposome constructs was successful in improving EAE when IL-4, TGF-β, IFN-β, p75TNF receptor but not IL-10 were delivered.[50] The results obtained in EAE mice after intravenous injection of VV-derived vectors showed that EAE was ameliorated when

IL-6, TNF-α, IL-1β, IL-2 and IL-10 (but not IL-4 or IFN-γ) were administered.[51] The results obtained so far are encouraging, although the gene therapy techniques used to deliver cytokine genes might have major limitations when transferred to humans. This is because autoreactive T cells can be easily isolated in the animal model of MS but not in humans, where the MS antigen is still unknown, and because DNA–liposomes as well as VV have limited transfection efficiency when introduced into post-mitotic cells such as those resident in the CNS. As mentioned above, VV is also toxic and immunogenic.

A cytokine gene delivery system has been established based on a vector derived from HSV type 1, named d120; this is an HSV type 1 virus (Kos) strain that contains a deletion in both copies of the immediate early Infected Cell Protein or ICP4 gene.[52] The recombinant vectors expressing cytokines were generated by Cre–lox recombination, with a plasmid containing the HSV type 1 strong immediate early promoter ICP4 driving murine IL-4 or murine IFN-γ. β-Galactosidase, as a reporter gene, was also contained in the vector under the human cytomegalovirus promoter.[53] In vitro and in vivo preliminary experiments have been performed in order to test vector infectivity and toxicity. In vitro, umbilical vein endothelial cells (UVEC) as well as cerebellar neurons have been shown to be infectable.[54] In vivo, the d120–IFNγ–βgal vector was injected intracisternally in BALB–c mice. The ability of in vivo infected CNS cells to produce the reporter gene was evaluated from day 1 to day 28 after injection and the CNS cells that have been permanently infected by the vector were traced histologically.[55] It was found that the d120 is easily transferred within the CNS, diffuses consistently in all ventricular spaces (*Fig. 13.2*), can efficiently infect the layer of ependymal cells surrounding the ventricles (see *Fig. 13.2*) and, within the CNS, redirects the cell machinery of the infected CNS cells to produce certain amounts of the cytokine in the cerebrospinal fluid of the mice until day 28 post-injection. The IL-4-containing vector was then used as a therapeutic gene in EAE mice; IL-4 was administered intracisternally in Biozzi–ABH mice immunized with myelin– oligodendrocyte glycoprotein 40–55 before and after the appearance of EAE signs. No adverse effects on the peripheral immune system or toxic reactions have been observed. A significant improvement in the clinical and pathological CNS features of EAE was observed with both therapeutic protocols.[55]

These preliminary results indicate that vectors derived from HSV type 1 (e.g. d120) can be easily transferred within the CNS with no major reactions of resident cells, whose machinery can be used to express the gene of interest (e.g. cytokine genes). Cytokine gene delivery in the CNS of EAE mice using vectors derived from HSV type 1 is feasible and can be considered as an alternative to the common procedures of systemic cytokine delivery. The main advantages of this system are:

(a) the availability of high cytokine levels in the CNS;
(b) the persistent therapeutic effect (i.e. for 4 weeks) after a single vector administration;
(c) the lack of interference of this procedure with the proper functioning of the peripheral immune system.

These results also suggest that research into applicability of vectors derived for HSV type 1 as alternative therapeutic approach to diseases confined to the CNS is auspicious and favourable. Moreover, the possibility of accommodating multiple genes within the vectors suggests that this procedure might be useful for targeting multiple cytokines with synergistic activity within the CNS.

Fostering remyelination with gene therapy: future applications

The two major target candidates of the immune-mediated pathogenic process in MS are oligodendrocytes and myelin components.[3] Conceivably, both targets are involved in the disease, which would explain clinical heterogeneity of MS by virtue of target heterogeneity. In the chronic form of MS, oligodendrocytes seem to represent the primary target of the pathological process and are almost completely

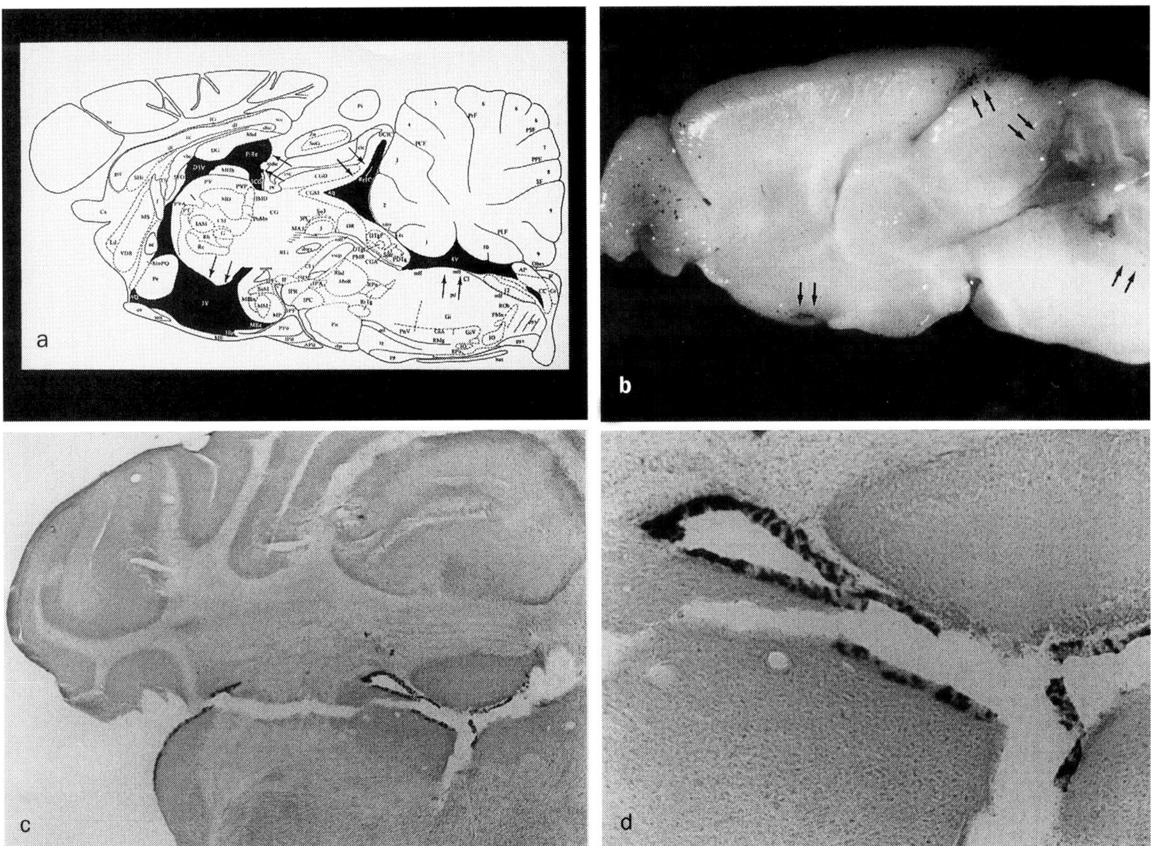

Figure 13.2 Distribution in the CNS of the d120 vector after intracisternal injection. (a) The ventricular spaces in the mouse CNS. The dark spaces represent ventricles (arrows). (b) The macroscopic appearance of a mouse CNS injected with the vector and stained for β-Gal (the d120 vector used contains the reporter gene LacZ); blue spots (arrows) indicate the presence of the vector and are visible in all the ventricular spaces. (c), (d) The preferential localization of the vector after intracisternal injection; the ependymal cells surrounding the ventricles are stained with β-Gal, indicating presence of the vector.

lost in demyelinating areas, so that no spontaneous remyelination takes place. In contrast, in the acute relapsing–remitting form of the disease, the persistence of oligodendrocytes in the demyelinating areas in which remyelination takes place suggests that the primary targets in this form of MS are myelin components, such as myelin basic protein, proteolipid protein or others. This form of MS, which accounts for more than 80% of MS patients, might therefore benefit from therapies aimed at stimulating oligodendrocytes to remyelinate. For a long time it was believed that repair of myelin

sheaths does not occur in MS. However, more recently a detailed analysis of MS pathology has provided evidence of extensive remyelination.[56,57] Remyelination is prominent during the early stage of disease evolution and apparently depends on the availability of oligodendrocytes or their progenitor cells within the lesions.[58,59] In the late, chronic stage of MS, repair of myelin is sparse and, if present at all, restricted to a small rim at the plaque edges. It is as yet unclear which cells in the CNS accomplish remyelination. The cells should be partly recruited from oligodendrocytes that have survived the acute phase of demyelination.[60] However, recent experimental data suggest that mature, terminally differentiated oligodendrocytes are incapable of synthesizing new myelin.[61] In contrast, in most experimental situations, remyelinating cells are derived from the pool of undifferentiated glial precursor cells, which are present even in the adult CNS tissue and can also be found in low numbers in demyelinated MS plaques. Thus, it is suggested that the failure of myelin repair in late chronic MS lesions is due to a depletion of this progenitor cell pool, which is likely to occur in areas of repeated demyelinating episodes.[56,61,62] On the other hand, some oligodendrocyte progenitor cells can be found even in old demyelinated scars of MS patients.

All these findings suggest that myelin repair in MS lesions could be therapeutically approached either by enhancing the transcription of genes that are involved in the maturation of myelin-forming cells or by introducing growth factors into the pathological tissue that prevent destruction of oligodendrocytes and stimulate undifferentiated glial precursor cells to divide, differentiate and remyelinate axons. The use of growth factors in humans should, however, take into consideration that growth factors may drive terminally differentiated mature oligodendrocytes into apoptosis[63] and that rescue of oligodendrocytes or their progenitor cells in demyelinating conditions depends on the mechanisms of myelin injury. Nevertheless, a gene therapy safety study using a growth factor named ciliary neurotrophic factor (CNTF) has already been performed in humans affected by amyotrophic lateral sclerosis, a neurodegenerative disease of the motor neurones.[66] This study showed that introduction of heterologous genes coding for CNTF into the cerebrospinal fluid using encapsulated genetically modified CNTF-producing myoblasts is feasible and non-toxic. Moreover, experiments aimed at delivering genes coding for other neurotrophic factors have been also performed in non-human primates affected by an experimental model of Parkinson's disease in which therapeutic effects have been observed without any side effects related to the procedure or to the

vector toxicity.[67] The authors have recently found that the introduction of vectors derived from HSV type 1 coding for basic fibroblast growth factor into mouse cerebrospinal fluid after the onset of myelin–oligodendrocyte glycoprotein 35–55-EAE induced by myelin–oligodendrocyte glycoprotein 35–55 is feasible and non-toxic. Tuohy and co-workers (personal communication) have showed that plasmid–DNA constructs coding for platelet-derived growth factor A (PDGF-A) and inserted into myelin-specific T cells improve EAE. Taken together, these studies, although preliminary, indicate that delivery of neurotrophic factor genes into the CNS can be approached using gene therapy systems without overt undesirable toxic effects.

CONCLUSION

MS is a heterogeneous disease in which different pathological mechanisms may operate to sustain the different clinicopathological forms of the disease. A successful therapeutic approach in MS should therefore be based on several strategies to be used in the different clinical and pathological conditions (*Fig. 13.3*). Since MS is characterized in its initial phase mainly by a prominent inflammatory process sustained by activated T cells (arising from the periphery and reaching the CNS where they initiate and regulate the myelinotoxic effector processes) and in its late stage by ongoing demyelination and axonal loss in the absence of overt inflammation, the therapeutic strategies should be flexible enough to allow the delivery of different 'drugs' into the CNS in the different stages of the disease (e.g. immunomodulatory molecules blocking T-cell activation in the early stage of the disease and 'drugs' promoting maturation of oligodendrocyte precursors in the late stage of the disease). Gene therapy using viral vectors represents a promising MS 'drug' since it shows a wide range of therapeutic flexibility. Different vectors can be used to deliver the above mentioned 'drugs' into the CNS; these vectors guarantee the required flexibility since they might have different life spans, tissue tropism and infectivity rate.

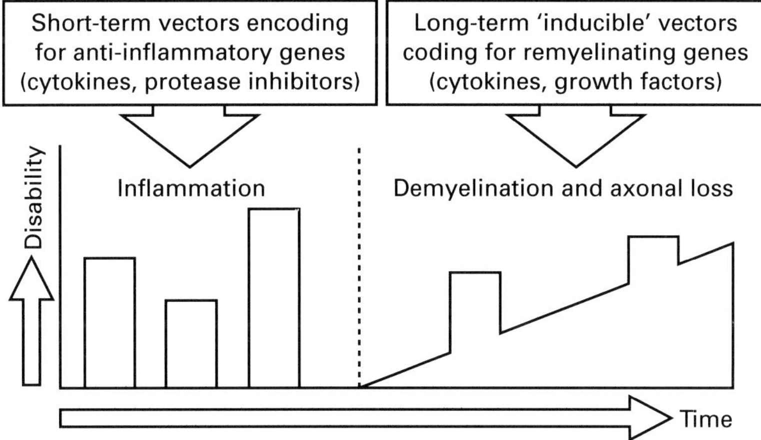

Figure 13.3 Synopsis of the possible future scenario of gene therapy approaches in MS. Considering the heterogeneity of the disease, the future gene therapy approaches should be flexible enough to be used in the different phases of the disease, as indicated. Short-term expressing vectors coding for anti-inflammatory cytokines might be useful in the early years of the disease, when the inflammatory component is prominent, while long-term expressing vectors coding for oligodendrocyte growth factors might be more useful in the late phases of the disease, when prominent demyelination and axonal loss take place.

The new improvements of viral vector technology should soon lead to:

(a) 'inducible' vectors in which the transcription of the heterologous gene contained in the vector can be exogenously induced or inhibited;

(b) chimeric vectors that are able to integrate into host DNA of post-mitotic cells (i.e. retrovirus combined with hepesvirus);

(c) short- and long-term expressing vectors

Moreover, the preliminary use of viral vectors in experimental animals and in humans have shown no toxic or undesirable effects for the host.

In conclusion, the establishment of new techniques to deliver therapeutic cytokine genes or genes promoting CNS remyelination should lead not only to better clarification of the role of each 'vector-injected' protein in the experimental demyelinating process but also to an understanding of whether gene therapy is a feasible and safe approach to treat demyelinating disorders in humans.

ACKNOWLEDGMENTS

This work has been supported in part by Telethon (Italy), Associazione Italiana della Sclerosi Multipla (AISM), and MURST. R Furlan is a recipient of a fellowship for TIGET (Italy).

REFERENCES

1. Martin R, McFarland HF, McFarlin DE. Immunological aspects of demyelinating diseases. *Annu Rev Immunol* 1992; **10**: 153–187.

2. Steinman L. A few autoreactive cells in an autoimmune infiltrate control a vast population of nonspecific cells: a tale of smart bombs and the infantry. *Proc Natl Acad Sci USA* 1996; **93**: 2253–2256.

3. Lucchinetti CF, Brück W, Rodriguez M, Lassmann H. Distinct patterns of multiple sclerosis pathology indicates heterogeneity on pathogenesis. *Brain Pathol* 1996; **6**: 269–274.

4. Goverman J, Woods A, Larson L et al. Transgenic mice that express a myelin basic protein-specific T cell receptor develop spontaneous

autoimmunity. *Cell* 1993; **72**: 551–560.

5. Lafaille JJ, Nagashima K, Katsuki M, Tonegawa S. High incidence of spontaneous autoimmune encephalomyelitis in immunodeficient anti-myelin basic protein T cell receptor transgenic mice. *Cell* 1994; **78**: 399–408.

6. Rudick RA, Cohen JA, Weinstock-Guttman B et al. Management of multiple sclerosis. *New Engl J Med* 1997; **337**: 1604–1611.

7. Ascadi G, Dickson G, Love DR et al. Human dystrophin expression in mdx mice after intra-muscular injection of DNA constructs. *Nature* 1991; **352**: 815–818.

8. Naldini L, Blomer U, Gallay P et al. In vivo gene delivery and stable transduction of nondividing cells by a lentiviral vector. *Science* 1996; **272**: 263–267.

9. Stewart MJ, Plautz GE, Del BL et al. Gene transfer in vivo with DNA-liposome complex: safety and acute toxicity in mice. *Hum Gene Ther* 1992; **3**: 267–275.

10. Wu GY, Wu CH. Receptor-mediated gene delivery and expression in vivo. *J Biol Chem* 1988; **263**: 14621–14624.

11. Sagot Y, Tan SA, Baetge E et al. Polymer encapsulated cell lines genetically engineered to release ciliary neurotrophic factor can slow down progressive motor neuronopathy in the mouse. *Eur J Neurosci* 1995; **7**: 1313–1322.

12. Aebischer P, Goddard M, Tresco PA. Cell encapsulation for the nervous system. In: Goosen MFA, ed. *Fundamentals of Animal Cell Encapsulation and Immobilization*. Boca Raton, Florida: CRC Press, 1993.

13. Kahn A, Haase G, Akli S, Guidotti JE. Gene therapy of neurological diseases. *C R Soc Biol (Paris)* 1996; **190**: 9–11.

14. Mulligan RC. The basic science of gene therapy. *Science* 1993; **260**: 926–932.

15. Scharfmann R, Axelrod JH, Verma IM. Long-term in vivo expression of retrovirus-mediated gene transfer in mouse fibroblast implants. *Proc Natl Acad Sci USA* 1991; **88**: 4626–4630.

16. Miller DG, Adams MA, Miller AD. Gene transfer by retrovirus vectors occurs only in cells that are actively x replicating at the time of infection. *Mol Cell Biol* 1990; **10**: 4239–4242.

17. Bandara G, Robbins PD, Georgescu HI et al. Gene transfer to synoviocytes: prospects for gene treatment of arthritis. *DNA Cell Biol* 1992; **11**: 227–231.

18. Naldini L, Blomer U, Gage FH et al. Efficient transfer, integration, and sustained long-term expression of the transgene in adult brains injected lentiviral vector. *Proc Natl Acad Sci USA* 1996; **93**: 11382–11388.

19. Schnell MJ, Buonocore L, Kretzschmar E et al. Foreign glycoproteins expressed from recombinant vesicular stomatitis viruses are incorporated efficiently into virus particles. *Proc Natl Acad Sci USA* 1996; **93**: 11359–11365.

20. Strauss SE. Adenovirus infection in humans. In: Ginsberg HS, ed. *The Adenoviruses*. New York: Plenum Press, 451–496.

21. Smith GM, Hale J, Pasnikowski EM et al. Astrocytes infected with replication-defective adenovirus containing a secreted form of CNTF or NT3 show enhanced support of neuronal populations in vitro. *Exp Neurol* 1996; **139**: 156–166.

22. Kozarsky KF, Wilson JM. Gene therapy: adenovirus vectors. *Curr Opin Genet Dev* 1993; **3**: 449–503.

23. Muzyczka N. Use of adeno-associated virus as a general transduction vector for mammalian cells. *Curr Top Microbiol Immunol* 1992; **158**: 97–123.

24. Moss B. Regulation of orthopoxvirus gene expression. *Curr Top Microbiol Immunol* 1990; **163**: 41–70.

25. Moss B, Flexner C. Vaccinia virus expression vectors. *Annu Rev Immunol* 1987; **5**: 305–324.

26. Glorioso JC, Goins WF, Meaney CA et al. Gene transfer to brain using herpes simplex virus vectors. *Ann Neurol* 1994; **35(suppl)**: S28–S34.

27. Lu B, Federoff HJ. Herpes simplex virus type 1 amplicon vectors with glucocorticoid-inducible gene expression. *Hum Gene Ther* 1995; **6**: 419–428.

28. Johnson PA, Friedman T. Replication-defective recombinant herpes simplex virus vectors. *Methods Cell Biol* 1994; **43**: 211–230.

29. Chou J, Roizman B. Herpes simplex virus 1 gamma(1)34.5 gene function, which blocks the host response to infection, maps in the homologous domain of the genes expressed during growth arrest and DNA damage. *Proc Natl Acad Sci USA* 1994; **91**: 5247–5251.

30. Spaete RR, Frankel N. The herpes simplex virus amplicon: analyses of cis-acting replication functions. *Proc Natl Acad Sci USA* 1985; **82**: 694–698.

31. Roizman B, Jenkins FJ. Genetic engineering on novel genome of large DNA viruses. *Science* 1985; **229**: 1208–1214.

32. Krisky DM, Marconi PC, Oligino T et al. Rapid method for construction of recombinant HSV-1 gene transfer vectors. *Gene Ther* 1997; **4**: 1120–1125.

33. Hay KA, Gaydos A, Tenser RB. The role of

herpes simplex thymidine kinase expression in neurovirulence and latency in newborn vs. adult mice. *J Neuroimmunol* 1995; **61**: 41–52.

34. Jonson PA, Miyanohara A, Levine F et al. Cytotoxicity of a replication-defective mutant of herpes simplex virus type 1. *J Virol* 1992; **66**: 2952–2965.

35. Wu N, Watkins SC, Schaffer PA, DeLuca NA. Prolonged gene expression and cell survival after infection by a herpes simplex virus mutant defective in the immediate-early genes encoding ICP4, ICP27, and ICP22. *J Virol* 1996; **70**: 6358–6369.

36. Marconi P, Krisky D, Oligino T et al. Replication-defective herpes simplex virus vectors for gene transfer in vivo. *Proc Natl Acad Sci USA* 1996; **93**: 11319–11320.

37. Krisky DM, Marconi PC, Oligino TJ et al. Development of herpes simplex virus replication defective multigene vectors for combination gene therapy applications. *Gene Ther* 1998; **5**: 1517–1530.

38. Unutmaz D, Pileri P, Abrignani S. Antigen-independent activation of naive and memory resting T cells by a cytokine combination. *J Exp Med* 1994; **180**: 1159–1164.

39. Tough DF, Borrow P, Sprent J. Induction of bystander T cell proliferation by viruses and type I interferon in vivo. *Science* 1996; **272**: 1947–1950.

40. Panitch HS, Hirsch RL, Haley AS, Johnson KP. Exacerbations of multiple sclerosis in patients treated with gamma interferon. *Lancet* 1987; **1**: 893–895.

41. Martino G, Grimaldi LME. The pathogenetic role of interferon-γ in multiple sclerosis. In: Reder A, ed. *Interferon Therapy of Multiple Sclerosis*. New York: Marcel Dekker, 1996, 193–214.

42. Abbas AK, Murphy KM, Sher A. Functional diversity of helper T lymphocytes. *Nature* 1996; **383**: 787–793.

43. Romagnani S, Human TH1 and TH2 subsets: doubt no more. *Immunol Today* 1991; **12**: 256–257.

44. The IFNB Multiple Sclerosis Study Group. Interferon beta-1b is effective in relapsing–remitting multiple sclerosis. I. Clinical results of a multicenter, randomized, double-blind, placebo-controlled trial. *Neurology* 1993; **43**: 655–661.

45. Weinstock-Guttman B, Ransohoff RM, Kinkel RP, Rudick RA. The interferons: biological effects, mechanisms of action, and use in multiple sclerosis. *Ann Neurol* 1995; **37**: 7–15.

46. The IFNB Multiple Sclerosis Study Group, The University of British Columbia MS/MRI Analysis Group. Neutralizing antibodies during treatment of multiple sclerosis with interferon beta-1b: experience during the first three years. *Neurology* 1996; **47**: 889–894.

47. Khan OA, Xia Q, Bever CT Jr et al. Interferon beta-1b serum levels in multiple sclerosis patients following subcutaneous administration. *Neurology* 1996; **46**: 1639–1643.

48. Shaw MK, Lorens JB, Dhawan A et al. Local delivery of interleukin 4 by retrovirus-transduced T lymphocytes ameliorates experimental autoimmune encephalomyelitis. Local delivery of interleukin 4 by retrovirus-transduced T lymphocytes ameliorates experimental autoimmune encephalomyelitis. *J Exp Med* 1997; **185**: 1711–1714.

49. Mathisen PM, Yu M, Johnson JM et al. Treatment of experimental autoimmune encephalomyelitis with genetically modified memory T cells. *J Exp Med* 1997; **186**: 159–164.

50. Croxford JL, Triantaphyllopoulos K, Podhajcer OL et al. Cytokine gene therapy in experimental allergic encephalomyelitis by injection of plasmid DNA–cationic liposome complex into the central nervous system. *J Immunol* 1997; **160**: 5181–5187.

51. Willenborg DO, Fordham SA, Cowden WB, Ramshaw IA. Cytokines and murine autoimmune encephalomyelitis: inhibition or enhancement of disease with antibodies to select cytokines, or by delivery of exogenous cytokines using a recombinant vaccinia virus system. *Scand J Immunol* 1995; **41**: 31–40.

52. DeLuca NA, McCarthy AM, Schaffer PA. Isolation and characterization of deletion mutants of herpes simplex virus type 1 in the gene encoding immediate-early regulatory protein ICP4. *J Virol* 1985; **56**: 558–570.

53. Kuklin NA, Daheshia M, Marconi PC et al. Modulation of mucosal and systemic immunity by enteric administration of non-replicating herpes simplex virus expressing cytokines. *Virology* 1998; **240**: 245–253.

54. Martino G, Furlan R, Galbiati F et al. A gene therapy approach to treat demyelinating diseases using non-replicative herpetic vectors engineered to produce cytokines. *Multiple Sclerosis* 1998; **4**: 222–227.

55. Furlan R, Poliani PL, Galbiati F et al. Central nervous system delivery of interleukin-4 by a non-replicative herpes simplex type 1 viral vector ameliorates autoimmune demyelination. *Hum*

Gene Ther 1998; **9**: 2605–2617.

56. Prineas JW, Barnard RO, Kwon EE et al. Multiple sclerosis: remyelination of nascent lesions. *Ann Neurol* 1993; **33**: 137–151.

57. Rodriguez M. Central nervous system demyelination and remyelination in multiple sclerosis and viral models of disease. *J Neuroimmunol* 1992; **40**: 255–263.

58. Brück W, Schmied M, Suchanek G et al. Oligodendrocytes in the early course of multiple sclerosis. *Ann Neurol* 1994; **35**: 65–73.

59. Ozawa K, Suchanek G, Breitschopf H et al. Patterns of oligodendroglia pathology in multiple sclerosis. *Brain* 1994; **117**: 1311–1322.

60. Targett MP, Sussman J, Scolding N et al. Failure to achieve remyelination of demyelinated rat axons following transplantation of glial cells obtained from the adult human brain. *Neuropath Appl Neurobiol* 1996; **22**: 199–206.

61. Ludwin SK. Central nervous system demyelination and remyelination in the mouse: an ultrastructural study of cuprizone toxicity. *Lab Invest* 1978; **39**: 597–612.

62. Linington C, Engelhardt B, Kapocs G, Lassmann H. Induction of persistently demyelinated lesions in the rat following the repeated adoptive transfer of encephalitogenic T cells and demyelinating antibody. *J Neuroimmunol* 1992; **40**: 219–224.

63. Muir DA, Compston DA. Growth factor stimulation triggers apoptotic cell death in mature oligodendrocytes. *J Neurosci Res* 1996; **44**: 1–11.

64. D'Souza S, Alinauskas KA, Antel JP. Ciliary neurotrophic factor selectively protects human oligodendrocytes from tumor necrosis factor-mediated injury. *J Neurosci Res* 1996; **43**: 289–298.

65. Scolding NJ, Compston DA. Growth factors fail to protect rat oligodendrocytes against humoral injury in vitro. *Neurosci Lett* 1995; **183**: 75–78.

66. Aebischer P, Schluep M, Deglon N et al. Intrathecal delivery of CNTF using encapsulated genetically modified xenogeneic cells in amyotrophic lateral sclerosis patients. *Nature Med* 1996; **2**: 696–699.

67. Zurn AD, Tseng J, Aebischer P. Treatment of Parkinson's disease. Symptomatic cell therapies: cells as biological minipumps. *Eur Neurol* 1996; **36**: 405–408.

14

The rationale for anti-viral therapies in multiple sclerosis

Oluf Andersen

GENETICS AND INFECTIONS ARE INTERACTIVE

Genetic factors are important in and probably necessary for the pathogenesis of multiple sclerosis (MS).[1,2] However, this in no way precludes important infectious factors. Both in a general sense and for issues that specifically concern MS, there is experimental and clinical evidence that individual susceptibility to viral infections may be influenced by polymorphic genes of the immune system:

(a) the Friend virus infection is an animal model for studying genetic resistance against a retroviral infection, and mice have a number of genes involved in immunological resistance to the Friend virus, including at least four major histocompatibility complex (MHC) genes and a further gene (Rfv-3);[3]

(b) susceptibility to demyelination induced by Theiler's virus, which is a model for MS, is genetically regulated, and multiple genes both in and outside the MHC seem to be involved;[4]

(c) the binding constant between the adenovirus E19 protein and different human leukocyte antigen (HLA) class I molecules differ up to 150-fold, suggesting that the pathogenicity of this virus, which has a possible relationship to MS bouts,[5] may be dependent on the HLA type of the infected person;[6]

(d) in a human twin study on hepatitis B virus carrier state, monozygotic twins were concordant for hepatitis B surface antigen carriage in 50% of cases, whereas only 20% of dizygotic twins and untwinned siblings were concordant;[7]

(e) specific HLA, tumor necrosis factor or chemokine genes were found to be associated with disease severity in widely different human infections caused by hepatitis B virus, hepatitis C virus, human immunodeficiency virus and malaria.[8,9]

Analogies between MS and other diseases reported as to provide clues on genetics and immunology often reveal dependency on infections as well. As discussed in other chapters in this book, experimental autoimmune encephalomyelitis, when elicited by particular myelin antigens, produces neuropathology similar to MS. Some experimental viral infections, including the disease elicited by Theiler's virus, also produces cellular pathology similar to that seen in MS.[4] Additional experimental studies have shown that a number of viral infections may interfere with and facilitate experimental autoimmune encephalomyelitis.[10] Deviating from the course of some experimental diseases, human MS disease seems to evolve slowly and subclinically for several years before clinical onset, as judged from cases in which the cerebrospinal fluid (CSF) has been investigated before onset.[11] Even genetically determined autoimmune diseases may be influenced by the environment. Diabetes mellitus is supposed to have an aetiology similar to that of MS. A survey of colonies of mice with non-obese diabetes (NOD) throughout the world revealed that there is a wide range in the frequency of diabetes in various NOD mouse colonies from the same ancestors, with an overall reciprocal relationship between the incidence of diabetes and the level of infection within the colony.[12] In a large prospective study, islet cell antibodies were assayed in schoolchildren and correlated to the later risk of insulin-dependent diabetes. Islet cell antibodies predicted insulin-dependent diabetes mellitus as powerfully in unrelated school-age children as in first-degree relatives.

The interaction between genetics and infections is a framework that fits with the reports of differences in the HLA types associated with MS in different parts of the world. It is well established that HLA-DR2 is associated with the highest relative risk factor known for MS (by a factor of 3–4), at least in northern Europe and North America. However, HLA-DR4 has been reported as prevailing or being important in some other areas, such as Sardinia[13] and Turkey,[14] and in Japanese patients with 'Western'-type MS without oligoclonal bands.[15]

THE HYPOTHESIS THAT MS IS CAUSED BY A SELF-REPLICATING VIRAL INFECTION IN THE CENTRAL NERVOUS SYSTEM IS LARGELY DISCOUNTED

Historically, a number of virus isolations have allegedly been achieved in MS patients but never confirmed, and negative reports include polymerase chain reaction (PCR) studies on MS autopsy material concerning candidate childhood diseases.[16] Because the first reports of human T-cell leukemia virus (HTLV)-1 as a candidate virus for MS[17,18] were followed by negative reports,[19,20] some researchers suggested that another human retrovirus could be a candidate agent. After the human spumaretrovirus (HSRV) and its ribonucleic acid sequence was characterized,[21] the author investigated plasma and CSF cell cultures obtained by PCR and liquid hybridization from patients with relapsing–remitting MS in exacerbation. These materials were negative for HTLV-1 and HTLV-2 and HSRV. Reverse transcriptase assays on the supernatant were also negative.[22] Furthermore, a group analysis of 60 patients with relapsing–remitting MS showed no difference between MS and healthy controls in reactivity against a recombinant HSRV envelope antigen. Antibody reactivity against the HSRV antigen in blood and CSF from seven patients was examined every 4 months for 2 years. There was no significant change, either during latent periods or relapses.[23] Recently, an extensive brain autopsy material was examined with PCR (using reverse transcriptase) for enteroviruses and cardioviruses (a group of viruses, including Theiter's virus, used in experimental MS models), as well as specimens from 25 MS patients, all of which were negative.[24] PCR studies in MS autopsy material were also essentially negative for coronavirus (Dessau R, dissertation, University of Copenhagen, 1997). Human herpes (HHV)-6 deoxyribonucleic acid (DNA) was reported to be present in active MS plaques but also in controls and was therefore considered to be commensal in the human brain. However, it was reported to have a specific nuclear localization in MS oligodendrocytes,[25] but this finding and the later report of HHV-6 DNA in serum samples from MS patients[26] seem to be unconfirmed. A direct causal role of self-replicating infection in the central nervous system in MS has largely been discounted.

EVIDENCE THAT A HISTORY OF PREVIOUS ACUTE INFECTIONS DIFFERS BETWEEN MS PATIENTS AND CONTROLS

Although data used in epidemiological studies, such as disease prevalences, are innately unprecise, the extensiveness of these data in MS should partially compensate for this. Several studies agree that both genetic and exogenous factors may contribute to the global distribution of MS. Some migration studies indicate that migration early in life tends to produce the MS risk of the new environment, whereas persons migrating in their teenage years tend to retain the risk of the area that they have migrated from. However, the precise age limits for this environmental influence on subsequent individual MS risk have not been settled. Data from north–south migration in the USA suggest that the age frame when the new environment may still influence the subsequent MS risk extends up to 20 years,[27] not far from the stage of manifest MS where a relationship exists between common infections and relapses. Several studies performed in high-risk areas indicate that the risk for later development of MS increases if the childhood diseases occur at a later age.[28] Although neurotropism of childhood diseases generally increases with age, there is no generally accepted explanation to the effect of age on subsequent MS risk; however, the potential neurotropism of most childhood diseases may be important. In a prospective study on uncomplicated measles infection, there was a CSF pleocytosis in 30% of cases.[29]

There is an individual relationship between infectious mononucleosis and subsequent MS; this may also be an effect of a relatively late infection, since infectious mononucleosis is indicative of a late (teenage) infection with Epstein–Barr virus (EBV). The first indication of this relationship came from a case–control study.[30] The author cross-matched his MS register with the diagnosis register of the Department of Infectious Disease in Göteborg. There was a three-fold increase in the risk of contracting MS after infectious mononucleosis. The latency was, on average, 12 years.[31] This three-fold surplus risk was confirmed in a larger study, using the central Danish MS and Epstein–Barr virus (EBV) registers.[32] A further study confirmed this general risk, with a teenage subgroup having an eight-fold surplus risk.[33]

EVIDENCE THAT COMMON VIRAL INFECTIONS TRIGGER RELAPSES IN MANIFEST MS

Six studies have indicated that relapses in established MS cases are triggered by systemic viral infections (*Table 14.1*), although they have not provided an unanimous answer about the agent responsible. In some of the studies, there is an overall relationship between infection and relapse, with more infections in cases with more relapses, but these studies were also evaluated with better temporal resolution. An 'at-risk' period was defined in relation to the day of onset of a common viral infection (usually an upper respiratory tract infection (URTI), but sometimes a gastrointestinal infection), usually including the period from 1 week before to 3 weeks after the infection. At-risk periods including 2 weeks before and 5 weeks after the day of onset day of the UTRI or only 2 weeks after the day of onset were also used. The remaining observation time is the 'not-at-risk' period. In principle, the at-risk period is a statistical parameter that should be conceived as the time interval when the immune defence against the infection sets the stage for the immune attack that elicits the bout of MS. Thus, the at-risk period encompasses the mean latency period between onset of the URTI onset and the onset of the MS relapse. The relative risk of relapse after an URTI is calculated from the ratio between the frequency of MS relapses during at-risk and the not-at-risk periods.

In the first-study, the authors tested 243 sera from 34 patients. The sera were obtained at intervals of 6–8 weeks, not in relationship to upper respiratory tract infections (URTI). They performed analysis of antibodies to mumps virus, adenovirus, respiratory syncytial virus (RSV), herpes simplex virus (HSV) and measles virus. Only a few significant changes in titre were found: three related to herpes simplex virus, three related to RSV, and one to heterophile antibodies, mostly unrelated to bouts. No relationship was found between MS activity and vaccinations to influenza, polio or measles. This prospective study introduced the at-risk

Table 14.1 Viral infections and MS relapses. Four prospective studies on the temporal relationship between URTI and MS relapses. There is on the average 2–3 times increased risk of an MS relapse in the at-risk period encompassing the onset of an URTI.

Reference	At-risk/not-at-risk relapse rates
Sibley et al 1985[35]	0.64/0.23 (p < 0.001)
Andersen et al 1993[5]	1.7/1.29 (p = 0.048)
Panitch 1994[37]	2.92/1.16 (p < 0.001)
Edwards et al 1998[38]	3.3/1.6 (p = 0.004)

and not-at-risk statistics using a 4-weeks at-risk period during 461 patient–months. Of 82 infections, 33 were associated with an exacerbation. Gastrointestinal symptoms were manifest in 27% of infections associated with an MS exacerbation, but only in 6% of infections without such association. The periannual distribution of URTI showed a bi-modal peak, in April and August.[34] In a subsequent prospective study by the same group, a 7-week at-risk period was used, from 2 weeks before to 5 weeks after the onset of the common infection. Common viral infections (including colds, 'flu', enteric infections and herpes) were significantly less frequent in MS patients than in controls. There was a linear drop with advancing disability, which could suggest an effect of isolation, but the frequency of common infections was also significantly lower in the MS patient group with expanded disability status scale (EDSS) between 0 and 2. A questionnaire was sent each month to 170 patients, who were examined neurologically every 3 months. The exacerbation rate per year was 0.23 in the not-at-risk periods and 0.64 in the at-risk periods. There was also a significant correlation, seen also in the mildly disabled patients, between infection and bout frequency. The mean delay in the onset of relapse after the onset of infection was 10 days. No relationship was found between urinary tract infections which are generally bacterial, and MS relapses.[35] In another study, a

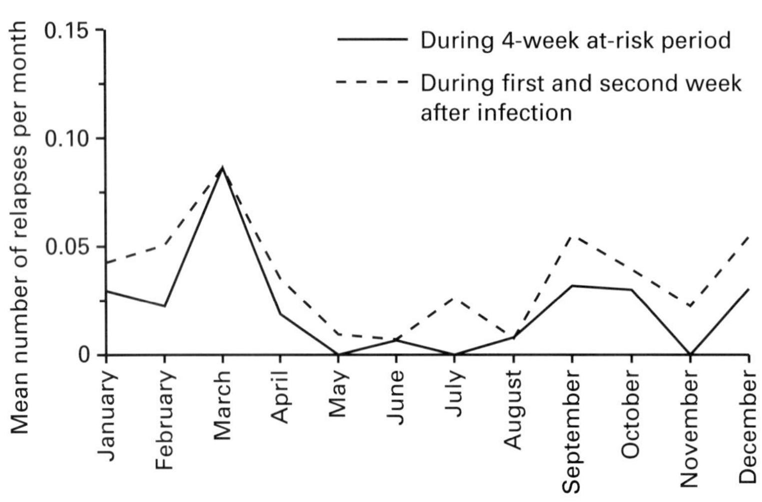

Figure 14.1 Number of at-risk relapses per month using 4- and 2-week at-risk periods, showing a winter maximum. Reproduced, with permission of the publishers, from Andersen et al 1993.[5]

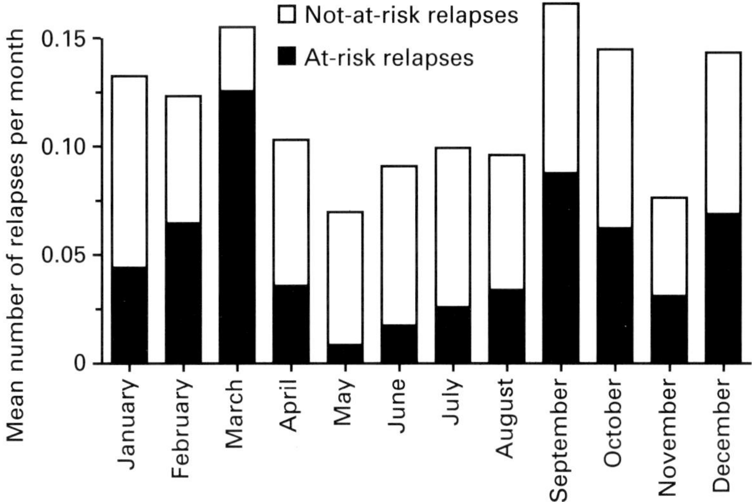

Figure 14.2 Not-at-risk and at-risk relapses per month using 7-week at-risk periods from a prospective seroepidemiological study in relapsing–remitting MS. There is a statistically significant periannual variation of the at-risk bouts but no statistically significant periannual variation of the not-at-risk bouts. Reproduced, with permission of the publishers, from Andersen et al 1993.[5]

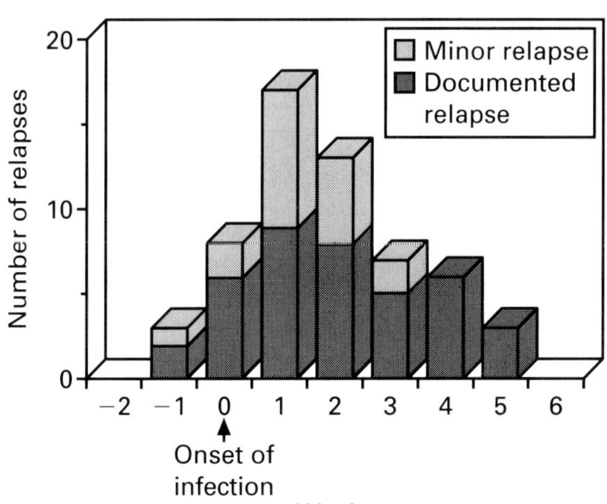

Figure 14.3 The relapse risk was at a maximum 2 weeks after the onset of the URTI in patients in an interferon-β trial. Reproduced, with permission of the publishers, from Panitch 1994.[37]

MS relapses with a significant relationship for the 4-weeks at-risk period and a tendency for the 7-week at-risk period. There was a significant periannual variation in at-risk MS relapses, but no significant periannual variation of the not-at-risk MS relapses (*Figs. 14.1* and *14.2*). The serological data suggested that there was a significant risk for an adenovirus infection to be followed by an at-risk relapse, but no significant relationship between influenza virus infection and relapses. For the other serologies tested (parainfluenza, RSV and mycoplasma) there were not enough at-risk bouts for conclusive statistics. The inference from this data set is that adenovirus has (or at least belongs to a group of viruses that has) a relationship with MS relapses, but that influenza virus does not (*Tables 14.2* and *14.3*).[5] The serological method used (complement fixation) did not allow any differentiation between new adenovirus infections and reactivations. Adenovirus establishes long or latent infections in the human host; 30% of healthy adults excrete adenovirus in the faeces, the virus probably originates from lymphoid tissues in Peyer's patches.[39]

three-fold higher relapse rate was reported in months where an URTI occurred.[36]

A prospective study performed in Göteborg confirmed the relationship between URTI and

In a subsequent study[37] there was a similar relationship between season and URTI, with a winter

Table 14.2 Statistics on the occurrence of a subsequent MS relapse after an adenovirus infection, showing a significant association. Data from a prospective seroepidemiological study in relapsing–remitting MS. Reproduced, with permission of the publishers, from Andersen et al 1993.[5]

	Yes	No	Total	Two-tailed P
Infections with major relapses	7	8	15	
Infections without relapses	0	23	23	0.001
Total	7	31	38	

Yes: significant increase in adenovirus titer in convalescent serum;
No: no significant increase in adenovirus titer in convalescent serum

Table 14.3 Statistics on the occurrence of a subsequent MS relapse after an influenza A infection, showing absence of association. Reproduced, with permission of the publishers, from Andersen et al 1993.[5]

	Yes	No	Total	Two-tailed P
Infections with major relapses	0	15	15	
Infections without relapses	5	18	23	0.134 (not significant)
Total	5	33	38	

Yes: significant increase in influenza A titer in convalescent serum;
No: no significant increase in influenza A titer in convalescent serum

peak, but there was no such periannual variation in MS relapse frequency. Since this study was part of an interferon-β (Betaseron®) trial, this finding gives rise to the interesting possibility that interferon-β weakens the relationship between URTI and MS relapses. The annual MS relapse rate was 2.92 in the at-risk periods and 1.16 per year in the not-at-risk periods, again showing a significant relationship between infections and MS relapses (*Fig. 14.3*). Antibodies against EBV (EBV-VCA antibodies) increased with attacks, but this was felt to be due to non-specific activation of the immune system. Titres against HSV type 1, HSV type 2, influenza viruses A and B, para-influenza virus and adenovirus fluctuated independently of MS attacks. Interferon-β did not prevent URTI, but it did seem to prevent some of the URTIs from triggering attacks.

A recent study[38] confirmed a two-fold increase in exacerbations during at-risk periods. Eight of 64 clinical URTIs were accompanied by a rise in antibodies. When at-risk periods were redefined by positive serology, they were associated with a 3.4-fold increase in MS relapse frequency. Magnetic resonance imaging showed a mean of/scan 1.125 lesions during the at-risk period compared with 0.69 during the not-at-risk period, which was not a significant result. Only eight instances of positive serology were found, without any consistent pattern. This was felt to support that several viruses may be implicated.

These studies were fairly consistent in showing an increased risk of MS relapse immediately after common viral infections. Why then does the serological part of the studies provide vague and divergent results? The choice of serological methods may influence the results. Complement fixation methods were generally used, and these are insensitive. Moreover, genetic variability may contribute to regional differences. One further reason may be that the specimens for serology were usually obtained at pre-set regular intervals. In the Göteborg study,[5] the time of obtaining blood specimens for serology was determined by the time of infections (as acute and convalescence specimens). Patients were instructed to come to the clinic for venepuncture immediately when the signs of a cold appeared.

MS MAY BE RELATED TO UNUSUAL VARIANTS OF COMMON VIRUSES

The authors isolated an HSV type 1 from the CSF of a patient during an acute myelopathy, which turned out to be the first bout of clinically definite MS; there was later secondary progression. This virus was unusual: it had, compared to other HSV type 1, a low neurovirulence and a high immunogenicity, and it produced few lesions in three different types of cell cultures (neuroblastoma, monkey kidney and fibroblasts).[40,41] Its DNA sequence was that of an HSV type 1, but mutations were detected in the immunoevasion region of an envelope glycoprotein. Adding to the complexity, a human host may exert selection pressure on the viral strains that are chronically infecting the host.

SYSTEMIC INFECTIONS HAVE THE CAPACITY TO TRIGGER LOCAL INFLAMMATION FROM LOCAL CNS IMMUNOLOGICAL MEMORY

One hypothesis is that MS depends on a local memory of previous infections that is activated later when the appropriate systemic infection occurs; at that time, specific, activated T cells crossing the blood–brain barrier find the local expression of the previous infection. Three types of experiments show that such basic mechanisms exist.

(a) Heat-killed bacillus Calmette–Guérin injected into the brain becomes sequestered for months in phagocytes behind the blood–brain barrier and is undetected by the immune system. However, independent peripheral sensitization of the immune system to the ballicus results in the induction of focal chronic lesions. Between 8 and 14 days after the subcutaneous challenge there was a conspicuous cellular infiltration at the site of the Calmette–Guérin deposits, consisting mostly of lymphocytes and macrophages. Dendritic cells were seen in close contact with lymphocytes. Between 2 and 3 months after the subcutaneous challenges, there was a lower number of cells and signs of demyelination.[42]

(b) Human adenovirus vectors were deleted in the E1 (early 1) region, which makes them replication-deficient, and were injected into the caudate nucleus of rats. After 2 months, expression of protein from the vector was still evident and histology revealed little inflammation. A subcutaneous injection of adenovirus vector at this time, however, led within 2 weeks to severe mononuclear inflammation, microglial activation, demyelination in the caudate and a decrease in protein expression from the vector. Cellular infiltration was also seen in brain areas containing neurones capable of retrograde transport of the adenovirus vector from the caudate, supporting the notion that viral antigens that are retrogradely transported by neurones can also be the target of a T-cell attack.[43]

(c) In an experimental model, the nucleoprotein or the glycoprotein of lymphocytic choriomeningitis virus (LCMV) was expressed in oligodendrocytes, the cell type that bears the brunt of the MS attack. When replicating LCMV was given parenterally to these experimental animals, LCMV-specific T lymphocytes were activated systemically, crossed the blood–brain barrier, entered the central nervous system and caused disease.[10,44]

Immunological memory may reside in memory T cells or, according to recent theories, as complexed epitopes (iccosomes) in dendritic cells, particularly in the case of B cells.[45] Dendritic cells, although of a different type, may migrate into perivascular sites of the CNS.[46] Although the origin of the oligoclonal IgG response in MS is outside the scope of this chapter, its origin may be mainly genetic or mainly infectious, and effects of a polyclonal stimulation is possible. However, some arguments can be raised against a polyclonal reaction. The reaction was reported to be specific against one but not another structural protein in the rubella virus.[47] Furthermore, two-dimensional electrophoresis shows a persistent homogeneous reaction in longitudinal studies.[48] The oligoclonal band pattern was reported to differ in IgG extract from two plaque regions in the same patient, which may be a suggestion that more than one antigen existed.[49]

Immunological memory may persist from inflammations during adolescence. A pleocytosis in the CSF accompanies 30% of cases of common measles, but the prospective study showed that this acute pleocytosis was transient.[29] The latency between infections that constitute a risk for MS and MS onset (12 years for infectious mononucleosis)[31] seems to be moderately long. Two hypotheses seem justified. First, a systemic infection with a virus presenting the same epitope elicits a focal CNS inflammation at the site of local immunological memory. Secondly, molecular mimicry with similar viruses or human epitopes occurs. The cross-reactivity of a known myelin basic protein-reactive T-cell clones derived from MS patients by peptides from HSV, EBV, adenovirus and influenza A virus was tested. Peptides were selected that would fit into the HLA groove. These viral peptides were able to activate T cells with an affinity at least as great as that of a known myelin basic protein peptide.[50]

However, a larger number of sequence homologies are found in databases than there are relevant diseases. Obviously, a DNA sequence homology is not sufficient to elicit disease. There are inhibitory principles in the immune system (e.g. the absence of co-stimulatory molecules, which induces antigen-specific anergy). There are preliminary data suggesting the such anergy or tolerance is to some degree broken in MS, since expression of co-stimulatory molecules seems to be increased in MS,[51] although this was not shown for specific antigens. Moreover, viruses may activate inflammation by eliciting the production of particular cytokines. One example is that rhinovirus induces IL-8.[52] A further possibility is that viral infections attack the endothelial cells and produce the lesion in the blood–brain barrier that is the first sign of the MS plaque.[53] The common denominator for this complex of theories is the insight that systemic infections in some circumstances have the capacity to break the immunological privilege of the CNS and elicit a local inflammation, provided there is, in some sense, a local immunological memory from previous infections.

ANTI-VIRAL DRUG TRIALS IN MS

Table 14.4 shows approved anti-viral drugs that are relevant for the theories mentioned in the previous section (they are not approved in all countries). Particularly non-toxic among them is acyclovir, a nucleoside analogue that is active against HSV infections; there have been only 100 serious adverse events reported after treating between 10 million and 15 million people. The study[54] was prompted by the intermittent time course and relative symmetry of MS lesions, reminiscent of the behaviour of HSV in several experimental models, including its axonal transport both in the peripheral nervous system and the CNS, which is sometimes symmetrical. Moreover, an unusual HSV was isolated from the CSF during an MS onset bout.[40] *Figure 14.4* shows the results of the Göteborg acyclovir trial in relapsing–remitting MS.[54] In all, 60 patients were divided into two parallel groups and treated for 2 years. A pharmacokinetic study showed a steady-state concentration of 3–4 µmol/l in serum and 1 µmol/l in the CSF, enough to inhibit the α-herpesviruses (HSV types 1 and 2 and varicella-zoster virus). The reduction in relapse frequency was one-third. This was close to significance when calculated according to the protocol. With additional calculations, using the patients as their own controls during the 2-year pre-study and 2-year

Table 14.4 Approved anti-viral drugs against herpesviruses and viral upper respiratory tract infections.

Drug	Viruses
Acyclovir	Herpes simplex virus, varicella-zoster virus
Valacyclovir	Herpes simplex virus
Cidofovir, ganciclovir	Cytomegalovirus
Other nucleoside analogues	Herpesviruses
Ribavirin	Respiratory syncytial virus (severe infections)
Amantadine, rimantidine	Influenza A virus

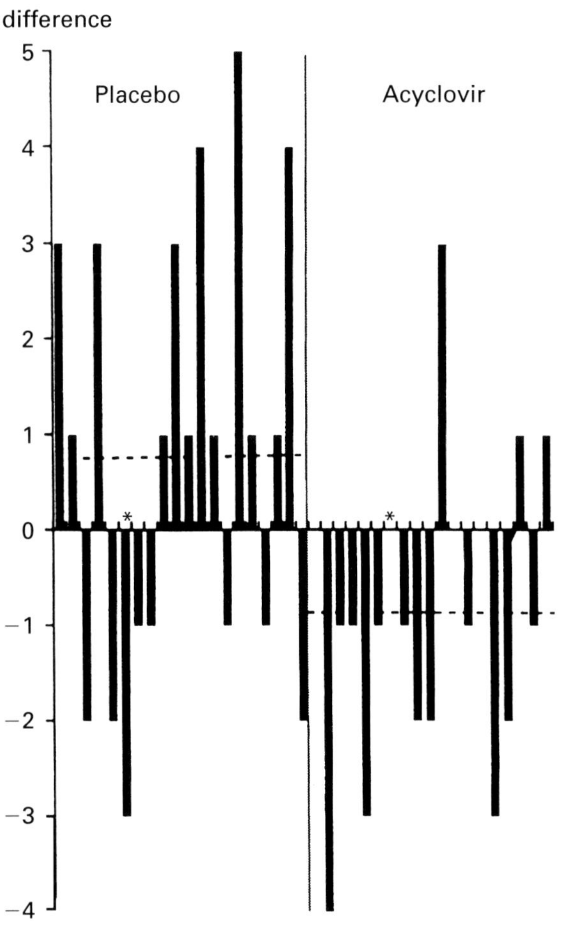

Figure 14.4 Exacerbation differences in MS patients between the two pre-study years and during the two-year trial. A subgroup of 20 placebo and 19 acyclovir patients, consisting of all patients with a duration of MS of at least 2 years before entry, was selected. Positive bars indicate increased and negative bars indicate reduced number of exacerbations. Dotted lines indicate mean exacerbation differences per 2 years. Patients whose disease course changed to progressive MS during the study are indicated by an asterisk. Reproduced, with permission of the publishers, from Lycke et al 1996.[54]

Table 14.5   Valacyclovir in multiple sclerosis. Design of a valacyclovir study.

75 clinically definite MS patients, randomized to oral valacyclovir 1000 mg tid or placebo

Two centres

MRI once a month; 1 month pre-study, 6 months intervention, 1 month post-study follow-up; quantitative neurology in months 1 and 7 and during relapses

Primary endpoint: cumulative number of active MRI lesions

Secondary endpoints: enhancing MRI lesions, EDSS and RFSS quantitative neurology and others

Clean file expected in 1999

EDSS: expanded disability status scale; RFSS: regional functional scoring system.

trial periods, the results were significant. However, there was no difference between groups in the deficit which increased gradually in both groups. After the encouraging results of this acyclovir trial, a two-centre study of 75 patients with relapsing–remitting MS was performed using the analogous drug valacyclovir, an acyclovir prodrug with a superior tissue concentration. The use of this prodrug gives a three-fold increase in CSF acyclovir concentrations (approximately 3 μmol/l, only approaching inhibitory levels for EBV in the CSF (6–7 μmol/l). However, the serum concentration is inhibitory for EBV replication, and according to the main theory presented in this chapter, the serum concentration may be more important than the CSF level. *Table 14.5* shows the design of the valacyclovir study, for which results are expected during 1999.

RATIONALE FOR FUTURE ANTI-VIRAL DRUG TREATMENTS IN MS

A number of viral infections are treated with interferons, e.g. interferon-α has been proposed as a treatment for rhinovirus. Are infections inhibited with interferon-β at the same time as MS is treated? The trials do not support that. Common infections have been found to be as frequent in the placebo-treated patients as in those receiving interferon-β.[55] However, the Betaseron® results support the notion that the infections do not elicit relapses during therapy with interferon-β.[37] A new development that

may be decisive is the capability of diagnosing almost all URTIs, with a diagnostic yield of 60–85%, using nasal washings and polymerase chain reaction.[56,57] The use of these methods during surveillance should enable us to diagnose almost all viral infections and so define the at-risk periods. And there are many emerging therapies for URTI, using principles such as nucleoside analogues, local interferons and vaccinations, as well as other, new principles.[58] For example, a new invention for the treatment of rhinovirus is stiffening of the pentamer channel; this inhibits the release of RNA from the rhinovirus particle. Clinical trials have been started.[59]

Thus, the possibility of diagnosing almost all URTIs by polymerase chain reaction and correlating them with MS activity, and of using new drugs that inhibit systemic viral infections that trigger MS relapses should be explored. There is a potential to influence a substantial part of all MS relapses.

REFERENCES

1. Sadovnick AD, Armstrong H, Rice GPA et al. A population-based study of multiple sclerosis in twins: Update. *Ann Neurol* 1993; **33**: 281–285.
2. Karpuj MV, Steinman L, Oksenberg JR. Multiple sclerosis: a polygenic disease involving epistatic interactions, germline rearrangements and environmental effects. *Neurogenetics* 1997; **1**: 21–28.
3. Hasenkrug KJ, Chesebro B. Immunity to retroviral infection: the Friend virus model. *Proc Natl Acad Sci USA* 1997; **94**: 7811–7816.

4. Dal Canto MC, Kim BS, Miller SD, Melvold RW. Theiler's murine encephalomyelitis virus (TMEV)-induced demyelination: a model for human multiple sclerosis. *Methods: Comparision to Methods Enzymol* 1996; **10**: 453–461.

5. Andersen O, Lygner PE, Bergström T et al. Viral infections trigger multiple sclerosis relapses: a prospective seroepidemiological study. *J Neurol* 1993; **240**: 417–422.

6. Beier DC, Cox JH, Vining DR et al. Association of human class I MHC alleles with the adenovirus E3/19K protein. *J Immunol* 1994; **152**: 3862–3872.

7. Lin TM, Chen CJ, Wu MM, Furthermore AA. Hepatitis B virus markers in Chinese twins. *Anticancer Res* 1989; **9**: 737–741.

8. Martin MP, Dean M, Smith MW et al. Genetic acceleration of AIDS progression by a promoter variant of CCR5. *Science* 1998; **282**: 1907–1911.

9. Thursz MR, Thomas HC. Host factors in chronic viral hepatitis. *Semin Liver Dis* 1997; **17**: 345–350.

10. von Herrath MG, Oldstone MB. Virus-induced autoimmune disease. *Curr Opin Immunol* 1996; **8**: 878–885.

11. Xu XH, Mcfarlin DE. Oligoclonal bands in CSF: twins with MS. *Neurology* 1984; **34**: 769–774.

12. Singh B, Prange S, Jevnikar AM. Protective and destructive effects of microbial infection in insulin-dependent diabetes mellitus. *Semin Immunol* 1998; **10**: 79–86.

13. Marrosu MG, Murru MR, Costa G et al. DRB1–DQA1–DQB1 loci and multiple sclerosis predisposition in the Sardinian population. *Hum Mol Genet* 1998; **7**: 1235–1237.

14. Saruhan-Direskeneli G, Esin S, Baykan-Kurt B et al. HLA-DR and -DQ associations with multiple sclerosis in Turkey. *Hum Immunol* 1997; **55**: 59–67.

15. Fukazawa T, Kikuchi S, Sasaki H et al. The significance of oligoclonal bands in multiple sclerosis in Japan: relevance of immunogenetic backgrounds. *J Neurol Sci* 1998; **158**: 209–214.

16. Godec MS, Asher DM, Murray RS et al. Absence of measles, mumps, and rubella viral genomic sequences from multiple sclerosis brain tissue by polymerase chain reaction. *Ann Neurol* 1992; **32**: 401–404.

17. Koprowski H, DeFreitas EC, Harper ME et al. Multiple sclerosis and human T-cell lymphotrophic retroviruses. *Nature* 1985; **318**: 154–160.

18. Reddy EP, Sandberg-Wollheim M, Mettus RV et al. Amplification and molecular cloning of HTLV-1 sequences from DNA of multiple sclerosis patients. *Science* 1989; **243**: 529–533.

19. Richardson JH, Wucherpfennig KW, Endo N et al. PCR analysis of DNA from multiple sclerosis patients for the presence of HTLV-1. *Science* 1989; **246**: 821–823.

20. Lycke J, Andersen O, Svennerholm B et al. Use of immunoreactive synthetic HTLV-1 peptides in search for antibody reactivity in multiple sclerosis. *Acta Neurol Scand* 1992; **85**: 44–45.

21. Flügel RM. Spumaviruses: a group of complex retroviruses. *J Acquir Immune Defic Syndr* 1991; **4**: 739–750.

22. Svenningsson A, Lycke J, Svennerholm B et al. No evidence for spumavirus or oncovirus infection in relapsing–remitting multiple sclerosis. *Ann Neurol* 1992; **32**: 711–714.

23. Lycke J, Svennerholm B, Svenningsson A et al. Human spumaretrovirus antibody reactivity in multiple sclerosis. *J Neurol* 1994; **241**: 204–209.

24. Dessau RB, Nielsen LP, Frederiksen JL. Absence of entero- and cardioviral RNA in multiple sclerosis brain tissue. *Acta Neurol Scand* 1997; **95**: 284–286.

25. Challoner PB, Smith KT, Parker JD et al. Plaque-associated expression of human herpesvirus 6 in multiple sclerosis. *Proc Natl Acad Sci USA* 1995; **92**: 7440–7444.

26. Soldan SS, Berti R, Salem N et al. Association of human herpes 6 (HHV-6) with multiple sclerosis: increased IgM response to HHV-6 early antigen and detection of serum HHV-6 DNA. *Nature Med* 1997; **3**: 1394–1397.

27. Detels R, Visscher B, Haile R et al. Multiple sclerosis and age at migration. *Am J Epidemiol* 1978; **108**: 386–393.

28. Bachmann S, Kesselring J. Multiple sclerosis and infectious childhood diseases. *Neuroepidemiology* 1998; **17**: 154–160.

29. Hänninen P, Arstila P, Lang H et al. Involvement of the central nervous system in acute, uncomplicated measles virus infection. *J Clin Microbiol* 1980; **11**: 610–613.

30. Operskalski EA, Visscher BR, Malmgren RM, Detels R. A case-control study of multiple sclerosis. *Neurology* 1989; **39**: 825–829.

31. Lindberg C, Andersen O, Vahlne A et al. Epidemiological investigation of the association between infectious mononucleosis and multiple sclerosis. *Neuroepidemiology* 1991; **10**: 62–65.

32. Haahr S, Koch-Henriksen N, Möller-Larsen A et al. Increased risk of multiple sclerosis after late Epstein–Barr virus infection: a historical

prospective study. *Multiple Sclerosis* 1995; **1**: 73–77.

33. Martyn CN, Cruddas M, Compston DAS. Symptomatic Epstein–Barr virus infection and multiple sclerosis. *J Neurol Neurosurg Psychiatry* 1993; **56**: 167–168.

34. Sibley WA, Foley JM. Infection and immunization in multiple sclerosis. *Ann N Y Acad Sci* 1965; **122**: 457–468.

35. Sibley WA, Bamford CR, Clark K. Clinical viral infections and multiple sclerosis. *Lancet* 1985; **1**: 1313–1315.

36. Narod S, Johnson-Lussenburg CM, Zheng Q et al. Clinical viral infections and multiple sclerosis. *Lancet* 1995; **ii**: 165–166.

37. Panitch HS. Influence of infection on exacerbations of multiple sclerosis. *Ann Neurol* 1994; **36**(suppl): S25–S28.

38. Edwards S, Zvartau M, Clarke H et al. Clinical relapses and disease activity on magnetic resonance imaging associated with viral upper respiratory tract infections in multiple sclerosis. *J Neurol Neurosurg Psychiatry* 1998; **64**: 736–741.

39. Allard A, Albinsson B, Wadell G. Detection of adenoviruses in stools from healthy persons and patients with diarhoea by two-step polymerase chain reaction. *J Med Virol* 1992; **37**: 149–157.

40. Bergström T, Andersen O, Vahlne A. Biological properties of a herpes simplex virus type 1 strain isolated from cerebrospinal fluid of an MS patient. In: Battaglia MA, Crimi G, eds. *An Update on Multiple Sclerosis*. Bologna: Monduzzi, 1988, 97–100.

41. Bergström T, Andersen O, Vahlne A. Isolation of herpes virus type 1 during first attack of multiple sclerosis. *Ann Neurol* 1989; 283–285.

42. Matyszak MK, Townsend MJ, Perry VH. Ultrastructural studies of an immune-mediated inflammatory response in the CNS parenchyma directed against a non-CNS antigen. *Neuroscience* 1997; **78**: 549–560.

43. Byrnes AP, MacLaren RE, Charlton HM. Immunological instability of persistent adenovirus vectors in the brain: peripheral exposure to vector leads to renewed inflammation, reduced gene expression, and demyelination. *J Neurosci* 1996; **16**: 3045–3055.

44. Selin LK, Nahill SR, Welsh RM. Cross-reactivities in memory CTL recognition of heterologous viruses. *J Exp Med* 1994; **179**: 1933–1943.

45. Tew JG, Wu J, Qin D et al. Follicular dendritic cells and presentation of antigen and costimulatory signals to B cells. *Immunol Rev* 1997; **156**: 39–52.

46. Matyszak MK, Perry VH. The potential role of dendritic cells in immune-mediated inflammatory diseases in the central nervous system. *Neuroscience* 1996; **74**: 599–608.

47. Nath A, Wolinsky JS. Antibody response to rubella virus structural proteins in multiple sclerosis. *Ann Neurol* 1990; **27**: 533–536.

48. Walsh MJ, Tourtellotte WW. Temporal invariance and clonal uniformity of brain and cerebrospinal IgG, IgA, and IgM in multiple sclerosis. *J Exp Med* 1986; **163**: 41–53.

49. Olsson T, Link H, Kostulas V, Henriksson KG. Direct tissue isoelectric focusing of nervous system and muscle sections for detection of IgG patterns. *Acta Neurol Scand* 1983; **67**: 202–209.

50. Wucherpfennig KW, Strominger JL. Molecular mimicry in T-cell mediated autoimmunity: viral peptides activate human T-cell clones specific for myelin basic protein. *Cell* 1995; **80**: 695–705.

51. Svenningsson A, Dotevall L, Stemme S, Andersen O. Increased expression of B7 costimulatory molecule in cerebrospinal fluid and blood of patients with multiple sclerosis. *J Neuroimmunol* 1997; **75**: 59–68.

52. Zhu Z, Tang W, Gwaltney JM Jr et al. Rhinovirus stimulation of interleukin-8 in vivo and in vitro: role of NF-kB. *Am J Physiol* 1997; **273**: L814–L824.

53. Allen I, Brankin B. Pathogenesis of multiple sclerosis—the immune diathesis and the role of viruses. *J Neuropathol Exp Neurol* 1993; **52**: 95–105.

54. Lycke J, Svennerholm B, Hjelmquist E et al. Acyclovir treatment of relapsing–remitting multiple sclerosis. A randomized, placebo-controlled, double-blind study. *J Neurol* 1996; **243**: 214–224.

55. PRISMS Study Group. Randomized double-blind placebo-controlled study of interferon beta-1a in relapsing–remitting multiple sclerosis. *Lancet* 1998; **352**: 1498–1504.

56. Mäkelä MJ, Puhakka T, Ruuskanen O et al. Viruses and bacteria in the etiology of the common cold. *J Clin Microbiol* 1998; **36**: 539–542.

57. Arruda E, Pitkaranta A, Witek TJJ, Doyle CA. Frequency and natural history of rhinovirus infections in adults during autumn. *J Clin Microbiol* 1997; **35**: 2864–2868.

58. Johnston SL. Problems and prospects of developing effective therapy for common cold viruses. *Trends Microbiol* 1997; **5**: 58–63.

59. Vaidehi N, Goddard WA. The pentamer channel stiffening model for drug action on human rhinovirus HRV-1A. *Proc Natl Acad Sci USA* 1997; **94**: 2466–2471.

PART V

Organization of multiple sclerosis care

15

Multiple Sclerosis Clinical Practice Guidelines

Michele Messmer Uccelli, Deborah M Miller and Steve Shindell

Clinical practice guidelines are a useful and important way of ensuring that people with a given condition receive consistently good and cost-effective care throughout all stages of the illness. People with multiple sclerosis (MS) come from all walks of life and live with a broad range of disabilities. Their care is provided by many types of health-care professionals in varied settings in many countries. The Multiple Sclerosis Council for Clinical Practice Guidelines is an international collaboration of 22 member organizations that develops guidelines for use with the MS population across the full range of patients, clinicians and settings. The Council, which was established in 1997 and has produced two guidelines to date, accepts the need for adaptability by implementing treatment recommendations that are based on the best available scientific evidence and systematically developed expert consensus. This chapter provides some historical background on guidelines in health care in general and for MS in particular as well as information on the structure of the Council and of its guideline development panels. The chapter also describes the guidelines that have been finished and those that are under development, and it presents a plan for international dissemination and assessment of the guidelines.

BACKGROUND

Professional organizations from all sectors of the health-care community have embraced the development, use and evaluation of practice guidelines with which they collate and evaluate empirical evidence and expert opinion. Generally, the goals of these practice guidelines are to reduce inappropriate care and improve patient outcomes, to reduce health care cost, to enhance quality assurance and to improve medical education. Their benefit is in documenting the advice of clinical experts, documenting clinical research and assessing the clinical significance of conflicting research findings.[1] There are many public and private health-care organizations involved in developing practice guidelines, and the scope of their topics and the development methodologies they use are diverse. The choices of topics and methods reflect the major practice concerns of each organization, the empirical evidence available on those topics and, just as importantly, the resources available to the organization for developing guidelines. Whenever possible, clinical practice guidelines are based on empirical evidence and, in these cases the recommendations are graded on the quality of evidence. Although the highest reliance is placed on empirical evidence, expert opinion remains an

Table 15.1 Organizations and representatives on the Multiple Sclerosis Council for Clinical Practice Guidelines.

Organization	Representative
American Academy of Neurology	Michael K Greenberg, MD
American Academy of Physical Medicine and Rehabilitation	George H Kraft, MD
American Congress of Rehabilitation Medicine	Doug Jeffrey, MD, PhD
American Neurological Association	Fred Lublin, MD
American Occupation Therapy Association	Lois F Cooperman, PhD, OTR/L
American Physical Therapy Association	Lucinda L Hugos, MS, PT
American Psychological Association	David C Mohr, PhD
American Society of Neuroradiology	Craig Bash, MD
American Society of Neurorehabilitation	Jack Burks, MD
American Speech–Language–Hearing Association	Pam Sorensen, MA, CCC-SLP
Association of American Psychiatrists	Ronald S Taylor, MD
Association of Rehabilitation Nurses	Ismari M Clesson, RN
Canadian Neurological Association	TJ Murray, MD
Consortium of Multiple Sclerosis Centers	Deborah M Miller, PhD
Eastern Paralyzed Veterans Association	Vivian Beyda, Dr PH
International Federation of Multiple Sclerosis Societies	Robert Herndon, MD
Kaiser–Permanente Health Maintenance Organization	Jay Rosenberg, MD
National Institute of Neurological Disorder and Stroke	Henry McFarland, MD
National Multiple Sclerosis Society	Nancy J Holland, Ed D
Paralyzed Veterans of America	Suzanne Diffley, RN
Rehabilitation in Multiple Sclerosis (RIMS)	Michele Messmer Uccelli, BA
US Department of Veterans' Affairs	John Booss, MD

integral part of guideline development 'because reliable scientific evidence is lacking for most clinical practices'.[2] Whether the process used to develop a guideline is more reliant on empirical evidence or on expert consensus, it is essential that it is explicitly reported.

Two separate organizational efforts stimulated the 1997 formation of The Multiple Sclerosis Council for Clinical Practice Guidelines. The first of these efforts was formalized in 1995 when the Consortium of Multiple Sclerosis Centers, the American Academy of Neurology and the National Multiple Sclerosis Society established the inter-organizational Collaborative Group for Multiple Sclerosis Management Strategies (CGMSMS). In that same year the CGMSMS formed a steering committee, which established criteria for topic selection and management strategy development and which convened management strategies development panels on two topics, fatigue and bladder dysfunction.

The second organizational effort was initiated by the Paralyzed Veterans of America (PVA) in order to better serve the approximately 30% of PVA members who experience MS, the PVA made a board-level decision in 1997 to commit resources for developing MS practice guidelines. This commitment paralleled the guideline support that the PVA had been providing to the spinal cord injury community since 1995 to the Consortium of Spinal Cord Medicine. By making these resources available, the PVA also ensured that its only influence on the recommendations generated through the MS guideline effort would be through its one voting member on the Council. In 1997 the two organizational efforts were integrated and the Multiple Sclerosis Council for Clinical Practice Guidelines was established. This merger allowed for the inclusion of a greater number of participating organizations and a more ambitious schedule for producing guidelines.

STRUCTURE OF THE COUNCIL

The Multiple Sclerosis Council for Clinical Practice Guidelines is made up of 22 representatives from key MS professional and consumer organizations. It is multidisciplinary and includes civilian and military representatives with experience in fee-for-service and managed care payment systems, as well as those with experience in academic, group and individual practice settings. These representatives and their organizations are listed in *Table 15.1*. Each member organization is responsible for providing the following:

1. Appointment of one member on the Council.
2. Recommendation of experts from their organization to participate in guideline development panels.
3. High level professional and technical peer review of materials associated with the guidelines development process.
4. Dissemination and application of guidelines through the organization's educational offerings.
5. Organizational endorsement of the completed practice guidelines and related products.

Each member of the Council participates in one of three advisory sub-committees.

Methodological and Scientific Review Advisory Subcommittee

This subcommittee:

(a) recommends methodological experts;
(b) recommends levels of evidence required for each type of recommendation; and
(c) recommends how to substantiate expert consensus given inadequate empirical evidence.

Topic Selection and Panel Recruitment Advisory Subcommittee

This subcommittee:

(a) establishes and oversees the process for guideline topic selection; and
(b) recommends guideline development panel chairs and members;
(c) assures that guideline development panels comply with timetable for completing recommendations.

Peer Review, Dissemination and Outcomes Evaluation Advisory Subcommittee

This subcommittee:

(a) establishes and oversees the process for peer review of draft guidelines;
(b) monitors the implementation and impact of guidelines; and
(c) monitors the need for review and update of guidelines.

Although the members of the Council, through these subcommittee activities, are responsible for overseeing the development of guidelines as well as for approving and disseminating the recommendations, members of the Council do not write the guidelines. Instead, they are written by Guideline Development Panels, which are multidisciplinary and are composed of people who are experts in the topic field. These experts include MS specialists from a variety of clinical and research backgrounds and, as warranted by the topic,

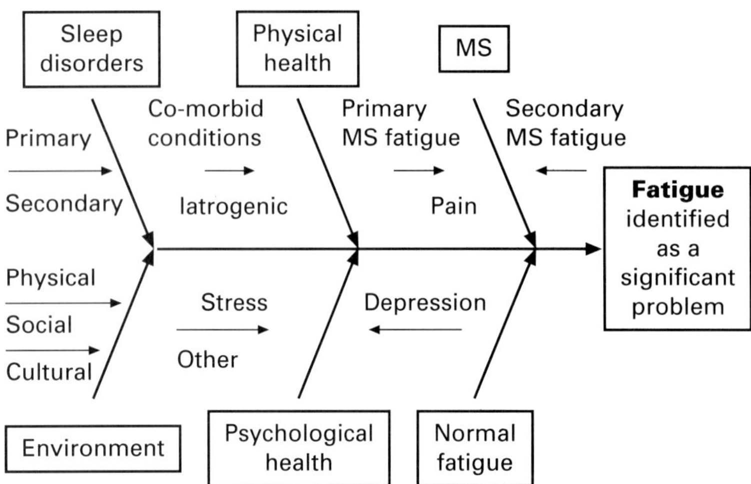

Figure 15.1 A potential cause and effect diagram for fatigue.

consumers and non-MS specialists such as epidemiologists, general practitioners or surgeons. Each development panel has a chairperson who is not a member of the Council and a liaison person who is a Council member. The chairperson leads the group in developing the recommendations while the liaison person ensures that the methods and timetable of the Council are maintained. The types of expertise needed for the guideline development panel is recommended by the Council. The chairperson and liaison person of each panel is responsible for recruiting the individual members of the panel, who are approved by the Council.

DEVELOPMENTAL PROCESS

Guideline Development Panels follow a process that integrates empirical evidence and expert opinion. The framework for a guideline is established when the development panel constructs a potential cause-and-effect diagram (*Fig. 15.1*). This allows the panel members to identify a comprehensive list of factors that can have either a positive or a negative impact on the target condition. This technique, taken from the Continuous Quality Improvement literature, helps the Guideline Development Panel to specify the scope of care that will be included

in the guideline and to indicate explicitly what will be excluded.

The next step in setting the framework is specifying the outcomes, both positive and negative, that are expected from the recommendations to be included in the guidelines. This specifying of expected outcomes is important for three reasons: first, it helps to direct the development panel in selecting the interventions included in the guidelines; secondly, it helps clinicians using the guidelines to assess the impact of treatment on individual patients; and thirdly it allows health researchers to evaluate the benefit of the guideline. The development panel next constructs a proto-algorithm of the treatment process that they believe, based on their expert opinion, will maximize the preferred outcomes and minimize negative ones (*Fig. 15.2*).

The literature review strategy is subsequently developed and documented by the Guideline Development Panel and by process methodologists with expertise in medical literature review, data extraction and data synthesis. Potentially relevant original research articles are collected through electronic search procedures, review of research and survey article bibliographies, and recommendations from experts in the field. Relevant original research articles are identified and levels of evidence are assigned. The levels of evidence and strength of

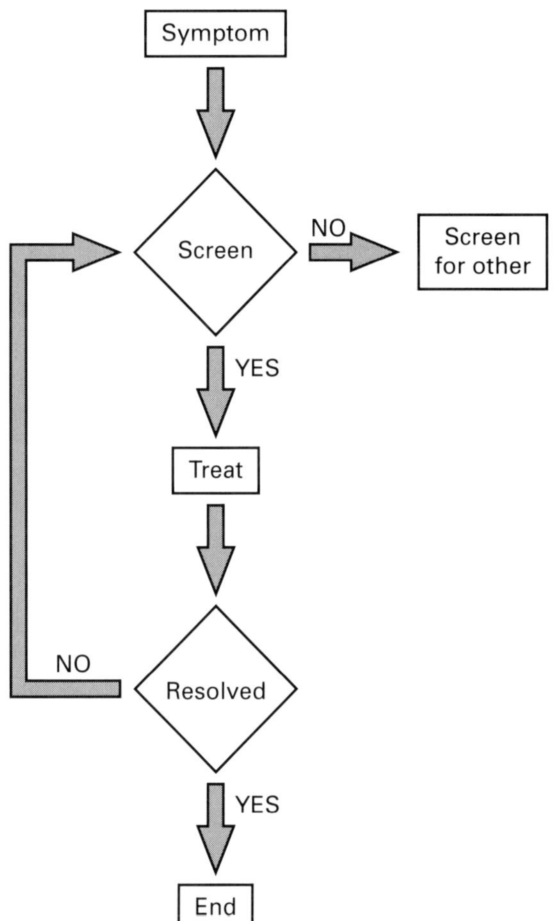

Figure 15.2 Example of a generic proto-algorithm.

Table 15.2 Grades of recommendations and levels of evidence.

Class A recommendations require:
one level 1 study: randomized controlled trial
  with significant statistical power and duration
OR
two or more level 2 studies: randomized
  controlled trials of smaller magnitude and/or
  duration

Class B recommendations require:
one or more level 3 studies: prospective cohort
  design

Class C recommendations require:
one or more level 4 studies: cross-sectional
  controlled studies or retrospective cohort
OR
two or more level 5 studies: case series of any
  size

recommendations used in this process are listed in *Table 15.2*.[3,4] All members of the Guideline Development Panel read all relevant articles.

The guideline writing process occurs as the development panel expands the proto-algorithm and writes supporting annotations based on the available literature. This process may take several iterations between the Guideline Development Panel and the process methodologist who conducts the literature review. Integrated in this process, the development panel identifies aspects of care that are recommended on the basis of their own expertise but that are not supported by empirical research.

This documenting of the Guideline Development Panel's expert opinion begins the expert consensus process. When possible to arrange, the second step in the consensus is to present these expert opinions at a consensus conference held in conjunction with a major MS professional meeting. The final step in the consensus process consists of a review of the document by the 22 members of the Multiple Sclerosis Council for Clinical Practice Guidelines and as many as three additional reviewers from each of the member organizations. Endorsement of each guideline is made by each organization of the Multiple Sclerosis Council for Clinical Practice Guidelines according to their own rules of governance. Documents are also disseminated through the member organizations and other key societies as indicated by the guideline topic.

Conducting evaluations of the guidelines is a goal of the Multiple Sclerosis Council for Clinical Practice Guidelines, which intends to assess the utility of each guideline, its impact on practice and the need for revision resulting from new empirical research. All interested parties are invited to initiate their own evaluation efforts, and reports of their findings are welcomed by the Multiple Sclerosis Council for Clinical Practice Guidelines.

EUROPEAN COLLABORATION

It is the aim of the Multiple Sclerosis Council for Clinical Practice Guidelines to advance collaboration with European colleagues in the field of MS. The interest of European MS groups in the work of guideline development is apparent, as expressed by the representation of two respected MS organizations on the Multiple Sclerosis Council for Clinical Practice Guidelines: Rehabilitation in Multiple Sclerosis (RIMS) and the International Federation of Multiple Sclerosis Societies (IFMSS). Thus far, involvement of European experts in the development of guidelines has included participation in the peer review process of the first two guidelines (fatigue management and bladder management). Various opportunities for the involvement of European MS professionals in the development of subsequent guidelines include the role of panel chairperson or panel member, as well as involvement in the peer review process, in the application of the guideline and in the assessment of outcomes.

Guidelines will be systematically distributed throughout Europe via the organizations that are represented on the MS Council. These organizations will describe to the Council the methodology used for distributing the guidelines to its members or affiliates. RIMS is composed of MS rehabilitation centre members from 18 countries. RIMS members will receive the guidelines as they become available and will have the opportunity of discussing and responding to practical and other issues during the annual conference sponsored by RIMS, as well as through survey and similar types of information-gathering techniques, in order to assess guideline utilization. The IFMSS is composed of 35 national multiple sclerosis societies from around the world. The IFMSS will be formally approached to use its member societies in the translation and dissemination of the guidelines.

REFERENCES

1. American Medical Association. *Principles of Practice Parameters.* Chicago: American Medical Association, 1995.
2. Woolf S. Practice guidelines, a new reality in medicine: II. Methods of developing guidelines. *Arch Intern Med* 1992; **52**: 946–952.
3. Cook DJ, Guyatt GH, Laupacis A et al. Rules of evidence and clinical recommendations on the use of thrombotic agents. Antithrombotic Therapy Consensus Conference. *Chest* 1992; **102**(suppl 4): 305S–311S.
4. Sackett DL. Rules of evidence and clinical recommendations on the use of antithrombotic agents. *Chest* 1989; **95**(suppl 2): 2S–4S.

16

Advances in multiple sclerosis rehabilitation

Alan J Thompson

INTRODUCTION

It has been very encouraging to watch the growing importance of rehabilitation in multiple sclerosis (MS) over recent years. Rehabilitation is now considered an essential component of any scientific MS meeting, which has in turn underlined the need for a sound evidence base for its practice. On reviewing the recent developments in MS rehabilitation, the key theme that emerges is 'co-ordinated involvement'—across disciplines, across patients, carers and their families and across continents.

When considering rehabilitation it is useful to begin with its definition, one of the better of which is that of the Royal College of Physicians: 'an active process of change by which a person who has become disabled acquires and uses the knowledge necessary for optimal physical, psychological and social function'. The most important components then are the focus on the impact of disease on the patient and the encouragement of self-management.

The key areas of development that are reviewed briefly in this chapter include

(a) understanding mechanisms of disability and recovery;
(b) measuring the full impact of the disease;
(c) management of symptoms and rehabilitation;
(d) service provision; and
(e) the development of standards of care.

MECHANISMS OF DISABILITY AND RECOVERY

Managing the impact of disease must be based on an understanding of the underlying pathology in terms of mechanisms of disability and the potential for recovery, if the former is to be prevented and the latter encouraged. This is clearly important in an area such as MS, which has a complex, diffuse pathology that continues over many decades. In recent years, there has been improved understanding of the pathology of MS, resulting both from direct pathological studies and from the application of magnetic resonance imaging (MRI). In the most comprehensive study of its kind, Hans Lassman and co-workers in the Mayo Clinic have identified a number of immunopathogenic mechanisms, ranging from T cell–antibody mediated destruction of oligodendrocytes to primary oligodendrogliopathy, and have looked at the relative occurrence of these processes in the clinical subtypes of MS.[1] Another major development has been the increased awareness of the importance

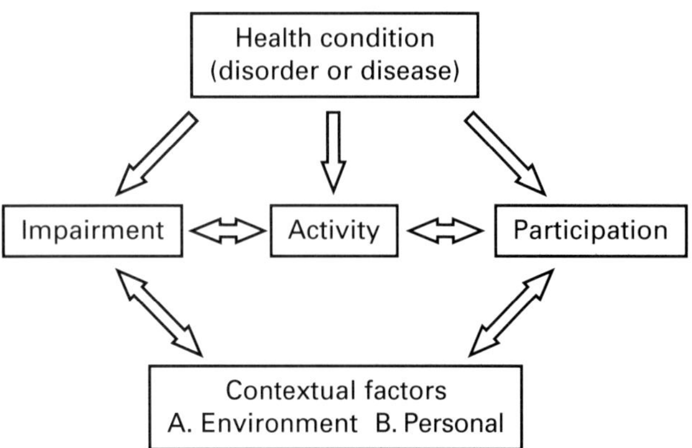

Figure 16.1 New ICDH-2 classification.

of axonal loss in MS. These reminders have come both from MRI and from pathology studies.[2] Axonal loss has been seen both within the lesion and, albeit to a lesser extent, in the normal-appearing white matter (NAWM), and it has been particularly well demonstrated in a collaborative study between the Cleveland Clinic, USA, and Bergen, Norway.[3] The clinical importance of axonal loss in relation to irreversible disability has been highlighted by the strong correlation between MRI measures of atrophy, of both cord and brain,[4,5] and disability. It has been specifically identified by studies using magnetic resonance spectroscopy. Reduction in N-acetyl aspartate, a marker of axonal dysfunction, has been shown in MS lesions but also in the NAWM of both primary and secondary progressive MS.[6–8] Finally, a recent pathological study of hypointense lesions, or black holes, on T1-weighted scans, which are known to correlate with disability, has shown that they reflect destructive lesions with marked axonal loss.[9]

Other MRI approaches that may tell us more about the underlying mechanisms of disability include measures that give better structural information, such as diffusion tensor imaging, which allows accurate demonstration of individual fibre tracts and an indication of the severity of damage.[10] Finally, the exciting prospect of being able to study the process of recovery, particularly in relation to cortical plasticity or adaptation, is possible through the use of functional MRI and, although studies need to be carried out with considerable care in MS, the potential for advances is considerable.[11,12]

MEASUREMENT OF DISEASE IMPACT

The issues surrounding the measurement of the impact of MS on patients have received considerable attention, particularly as a result of recent therapeutic trials and the acknowledged limitations of Kurtzke's Expanded Disability Status Scale (EDSS). The importance of measurement is now fully appreciated (see Chapter 17), as is the need for scientifically sound measurement instruments[13] that are valid, reliable and responsive to change.[14] There is also increasing awareness of the importance of incorporating the patient's perspective[15] and of using clinically appropriate measures.

A further development, which may take some time to get used to, is the recent revision of the International Classification of Impairments, Disability and Handicap by the World Health Organization; it now uses the terms 'activity' and 'participation' in place of 'disability' and 'handicap' and has been designed to underline the importance of the interactions between each of these elements and the role of environmental and personal factors

(*Fig. 16.1*).[16] It also underlines the positive aspects of function rather than dysfunction.

MANAGEMENT OF MS

Symptomatic management

The diversity of symptoms in MS and their complex interactions are well known. It is also apparent that there is very little evidence base for the way in which these symptoms are managed and certainly little consensus among MS physicians.[17] This issue is currently being addressed by a major new international initiative, namely the establishment of an MS Council for Clinical Practice Guidelines (see Chapter 15). This is a serious attempt to develop evidence-based consensus in the management of many symptoms, including fatigue and bladder dysfunction, using a well-established scientific methodology. These two guidelines have now been completed. Another recent and complementary initiative has been the establishment of the Cochrane Collaboration for Multiple Sclerosis, led by Dr Filippini in Milan. This is carrying out systematic reviews on a number of topics, including the use of steroids, 4-aminopyridine and interferon-β in MS.

Rehabilitation

The potential value of rehabilitation in MS is well recognized.[18] However, it is also appreciated that there is an urgent need to standardize input and to evaluate outcome, even to the extent of carrying out randomized, controlled trials. A major component of this standardization is the participation of the multidisciplinary team. In this regard, one of the key developments in rehabilitation, and indeed MS management in general, has been the evolution of the nursing role.[19] Within the rehabilitation setting the unique relationship, expertise and amount of time the nurse spends with the patient provides great potential for expanding the role of the nurse in facilitating the rehabilitation process.

When considering the evaluation of rehabilitation in MS there are three 'simple' questions:

(a) Does it work?
(b) Do the benefits carry over?
(c) How is rehabilitation best carried out?

Although these questions appear relatively straightforward they are far from easy to address, particularly if one considers the potential difficulties in carrying out therapeutic trials in MS, with its varying and unpredictable course and its potential for spontaneous recovery, and then adds the difficulties implicit within rehabilitation. These difficulties include:

(a) the lack of standardization of input;
(b) the lack of consensus on location and duration of input;
(c) difficulty with identifying appropriate outcomes;
(d) reluctance to use a control group;
(e) difficulty with blinding (almost impossible);
(f) the decision on whether or not to evaluate a component of the rehabilitation process or the entire package.

Despite these difficulties an encouraging number of collaborative studies have been published within the last 2 years. Components of the rehabilitation process have been studied, including aerobic training,[20] inpatient physiotherapy[21] and pelvic floor exercises for bladder dysfunction.[22] The entire rehabilitation package has also been evaluated[23] in a stratified, randomized, wait-list controlled study involving 66 patients with progressive MS. The treatment group underwent a short period (28 days) of multidisciplinary rehabilitation. All patients were assessed at 0 and 6 weeks with the EDSS, Functional Systems, Functional Independence Measure (FIM) and the London Handicap Scale (LHS). At the end of 6 weeks, although the impairment of both groups remained the same, the treatment group showed significantly improved levels of disability (p = <0.001) and handicap (p = <0.01) (*Fig. 16.2*).

In a more recent randomized, single-blind, controlled trial, 50 ambulatory patients with MS were involved in a study comparing inpatient

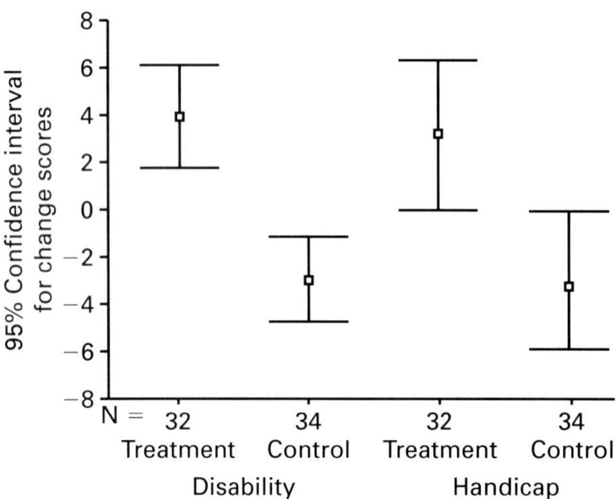

Figure 16.2 Error-bar chart comparing the disability and handicap change scores in the treatment and control groups.

rehabilitation (3 weeks) with a home exercise programme. Evaluation with the EDSS, FIM and SF-36 (a generic quality of life measure) was carried out at baseline, 3 weeks and 15 weeks, and a persistent benefit in disability, with improvement in some aspects of health-related quality of life, was seen in the treated group.[24]

The more difficult evaluation of outpatient rehabilitation has also been carried out.[25] The authors studied 46 patients with progressive MS, 20 of whom received 5 hours of outpatient rehabilitation per week (1 day) for 1 year, while the other 26 were wait-list controlled. Outcome measures included the MS-related Symptom Check List, Composite Score, Fatigue Frequency, and items from the Rehabilitation Institute of Chicago Functional Assessment Scale. The study demonstrated a reduction in fatigue and MS-related symptoms in the treatment group.

The second question relating to carry-over of benefit is also difficult to address. Some attempts have been made with single group studies, the most recent of which followed 50 patients for 12 months after inpatient rehabilitation.[26] The patients were assessed at the onset of the rehabilitation process and at the end, and then at 3 month intervals; measurements included the EDSS, the FIM, the London Handicap Scale, Short Form-36 (SF-36) and the eight-item General Health Questionnaire. Improvements in disability following rehabilitation were maintained for approximately 6 months. Handicap actually improved further following discharge and this improvement was maintained for over 6 months. Similar patterns were seen in both physical and mental components of quality of life and emotional well-being. There was a strong correlation between the extent of benefit during the rehabilitation programme and the duration of carry over.

There remains a need to carry out a more rigorous study of carry-over in MS and also to compare different models of rehabilitation (e.g. inpatient versus outpatient) with appropriate scientific rigour. The methodological issues involved in such studies are considerable but not insurmountable.

SERVICE PROVISION

Information from a number of areas are essential when planning the provision of services in MS. These include:

(a) assessment of need;
(b) utilization of services;
(c) costs of services; and
(d) location of services (see Chapter 19).

Recent efforts to address the issue of assessment of need have resulted in the development of a new questionnaire addressing services and unmet needs, developed by Professor McLellan and Paula Kersten, as part of the Multiple Sclerosis and Rehabilitation, Care and Health Services in Europe (MARCH) programme.[27] This has been successfully applied in a number of European countries. There has also been encouraging and informative work on service utilization and the resulting costs.[28,29] These have highlighted, among other issues, the amount of input and support that comes from informal care, which up until recently has not been acknowledged.

STANDARDS

The lack of standardization of rehabilitation and agreed levels of service provision has resulted in inequality and inconsistency across services and countries. This has prompted an initiative to establish standards of care, both in relation to rehabilitation in general and to MS in particular. Although these initiatives are described as 'standards', they are not evidence based, but rather attempts to describe what might be considered expert consensus. It is hoped that they will encourage better practice and stimulate the provision of evidence to support them. Standards for rehabilitation have been produced by the European Federation of Neurological Societies and have identified key service values in neurological rehabilitation, including choice, consultation, information, participation, recognition and autonomy.[30] In the UK, standards for MS have been developed by the National Hospitals for Neurology and Neurosurgery and the MS Society of Great Britain and Northern Ireland, with input from a range of experts, including people with MS, their carers, families and service providers.[31] These standards cover the four main stages of MS (the diagnostic phase, the phase of minimum impairment, the phase of moderate disability and the phase of severe disability), and they have recently been adapted to create a measuring tool that will be used to evaluate MS

units and provide awards for those who meet the required standard.

Finally, the World Health Organization has identified MS as a condition in which it intends to take a particular interest and has had an initial meeting with the International Federation of MS Societies in order to establish a joint MS working group. The aims of this group are to promote awareness, develop educational material and encourage cross-cultural research.

CONCLUSION

Innovative studies over recent years have demonstrated that it is now possible to evaluate all aspects of rehabilitation in MS, and they emphasize the need to develop our practice along evidence-based guidelines and standards. There is still much work to be done and it is important that the momentum that has developed is maintained though active collaboration across discipline, patients and continents.

REFERENCES

1. Lucchinetti CF, Bruck W, Rodriguez M, Lassmann H. Distinct patterns of multiple sclerosis pathology indicates heterogeneity of pathogenesis. *Brain Pathology* 1996; **6**: 259–274.
2. McDonald WI, Rachelle Fishman-Matthew Moore Lecture. The pathological and clinical dynamics of multiple sclerosis. *J Neuropathol Exp Neurol* 1994; **53**: 338–343.
3. Trapp BD, Peterson J, Ransohoff RM et al. Axonal transection in the lesions of multiple sclerosis. *N Engl J Med* 1998; **338**: 278–285.
4. Losseff NA, Wang L, Lai HM et al. Progressive cerebral atrophy in multiple sclerosis. A serial study. *Brain* 1996; **119**: 2009–2019.
5. Losseff NA, Webb SL, O'Riordan JL et al. Spinal cord atrophy and disability in multiple sclerosis. A new reproducible and sensitive MRI method with potential to monitor disease progression. *Brain* 1996; **119**: 701–708.
6. Davie CA, Barker GJ, Webb S et al. Persistent functional deficit in multiple sclerosis and autosomal dominant cerebellar ataxia is associated with axon loss. *Brain* 1995; **118**: 1583–1592.

7. Leary SM, Davie CA, Parker GJM et al. 1H magnetic resonance spectroscopy of normal-appearing white matter in primary progressive multiple sclerosis (abstract). *Ann Neurol* 1998; **44**: 464.

8. Fu L, Matthews PM, De Stefano N et al. Imaging axonal damage of normal-appearing white matter in multiple sclerosis. *Brain* 1998; **121**: 103–113.

9. van Walderveen MAA, Kamphorst W, Scheltens P et al. Histopathologic correlate of hypointense lesions on T1-weighted spin-echo MRI in multiple sclerosis. *Neurology* 1998; **50**: 1282–1288.

10. Werring DJ. Diffusion MRI in multiple sclerosis. *Multiple Sclerosis* 1998; **4**: 281.

11. Clanet M, Berry I, Boulanouar K. Functional imaging in multiple sclerosis. *Multiple Sclerosis J* 1997; **4**: 26–32.

12. Werring DJ, Bullmore ET, Miller DH et al. Extensive brain activation following recovery from optic neuritis: a pilot study using functional magnetic resonance imaging (fMRI). Proceedings of the 7th Scientific Meeting of the International Society for Magnetic Resonance in Medicine 1999; in press.

13. Hobart JC, Lamping DL, Thompson AJ. Evaluating neurological outcome measures: the bare essentials (editorial). *J Neurol Neurosurg Psychiatry* 1996; **60**: 127–130.

14. Thompson AJ, Hobart JC. Multiple sclerosis: assessment of disability and disability scales. *J Neurol* 1998; **245**: 189–196.

15. Rothwell PM, McDowell Z, Wong CK, Dorman PJ. Doctors and patients don't agree: cross sectional study of patients' and doctors' perceptions and assessments of disability in multiple sclerosis. *Br Med J* 1997; **314**: 1580–1583.

16. World Health Organization. *ICIDH-2: International Classification of Impairments, Activities, and Participation. A Manual of Dimensions of Disablement and Functioning.* Geneva: World Health Organization, 1997.

17. Thompson AJ. Symptomatic treatment in multiple sclerosis. *Curr Opin Neurol* 1998; **11**: 305–309.

18. Thompson AJ. Rehabilitation solutions in multiple sclerosis. *Schweiz Arch Neurol Psychiatr* 1998; **148**: 182–186.

19. Johnson J. What can specialist nurses offer in caring for people with multiple sclerosis? In: Thompson AJ, Polman CH, Hohlfeld R, eds. *Multiple Sclerosis: Clinical Challenges and Controversies.* London: Martin Dunitz Ltd, 1997, 335–343.

20. Petajan JH, Gappmaier E, White AT et al. Impact of aerobic training on fitness and quality of life in multiple sclerosis. *Ann Neurol* 1996; **39**: 432–441.

21. Fuller KJ, Dawson K, Wiles CM. Physiotherapy in chronic multiple sclerosis: a controlled trial. *Clin Rehabil* 1996; **10**: 91–97.

22. Vahtera T, Haaranen M, Viramo-Koskela AL, Ruutiainen J. Pelvic floor rehabilitation is effective in patients with multiple sclerosis. *Clin Rehabil* 1997; **11**: 211–219.

23. Freeman JA, Langdon DW, Hobart JC, Thompson AJ. The impact of inpatient rehabilitation on progressive multiple sclerosis. *Ann Neurol* 1997; **42**: 236–244.

24. Solari A, Filippini G, Gasco P et al. Physical rehabilitation has a positive effect on disability in multiple sclerosis patients. *Neurology* 1999; **52**: 57–62.

25. Fabio RP, Soderberg J, Choi T et al. Extended outpatient rehabilitation: its influence on symptom frequency, fatigue, and functional status for persons with progressive multiple sclerosis. *Arch Phys Med Rehabil* 1998; **79**: 141–146.

26. Freeman JA, Langdon DW, Hobart JC, Thompson AJ. Inpatient rehabilitation in multiple sclerosis: do the benefits carryover into the community? *Neurology* 1999; **52**: 50–56.

27. Kersten P, McLellan DL, George S et al. A questionaire assessment of unmet needs for rehabilitation services and resources for people with MS: results of a pilot study in five European countries. *Clin Rehabil*; in press.

28. Carton H, Loos R, Pacolet J et al. Utilisation and cost of the professional care and assistance according to disability of patients with multiple sclerosis in Flanders (Belgium). *J Neurol Neurosurg Psychiatry* 1998; **64**: 444–450.

29. Stolp-Smith KA, Atkinson EJ, Campion ME et al. Health care utilization in multiple sclerosis. A population-based study in Olmsted County, MN. *Neurology* 1998; **50**: 1594–1600.

30. European Federation of Neurological Societies Task Force. Standards in neurological rehabilitation. *Eur J Neurol* 1997; **4**: 325–331.

31. Hatch J, Johnson J, Thompson AJ. Standards of health care for people with MS. *Multiple Sclerosis Management*; in press.

17

New trends in multiple sclerosis rehabilitation: update on outcome measurements

Jeremy Hobart

INTRODUCTION

In order to provide evidence that health care interventions are effective, the outcomes, or results, attributed to those interventions must be measured.[1,2] This chapter concerns the instruments or scales used to measure the outcomes of rehabilitation in multiple sclerosis.

The importance of rigorous measurement, and the crucial role played by the measurement instruments themselves, is emphasized by the following:

> The elegant design of a clinical study will not overcome the damage caused by unreliable or imprecise measurement. The requirement that one's data be of high quality is at least as important a component of proper study design as the requirement for randomization, double blinding, controlling when necessary for prognostic factors and so on.[3]

> All science is measurement. (Helmholtz, quoted by Bradford Hill.[4])

This chapter addresses new trends in outcomes measurement in MS rehabilitation under three headings: which outcomes are being measured? what new instruments have been developed, and what are the key methodological issues?

WHICH OUTCOMES ARE BEING MEASURED?

A recent advance in the measurement of rehabilitation outcomes is a recognition of the importance of patient-report data. A Medline search for published studies evaluating comprehensive rehabilitation programmes shows that there have been few studies in the last 17 years (*Table 17.1*). Most of these studies have based their outcomes measured on the WHO classification of impairments, disabilities, and handicaps. Only in the last two studies have self-report measures been used (London Handicap Score and Medical Outcome Study 36-Item Short Form Health Survey (SF-36).

The evidence that patient perception is considered an important assessment in MS is supported by a literature search using the keywords 'MS' and 'quality of life'. *Table 17.2* reports some of these published studies over the last 3 years along with the instruments used. However, it is important to note that none of these studies concern MS rehabilitation, indicating that quality of life measurement is not yet widely accepted as part of the assessment of this therapeutic intervention.

There is no consensus as to which outcomes measures should be used in MS rehabilitation. Clearly, the outcomes should measure the effects of the intervention. However, the choice

Table 17.1 Studies evaluating comprehensive rehabilitation programmes.

Year	Author	Outcomes measured and instruments used
1981	Feigenson[5]	Impairment + disability + handicap + cost (MS functional profile)
1987	Greenspun[6]	Disability (CRDS)
	Reding[7]	Disability (ISS) + re-admission rate + cost
1988	Carey[8]	Disability (LORS-II)
	Francabandera[9]	Disability (ISS)
1995	Kidd[10]	Impairment (EDSS) + disability (BI) + handicap (ESS)
1996	Cendrowski[11]	Disability (EDSS)
	Aisen[12]	Impairment (FS/EDSS) + disability (FIM)
	Vaney[13]	Disability (FIM)
1997	Kidd[14]	Impairment (EDSS) + disability (FIM) + handicap (ESS)
	Freeman[15]	Impairment (FS/EDSS) + disability (FIM) + handicap (LHS)
	Fabio[16]	Health-related quality of life (SF-36)

CRDS: Comprehensive Rehabilitation Disability Scale; ISS: Incapacity Status Scale; LORS-II: Level of Rehabilitation Scale (version II); EDSS: Kurtzke Expanded Disability Status Scale; FIM: Functional Independence Measure; BI: Barthel Index; ESS: Environmental Status Scale; FS: Kurtzke Function Systems; LHS: London Handicap Scale; SF-36: Medical Outcomes Study 36-Item Short Form 36 Health Survey.

of instruments is complex since people with MS undergoing rehabilitation have diverse problems and because rehabilitation programmes are multidisciplinary, variable in nature, and tailored to the specific needs of the individual. Since one definition of rehabilitation is 'an active process of change by which a person who has become disabled acquires and uses the knowledge and skills necessary for optimal physical, psychological, and social function', measurement of quality of life is intuitively sound.

WHAT NEW INSTRUMENTS HAVE BEEN DEVELOPED?

Outcome measurement instruments can be divided into disease- or condition-specific and

generic.[29] The former measures are designed for use in specific diseases and the latter measures are designed for use in any disease group. The theoretical advantages of disease-specific measures are that they are likely to be more relevant to, and more likely to detect change in, the disease under study than generic measures. The advantage of generic measures is that they allow different diseases to be compared on the outcome of interest.

In the past few years, six new MS-specific measures have been developed (*Table 17.3*). Three have been published in peer-review journals and three have yet to be subjected to peer review. It is notable that none of these instruments was specifically developed for or has been studied in MS rehabilitation. All instruments provide preliminary evidence supporting their reliability and validity, but there is

Table 17.2 Some studies using self-report measurement in MS.

Year	Author	Self-report measurement instrument
1996	Hermann et al[17]	SF-36
	Brunet et al[18]	SF-36
	Jonsson et al[19]	Laman/Lankhorst Questionnaire + BDI
	Cella et al[20]	FAMS
	Petajan et al[21]	SIP
1997	Rothwell et al[22]	SF-36+ EuroQoL (EQ-5D)
	Schwartz et al[23]	Q-TWiST
	Vickrey et al[24]	SF-36
	Lankhorst et al[25]	Disability and impact profile
1998	Gianino et al[26]	Ferrans and Powers Quality of Life index + SIP
	Plohman et al[27]	Self-report daily functioning
	Canadian Burden of Illness Study Group[28]	SF-36

SF-36: Medical Outcomes Study 36-Item Short Form 36 Health Survey; FAMS: Functional Assessment of MS Score; BDI: Beck Depression Inventory; FAMS: Functional Assessment of MS; SIP: Sickness Impact Profile; Q-TWiST: Quality-adjusted Time Without Symptoms and Toxicity of treatment.

little evidence supporting their responsiveness (i.e. their ability to detect change in the outcome of interest). Unpublished measures cannot be recommended for widespread use.

Published MS-specific measures

MS Impairment Scale (MSIS)

This instrument quantifies the abnormal findings during a standard neurologic examination.[30] It is based on the World Health Organization definition of impairments and is composed of 53 subscores, which may be divided into five functional groups: cognition, cranial nerve functions, limb motor functions, sensory functions, and complex functions. A total score is obtained by summing subscores (0 = minimum impairment, 209 = maximum

Table 17.3 Newly developed MS-specific measures.

Published	
Vickrey et al 1995[31]	MSQoL-54
Cella et al 1996[20]	FAMS
Ravnborg et al 1997[30]	MS impairment scale
Unpublished	
Sharrack	GNDS
Ford	LMSQoL
LaRocca	MSQLI

MSQoL-54: MS Quality of Life Instrument; FAMS: Functional Assessment of MS Scale; GNDS: Guy's Neurological Disability Scale; LMSQoL: Leeds MS Quality of Life Scale; MSQLI: MS Quality of Life Inventory.

impairment). Little detail is given on the development process. Preliminary data are provided for some aspects of reliability, validity, and responsiveness (i.e. sensitivity). Further studies of the psychometric properties of the MSIS are required.

Functional Assessment in MS (FAMS)

This is a self-report measure of health-related quality of life (HRQoL) in MS.[20] It was developed by adding 31 MS-specific items to the 28-item FACT-G (Functional Assessment in Cancer Therapy—General version). The 59 items are grouped into six subscales: mobility, symptoms, emotional well-being, general contentment, thinking and fatigue, family and social well-being, and additional concerns.

The MS-specific items were generated from semistructured interviews of 20 patients, expert opinion from five medical practitioners and nurses, and a literature review. An item-reduction stage was included. Evidence of reliability and validity is provided using standard techniques. Responsiveness is not examined and item-level statistics are not provided.

MS Quality of Life instrument (MSQoL-54)

This is a self-report measure of HRQoL in MS developed by adding 18 MS-specific items to the SF-36.[31] The MS-specific items were selected by literature review and the expert opinion of two MS physicians and an MS nurse specialist. Reliability and validity is examined using standard methods. The authors of this study predict that the instrument takes 11–18 minutes to complete.[31]

Unpublished new MS-specific measures

Guy's Neurological Disability Scale (GNDS)

This is an interviewer-rated measure of disability in MS. Each of the 11 items is scored on an individualized six-point rating scale. A total score is generated by summing the item scores. Preliminary evidence for reliability, validity and responsiveness have been reported in conference proceedings.[32] No item-reduction stage was included in the development. Although the GNDS probably only takes a few minutes to complete and although data suggest that it can be easily administered by various health professionals, the interviewer-rated method of administration is more resource-consuming and less flexible than the self-report method and limits the types of studies in which it can be used.

Leeds MS Quality of Life Scale (LMSQoL)

This is a self-report measure of HRQoL in MS. Items were generated from patient interviews (in two focus groups) and reduced from 25 to 16. There are two eight-item scales, emotional and social functioning, generated by summing the item scores. The instrument takes only a few minutes to complete. Preliminary data for the reliability and validity of the LMSQoL have been reported in conference proceedings, but responsiveness has not been assessed.[33]

MS Quality of Life Inventory (MSQLI)

This instrument was developed largely by selecting, and in some cases adapting, existing health measures. Scales are organized according to the World Health Organization concept of health, with nine measures of impairment, eleven measures of disability, and seven measures of social handicap. Scores are generated by summing item scores. The instrument provides a profile of HRQoL and is said to take approximately 45 minutes to administer.[34]

Problems with the new instruments

Comparison of these new measures for MS illustrates an important point. Four of the above instruments are titled quality of life measures. However, they all assess different aspects of health, highlighting the lack of consensus concerning the type and number of dimensions that should be measured by a HRQoL instrument.[35,36] Although there is agreement that HRQoL concerns functioning and well-being, is multidimensional and subjective, self-report investigators are advised to examine carefully the content of instruments and their relevance to the sample and questions under study.

Generic instruments used in MS

Many generic measures have been used in MS. In this section three are examined: the Medical Outcomes Study 36-item Short-Form Health Survey (SF-36), EuroQoL, and the Functional Independence Measure (FIM). These measures have been chosen specifically as they are widely used and have been recommended for routine use.

SF-36

This is a self-report measure of health status in eight dimensions using multi-item scales: physical functioning (10 items), role limitations due to physical problems (four items), bodily pain (two items), general health perceptions (five items), energy and vitality (four items), mental health (five items), social functioning (two items), and role limitations resulting from emotional problems (three items). The remaining item assesses change in health over the previous year. The instrument takes approximately 5–10 minutes to complete. Scores are generated for each dimension,[37] and two summary scores (physical and mental component summary scores are arrived at).[38] There is also an even shorter form, the SF-12.[39]

The development of the SF-36 is a landmark in health measurement. The methods used provide an important model for investigators and there is extensive evidence to support the reliability and validity of the SF-36.[37] However, it is important to note that the SF-36 was not designed as a measure to evaluate the effectiveness of interventions, nor was it specifically designed for patients with MS undergoing rehabilitation. Awareness of these issues is important when examining its usefulness in MS rehabilitation.

The SF-36 has been used to study the impact of MS and has provided very useful information. These studies have demonstrated some of the advantages and disadvantages of the SF-36 in MS. Two useful studies have been the Canadian Burden of Illness study[28] and the study of Freeman et al[40] of the health-related quality of life of MS patients undergoing in-patient rehabilitation. Both studies indicate the

profound impact of MS, compared with norms and with other disorders, on all dimensions of health status measured by the SF-36. However, both studies also indicate a worrying floor effect (i.e. percentage of the sample scoring the worst possible score) in the physical functioning and physical role limitations dimensions for MS people with physical disability that is moderate or marked (expanded disability status score $\geqslant$ 6). These data mean that these dimensions of the SF-36 are unable to discriminate between patients with moderate disability and those with severe disability and are, in part, responsible for the limited responsiveness of this instrument in MS.[41] These factors limit the usefulness of the SF-36 for evaluating the effectiveness of rehabilitation in MS. Since it is important to use responsive instruments to evaluate health care interventions, the SF-36 is limited as an evaluative measure of rehabilitation outcomes.

EuroQoL Health Status Questionnaire

This is a self-report measure of health status.[42] It consists of two parts. In the first part there are five items (mobility, self-care, usual activities, pain and discomfort, and anxiety and depression). Each item is rated on a three-level scale (no problems, some problems, unable to do) and concerns the health state on the day of completion. Weights are used in scoring the responses. Scores for the five items are reported in two ways: first, as a profile of health status and second, as a total score by summation of the five item scores using a specified formula. The second half of the EuroQoL consists of a visual analogue scale drawn like a thermometer. Patients are required to rate their health state today on scale between 0 (worst imaginable health state) and 100 (best imaginable health state).

Evidence supporting the reliability and validity of the EuroQoL is largely from an earlier version of the instrument which had four dimensions. There are no studies formally examining the psychometric properties of the EuroQoL in MS. Unlike many other instruments, the EuroQoL asks about health status on the day of completion, which may limited reliability in MS, which is associated with notable day-to-day fluctuations. In addition, the imprecise rating scale for each item suggest that the EuroQoL may lack measurement precision[43] and be poorly responsive to changes induced by rehabilitation. Finally, when reported as a health profile, the items of the EuroQoL represent five single item measures. Since single item measures are less reliable, less valid and less responsive than multi-item measures,[44–47] use of the EuroQoL is theoretically of limited value in MS rehabilitation. In short, empirical evidence is needed to evaluate the usefulness of the EuroQoL as an outcome of MS rehabilitation.

Since both the SF-36 and EuroQoL are generic measures of health status is it reasonable to assume that they measure that same health constructs? Rothwell and co-workers[22] examined the SF-36 and EuroQoL in MS patients. They report correlations between the eight dimensions of the SF-36 and scores on the EuroQoL visual analogue scale (overall health status) ranging from 0.02 to 0.57 indicating that these two instruments are measuring very different health constructs.

FIM

This is an 18-item, observer-rated, generic measure of disability that is conceptualized as burden of care. It was designed specifically for evaluating the outcomes of rehabilitation programmes[48] and is used widely in the US, Europe and Australasia.

Each item has a seven-point rating scale. There is a common core to the rating of all items (1 = maximal dependence, 7 = fully dependent) but the rating of each item is individually defined. This creates some complexities for raters, results in a large manual (more than 40 pages) and detracts from the user-friendliness of the instrument. Despite these off-putting features, experienced users can rate the FIM in about 10 minutes.

Three scores can be generated by summation of item scores: a total score representing global disability (all items), a motor score representing physical disability (13 items), and a cognitive score representing cognitive disability (five items). Many publications from many authors

provide evidence to support the reliability and validity of the FIM. In addition, the psychometric properties of the FIM have been comprehensively studied in MS patients undergoing rehabilitation.[49–51]

Despite the empirical evidence for the scientific soundness of the FIM, its method of administration, the need for training raters and the costs imposed by the Uniform Data System (approximately US$1500 per annum) are likely to limit its usefulness in large studies of MS rehabilitation in Europe. The scientific properties of the FIM are further discussed in the next section of this chapter.

WHAT ARE THE KEY METHODOLOGICAL ISSUES?

Psychometric methods in health measurement

Psychometric methods are procedures for psychological measurement.[52] For the past century, psychologists and educators have wrestled with the measurement of constructs such as ability, personality, sentiments, and attitudes.[53] Their research has resulted in the development of methodologies enabling the reliable and valid measurement of abstract constructs.[54] Recent developments in health-care evaluation have indicated the importance of measuring health constructs such as disability, handicap and health-related quality of life. Like the psychological constructs mentioned above, these health constructs are abstract. Therefore, psychometric methods offer a method for the rigorous measurement of health outcomes. The increased awareness and use of psychometric principles in health measurement over the past few years is noticeable and represents a major advance.

An aspect of psychometrics that warrants further mention is the concept of incremental validity.[55] As well as demonstrating their psychometric soundness, new outcome measurement instruments must also demonstrate advantages over existing measures. These advantages must be empirical and not theoretical. The demonstration that the FIM is psychometrically equivalent to the Barthel Index[56] is an important point since one impetus behind the development of the FIM was an assumption that available measures, including the Barthel Index, were too simple and too crude to measure rehabilitation outcomes.[57]

Proxy measurement in neurological disease

The role of proxy measurements in MS has yet to be clearly determined. Since cognitive impairment is an important feature of MS, its influence on the reliability and validity of commonly used self-report measures is urgently required. However, proxy measurements are unable to provide an accurate assessment of patient perception.[58]

Cultural adaptations

The international nature of MS studies raises concerns about cultural adaptations of health measures. These concerns have been raised by others and there is an increasing literature of its importance. Although it is common to translate and back-translate an instrument, it is also necessary to study the measurement properties.[59] This means that measures developed in the UK, for example, must undergo reliability and validity testing in other cultures.

Individualized measurements

The individually tailored, goal-oriented nature of rehabilitation programmes has raised questions as to the relevance of standardized measures in the assessment of rehabilitation. Indeed, these questions have been raised about health-related quality of life measurement in general. Consequently, a number of individualized measurement methods have been developed over the past few years.[60–63] They have yet to be well studied.

CONCLUSIONS

Clinical scales are being increasingly used to evaluate health care interventions. In MS rehabilitation there is a move towards self-report measurement methods. The incorporation of psychometric methods in the development of health measures has improved, and will continue to improve measurement rigour. However, there are a number of important methodological aspects in need of investigation.

REFERENCES

1. Jenkinson C, ed. *Measuring Health and Medical Outcomes.* 1st edn. London: University College London Press, 1994.
2. Sackett DL, Rosenberg WM, Gray JM et al. Evidence based medicine: what it is and what is isn't. *Br Med J* 1996; **312**: 71–72.
3. Fleiss JL. *The Design and Analysis of Clinical Experiments.* New York: Wiley, 1986.
4. Bradford-Hill R. *Principles of Medical Statistics,* 9th edn. 1971.
5. Feigenson JS, Scheinberg L, Catalano M et al. The cost-effectiveness of multiple sclerosis rehabilitation: a model. *Neurology* 1981; **31**: 1316–1322.
6. Greenspun B, Stineman M, Agri R. Multiple sclerosis and rehabilitation outcome. *Arch Phys Med Rehabil* 1987; **68**: 434–437.
7. Reding MJ, La Rocca NG, Madonna M. Acute-hospital care versus rehabilitation hospitalisation for management of nonemergent complications in multiple sclerosis. *J Neurol Rehabil* 1987; **1**: 13–17.
8. Carey RG, Seibert JH. Who makes the most progress in inpatient rehabilitation? An analysis of functional gain. *Arch Phys Med Rehabil* 1988; **69**: 337–343.
9. Francabandera FL, Holland NJ, Wiesel-Levison P, Scheinberg LC. Multiple sclerosis rehabilitation: inpatient versus outpatient. *Rehabilitation Nursing* 1988; **13**: 251–253.
10. Kidd D, Howard RS, Losseff NA, Thompson AJ. The benefit of inpatient neurorehabilitation in multiple sclerosis. *Clin Rehabil* 1995; **9**: 198–203.
11. Cendrowski W, Kwolek A, Chmiel A et al. Multicenter study on rehabilitation in multiple sclerosis. *Eur J Neurol* 1996; **3** (Suppl 2): 16.
12. Aisen ML, Sevilla D, Fox N. Inpatient rehabilita-

tion for multiple sclerosis. *J Neurol Rehabil* 1996; **10**: 43–46.

13. Vaney C, Dubois S, Dehlinger A. Effectiveness of inpatient rehabilitation in multiple sclerosis (abstract). Atlanta: Multiple Sclerosis Consortium, 1996.

14. Kidd D, Thompson AJ. A prospective study of neurorehabilitation in multiple sclerosis. *J Neurol Neurosurg Psychiatry* 1997; **60**: 491–496.

15. Freeman JA, Langdon DW, Hobart JC, Thompson AJ. The impact of inpatient rehabilitation on progressive multiple sclerosis. *Ann Neurol* 1997; **42**: 236–244.

16. Fabio RP, Choi T, Soderberg J, Hansen CR. Health-related quality of life for patients with progressive multiple sclerosis: influence of rehabilitation. *Phys Ther* 1997; **77(12)**: 1704–1716.

17. Hermann BP, Vickrey BG, Hays RD et al. A comparison of health-related quality of life of patients with epilepsy, diabetes and multiple sclerosis. *Epilepsy Res* 1996; **125**: 113–118.

18. Brunet DG, Hopman WH, Singer MA et al. Measurement of health-related quality of life in multiple sclerosis patients. *Can J Neurol Sci* 1996; **23**: 99–103.

19. Jonsson A, Dock J, Ravnborg MH. Quality of life as a measure of rehabilitation outcome in patients with multiple sclerosis. *Acta Neurol Scand* 1996; **93**: 229–235.

20. Cella DF, Dineen K, Arnason B et al. Validation of the functional assessment of multiple sclerosis quality of life instrument. *Neurology* 1996; **47**: 129–139.

21. Petajan JH, Gappmaier E, White AT et al. Impact of aerobic training on fitness and quality of life in Multiple Sclerosis. *Ann Neurol* 1996; **39**: 432–441.

22. Rothwell PM, McDowell Z, Wong CK, Dorman PJ. Doctors and patients don't agree: cross sectional study of patients' and doctors' perceptions and assessments of disability in multiple sclerosis. *Br Med J* 1997; **314**: 1580–1583.

23. Schwartz CE, Coulthard-Morris L, Cole B, Vollmer T. The quality of life effects of interferon beta-1b in multiple sclerosis: an extended Q-TWIST analysis. *Arch Neurol* 1997; **54(12)**: 1475–1480.

24. Vickrey BG, Hays RD, Genovese BJ et al. Comparison of a generic to disease-targeted health–related quality of life measures for multiple sclerosis. *J Clin Epidemiol* 1997; **50(5)**: 557–569.

25. Lankhorst GJ, Jelles F, Smits RC et al. Quality of life in multiple sclerosis: the disability and impact profile (DIP). *J Neurol* 1996; **243(6)**: 469–474.

26. Gianino JM, York MM, Paice JA, Shott S. Quality of life: effect of reduced spasticity from intrathecal baclofen. *J Neurosci Nurs* 1998; **30(1)**: 47–54.

27. Plohmann AM, Kappos L, Ammann W et al. Computer assisted retraining of attentional impairments in patients with multiple sclerosis (abstract). *J Neurol Neurosurg Psychiatry* 1998; **64(4)**: 455–462.

28. The Canadian Burden of Illness Study Group. Burden of illness of multiple sclerosis; Part II: Quality of life. *Can J Neurol Sci* 1998; **25(1)**: 31–38.

29. Patrick D, Deyo R. Generic and disease-specific measures in assessing health status and quality of life. *Medical Care* 1989; **27**(suppl): S217–S232.

30. Ravnborg M, Gronbech-Jensen M, Jonsson A. The MS impairment scale: a pragmatic approach to the assessment of impairment in patients with multiple sclerosis. *Multiple Sclerosis* 1997; **3**: 31–42.

31. Vickrey BG, Hays RD, Harooni R et al. A health-related quality of life measure for multiple sclerosis. *Quality Life Res* 1995; **4**: 187–206.

32. Sharrack B, Hughes RAC, Soudain S. Guy's Neurological Disability Scale. *J Neurol* 1996; **243**(suppl 2): S32.

33. Ford HL, Tennant A, Johnson MH. The Leeds MSQoL scale: a disease specific measure of quality of life in multiple sclerosis (abstract). *J Neurol Neurosurg Psychiatry* 1997; **62**: 210.

34. LaRocca NG, Ritvo PG, Miller DM et al. 'Quality of life' assessment in multiple sclerosis clinical trials: current status and strategies for improving multiple sclerosis clinical trial design. In: Goodkin DE, Rudick R, eds. *Multiple Sclerosis: Advances in Clinical Trial Design, Treatment and Future Perspectives.* London: Springer-Verlag, 1996, 145–160.

35. Pfennings LEMA, Cohen L, Van der Ploeg HM. Assessing the quality of life of patients with multiple sclerosis. In: Thompson AJ, Polman C, Hohlfeld R, eds. *Multiple Sclerosis: Clinical Challenges and Controversies.* London: Martin Dunitz, 1997, 295–311.

36. Muldoon MF, Barger SD, Flory JD, Manuck SB. What are quality of life measurements measuring? *Br Med J* 1998; **316**: 542–545.

37. Ware JE Jr. SF-36 Health Survey Manual and Interpretation Guide. Boston, Massachussetts: Nimrod Press, 1993.

38. Ware JE Jr, Kosinski MA, Keller SD. *SF-36 Physical and Mental Health Summary Scales: a User's Manual.* Boston, Massachussetts: The

Health Institute, New England Medical Centre, 1994.

39. Ware JE Jr, Kosinski M, Keller SD. How to score the SF-12 physical and mental summary scales. Boston, Massachussetts: The Health Institute, New England Medical Centre, 1994.

40. Freeman JA, Langdon DW, Hobart JC, Thompson AJ. Health-related quality of life in people with multiple sclerosis undergoing inpatient rehabilitation. *J Neurol Rehabil* 1996; **10**: 185–194.

41. Hobart JC, Lamping DL, Freeman JA, Thompson AJ. The responsiveness of disabiliity measures in multiple sclerosis (abstract). *J Neurol Neurosurg Psychiatry* 1997; **62**: 213–214.

42. EuroQoL Group. EuroQoL: a new facility for the measurement of health-related quality of life. *Health Policy* 1990; **16**: 199–208.

43. McHorney CA, Ware JE Jr, Rogers W et al. The validity and relative precision of MOS short- and long-form health status scales and Dartmouth COOP charts. *Med Care* 1992; **30**: MS253–MS265.

44. Nunnally JC. *Psychometric Theory*, 2nd edn. New York: McGraw-Hill, 1978.

45. McIver JP, Carmines EG. Unidimensional scaling. *Sage University Paper Series on Quantitative Applications in the Social Sciences.* Newbury Park, California: Sage, 1981.

46. Stewart AL, Ware JE Jr, eds. *Measuring Functioning and Well-being: the Medical Outcomes Study Approach.* Durham, North Carolina: Duke University Press, 1992.

47. Spector PE. Summated rating scale construction: an introduction. In: Lewis-Beck MS, ed. *Quantitative Applications in the Social Sciences.* Newbury Park, California: Sage, 1992, 07–082.

48. Granger CV, Hamilton BB, Keith RA et al. Advances in functional assessment for medical rehabilitation. *Top Geriatr Rehabil* 1986; **1**: 59–74.

49. Hobart JC, Lamping DL, Freeman JA et al. Measuring neurology—is bigger better? Comparative measurement properties of the Functional Independence Measure (FIM) and the Barthel Index (BI). *J Neurol Neurosurg Psychiatry* 1997; **63**: 694–695.

50. Hobart JC, Langdon DW, Lamping DL et al. Can cognitive disability in multiple sclerosis be measured from behavioural observation? Validity of the Functional Independence Measure Cognitive Scale (FIM-c). *Multiple Sclerosis* 1997; **3**: 268.

51. Hobart JC, Lamping DL, Thompson AJ. Measuring disability in neurological disease: validity of the self-report Barthel Index. *J Neurol* 1996; **243**(suppl 2): S25.

52. Guilford JP. *Psychometric Methods*, 2nd edn. New York: McGraw-Hill, 1954.

53. Thurstone LL, Chave EJ. *The Measurement of Attitude.* Chicago, Illinois: University of Chicago Press, 1929.

54. Nunnally JC, Bernstein IH. *Psychometric Theory*, 3rd edn. New York: McGraw-Hill, 1994.

55. Sechrest L. Incremental validity. In: Jackson D, Messick S, eds. *Problems in Human Assessment.* New York: McGraw-Hill, 1967, 368–371.

56. Hobart JC, Lamping DL, Freeman JA et al. Measuring neurology – is bigger better? Comparative measurement properties of the Functional Independence Measure (FIM) and the Barthel Index (BI). *Neurology* 1997; **48**(suppl 3): A235.

57. Hamilton BB, Granger CV, Sherwin FS et al. A uniform national data system for medical rehabilitation. In: Fuhrer MJ, ed. *Rehabilitation Outcomes: Analysis and Measurement.* Baltimore, Maryland: Paul H Brookes, 1987, 137–147.

58. Sprangers MAG, Aaronson NK. The role of health care providers and significant others in evaluating the quality of life of patients with chronic disease: a review. *J Clin Epidemiol* 1992; **45**: 743–760.

59. Scientific Advisory Committee of the Medical Outcomes Trust. Instrument review criteria. *Med Outcomes Trust Bull* 1995; **3**: I–IV.

60. O'Boyle CA, McGee HM, Hickey A et al. *The Schedule for the Evaluation of Individual Quality of Life (SEIQoL): Administration Manual.* Dublin: Royal College of Surgeons in Ireland, 1993.

61. Ruta D, Garratt A, Leng M et al. A new approach to measurement of quality of life: the patient-generated index. *Med Care* 1994; **32**: 1109–1126.

62. Kiresuk TJ, Smith A, Cardillo JE eds. *Goal Attainment Scaling: Applications, Theory, and Measurement.* Hillsdale, New Jersey: Lawrence Erlbaum Associates, 1994.

63. Smith A, Cardillo JE, Smith SC, Amezaga AM. Improvement scaling (rehabilitation version): a new approach to measuring progress of patients in achieving their individual rehabilitation goals. *Med Care* 1998; **36**: 333–347.

18

Service location in multiple sclerosis: home or hospital

Carlo Pozzilli, Angela Pisani, Lucia Palmisano, Mario A Battaglia, Cesare Fieschi and the Roman Home Care Multiple Sclerosis Group

HOSPITAL-AT-HOME SCHEME

Improving the ability of the health-care system to respond to patient demands is one of the greatest challenges of our time. People affected by chronic disease, even those with considerable disability, often prefer to stay at home, and hospitals are shortening the lengths of stay. Community care has therefore acquired greater relevance. Increased provision of services in the community is also a proposed method for reducing the pressure on acute hospitals. Therefore, hospital-at-home schemes, which provide care in patients' homes that has traditionally been provided in hospital, have grown in importance in health services both in Europe and in North America.[1]

However, little research about hospital-at-home services have been done, and most of the studies have been small, with no consistency in outcome measures and little attempt at economic evaluation.[2,3] Recently, however, two separate randomized controlled trials have given an important contribution to our understanding of the potential for developing hospital-at-home schemes not least because they incorporate economic evaluations in their design. In both studies, hospital at home seems as effective and acceptable as routine hospital care.[4,5] There were no significant differences in patients' reported health outcome between the two services, although hospital-at-home patients have more days of care than their inpatient counterparts. Hospital-at-home teams may have difficulty discharging patients or discharge from inpatient care is sometimes premature.

The economic evaluations of the two services came to opposite conclusions, with reduced costs for hospital-at-home patients in one study[6] and higher costs in the other.[7] These results seem to be contingent on characteristics of local services that may have influenced the application of eligibility criteria sensitivity, recruitment to the study and timing of discharge from hospital at home.

Even if more trials are forthcoming soon, hospital at home may replace usual hospital care for some diagnostic groups without adverse effects and therefore potentially free up resources. Indeed, the type of patients admitted to this modality of care may significantly influence its cost effectiveness: early discharge from hospital at home probably implies a relatively short course of intensive and expensive treatments, whereas the admission of patients suffering from chronic conditions is likely to require a long-term provision of care, with less occurrence of 'emergencies' and more requests for social support and help to the caregivers.

HOSPITAL-AT-HOME SCHEME AND MULTIPLE SCLEROSIS

Multiple sclerosis (MS) is a chronic disabling disease that strikes early in life. The median age at onset is 30–32 years and there is a female preponderance. The initial course of MS is most often relapsing–remitting with accumulating deficit followed within 5–10 years by a secondary progressive course. In a minority of patients the disease is progressive from the onset. The mean time to reach a disability requiring aids for ambulation is 15 years.[8] Survival after onset is in the order of 35–40 years.[9] Apart from the personal suffering, the financial consequences for these patients and their family and the economic burden for society are enormous. Cost areas consist of medical treatments, lost earnings (for both patients and caregivers), provision for social security and social services, and private expenditure. According to a 'cost of illness' study, in England and Wales this corresponded to an estimated annual cost of MS to the community of £505.21 million.[10]

Therefore, MS may represent a proper target for the evaluation of home-care delivery systems as alternatives to the traditional health-care approach. Hospital-at-home care can provide support, nursing care, rehabilitation and administration of drugs and, most of all, can prevent admission to hospital.

MULTIPLE SCLEROSIS AND QUALITY OF LIFE

Most studies of people with MS have focused on either physiological outcome measure, such as neurological signs, neuroimaging and spinal fluid analysis, or on measure of physical disability only. Recently, health-related quality of life (HRQoL) (as well as functional status and general well-being) has been recognized as an important outcome, along with disease-specific measurements.

HRQoL is a multidimensional construct that explores physical, mental and social health as perceived by the patient. Physical health here refers to impairments and disabilities; psycho-logical health refers to measurement of anxiety–depression and fear; social functioning refers to social support, contacts with other people and to role fulfilment (the extent to which a person fulfils his or her role as a father, mother, husband, wife, etc).[11]

Medical Outcomes Study 36-Item Short Form Health Survey (SF-36),[12,13] Multiple Sclerosis Quality of Life (MSQoL),[14] Functional Assessment of Multiple Sclerosis (FAMS)[15] and the Disability of Impact Profile (DIP)[16] are some of the quality of life scales used in MS clinical trials.

The SF-36 includes one multi-item scale that assesses eight health concepts and produces two summary health status scores, a Physical Component Summary (PCS) score and a Mental Component Summary (MCS) score. Patients with MS reported significantly worse PCS scores and MCS scores compared to age- and sex-matched control populations[17] and to patients with chronic illness such as epilepsy and diabetes.[18]

Even if physical functioning seems to be an important factor of the HRQoL, several studies have pointed attention to the behavioural, mental and psychological aspects of MS. In this regard, patients and clinicians seem to disagree on which domains of health status are most important. Patients are significantly more likely than the physicians to rate mental health and emotional role limitations as important and significantly less likely to be concerned with physical functioning and physical role limitations.[19]

Patients with MS have been shown to score poorly in the HRQoL domains related to social activities.[14,17,18] A home-care delivery system, by preventing undue hospital admissions, may contribute to preserve their social dimension from further deterioration.

THE HOME-CARE PROJECT IN ROME

The authors conducted a randomized controlled trial comparing hospital-at-home care with inpatient hospital care in MS (*Fig. 18.1*). The aim of the study was threefold:

(a) to evaluate the health outcomes and costs of the hospital at home scheme compared to inpatient hospital care;

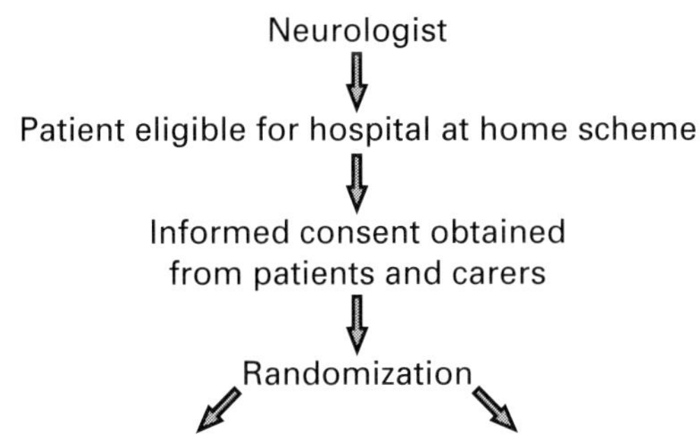

Figure 18.1　Study design of the Rome study.

(b) to identify medical, psychological and social factors that affect HRQoL of MS patients; and
(c) to analyse the impact of the hospital-at-home scheme on the HRQoL of caregivers.

Patients resident in Rome and suffering from clinically definite MS and referred either to the MS Centre of the Neurological Department, University of Rome ('La Sapienza') or other institutional centres for MS in Rome were considered eligible for the study. For each patient, a caregiver was identified, when possible, who was willing to be actively involved in the study. An informed consent was requested by eligible patients and carers.

Study design

An entry, patients suitable for the hospital-at-home scheme were randomized to hospital-at-home or hospital care in a ratio 2:1 in order to ensure that hospital-at-home population would be sufficiently represented. Randomization was stratified by age and expanded disability status score (EDSS). We hypothesized that both outcome and costs would differ according to disease disability and age and that valid conclusions could be drawn only by comparing similar patients.

Patients who were randomized to hospital-at-home care had access to a dedicated telephone number, on which an operator answered their calls and contacted the different specialists according to the specific requirement. The home-care multidisciplinary team included three neurologists, one urologist, one psychologist, one specialist in rehabilitation medicine, one physiotherapist, one nurse, one social worker and one co-ordinator.

Patients who were randomized to routine hospital care were followed as usual in their centres of referral. They were interviewed once monthly by a neurologist in order to collect information about medical visits, therapies, hospital admission and diagnostic procedures performed in the past month.

Patient assessment

After randomization and at the end of the 1-year follow-up period, all patients underwent an exhaustive interview that included socio-demographic information, neurological and psychological assessment, cognitive and functional abilities and HRQoL measures. The following scales were used: Functional System and EDSS,[20] Mini-Mental State (MMSE),[21] Standard Raven Progressive Matrices (SPM),[22] Functional Independence Measure (FIM),[23] Fatigue Severity Scale (FSS),[24] Illness Behavioural Questionnaire (IBQ),[25] State Trait Anger Expression Inventory (STAXI),[26] State Trait Anxiety Inventory (STAI),[27] Clinical Depression Questionnaire (CDQ),[28] Profile of Moods State (POMS)[29] (about caregivers' anxiety and stress), SF-36, Questionnaire on Family Problem (FP). *Table 18.1* shows the evaluating specialists and the functions covered by each scale.

Patient recruitment started in January 1996 and ended in December 1997. Since the length of follow-up period for each patient is 1 year

Table 18.1   Clinical interview at the baseline and after 1 year follow-up in the Rome study.

Specialist	Clinical assessment	Scale
Neurologist	Neurological assessment	EDSS
	Cognitive ability	MMSE
		SPM
Specialist in rehabilitation	Disability	FIM
	Fatigue	FSS
Psychologist	Illness behaviour	IBQ
	Anxiety	STAI
	Depression	CDQ
	Anger	STAXI
	Impact on caregivers	POMS
Social Worker	Sociodemographic characteristics	FP
	Quality of life	SF-36

EDSS: Expanded Disability Status Score; MMSE: Mini-Mental State Examination; SPM: Standard Raven Progressive Matrices; FIM: Functional Independence Measure; FSS: Fatigue Severity Scale; IBQ: Illness Behavioural Questionnaire; STAI: State Trait Anger Inventory; CDQ: Clincial Depression Questionnaire; STAXI: State Trait Anger Expression Inventory; POMS: Profile of Moods State; SF-36: 36-Item Short Form Health Survey.

and the study finished in December 1998, the time of writing this chapter, the results of the cross-sectional analysis on baseline data aimed at identifying the medical, psychological and social factors that affect quality of life in MS patients. Furthermore, it reports preliminary data on the number and type of interventions provided by the hospital-at-home team, as well as on a 'customer satisfaction questionnaire' that was mailed to patients randomized to the hospital-at-home scheme, at the end of their 1-year study period.

Results

A total of 201 consecutive patients were randomized (133 to the hospital-at-home scheme and 68 to routine hospital care). *Table 18.2* sum-

marizes the baseline sociodemographic and clinical characteristic of the patients. The two groups were broadly similar for all variables considered. The remarkably high mean value of EDSS (5.8) underlines the predominance of patients with primary and secondary progressive disease.

Factors affecting quality of life

The relationships between the two composite scores of HRQoL (PCS and MCS) and clinical variables were examined by multivariate regression analysis. Factors that significantly influenced ($p < 0.05$) the composite scores are shown in *Table 18.3*. The analysis revealed that disability and fatigue were significantly associated with physical problems (PCS), while mental health (MCS) was mainly influenced by anxiety and depression.

Table 18.2   Characteristics of patients at baseline in the Rome study.

	Hospital patients (n = 68)	Hospital-at-home patients (n = 133)
Male (%)	30.9	34.6
Female (%)	69.1	65.4
Age (mean, SD)	46.7 (2.2)	47 (10.3)
EDSS (mean, SD)	5.8 (2.2)	6.0 (2.0)
Disease duration (mean, SD)	18.6 (11.1)	18.4 (9.5)
Disease type (%)		
Relapsing–remitting	20.6	19.6
Primary progressive	20.6	20.5
Secondary progressive	58.8	59.9
FIM (mean, SD)	87.3 (28.6)	87.4 (27.7)
MMSE (mean, SD)	27 (4.5)	27.8 (3.1)

SD: standard deviation; FIM: Functional Independence Measure; MMSE: Mini-Mental State Examination.

Table 18.3   Multivariate regression analysis showing the variables that significantly influenced ($p < 0.05$) the quality of life measured by SF-36 in the Rome study.

	Covariate	β-Coefficient	p
Physical health composite score	Fatigue (FSS)	−0.11	0.04
	EDSS	−3.66	0.0001
Mental health composite score	Anxiety (STAI)	−0.32	0.001
	Depression (CDQ)	−0.25	0.01

FSS: Fatigue Severity Score; EDSS: Expanded Disability Status Score; STAI: State Trait Anger Inventory; CDQ: Clinical Depression Questionnaire.

Interventions

Between January 1996 and May 1998, 1069 requests of interventions from hospital-at-home patients were recorded. Only 6% of these were defined as 'urgent' (requiring attention within 4 hours of the call), 52% of home visits could be delayed, and an 'over-the-phone' intervention by the team specialist solved 42% of the calls. The distribution of interventions among the different specialists is shown in *Figure 18.2*. Intervention by the psychologist, physiotherapist and nurse was always part of short-term 'home treatment'.

Satisfaction questionnaire

A satisfaction questionnaire was mailed to the patients discharged from hospital-at-home scheme; the questionnaire (five sections, 21 individual items) was anonymous and was

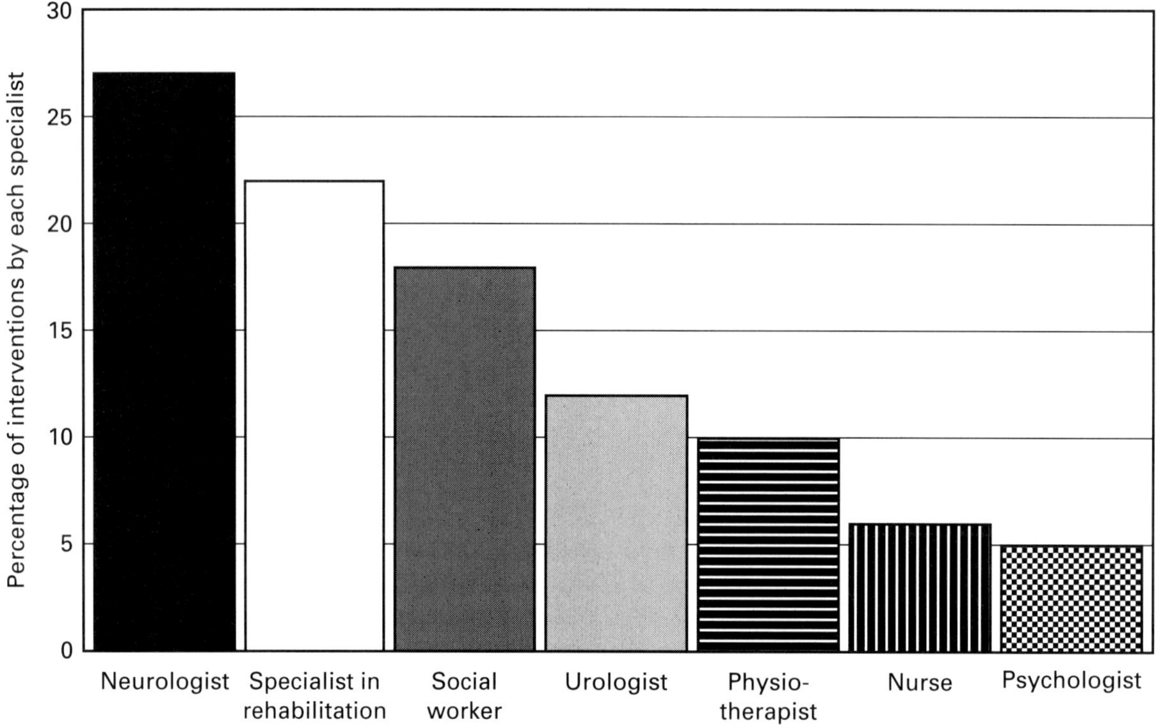

Figure 18.2 Distribution of interventions (n = 1069) among the various specialists in the Rome study.

filled by the patients or their caregivers. By May 1998, 80 questionnaires had been filled and posted back.

The survey showed that 94% of patients used the hospital-at-home care service whereas 6% didn't. The reason why patients did not use the service was:

(a) there was no need (65%);
(b) they preferred to be visited by other physicians (14%); and
(c) they did not know that they could (21%).

The quality and efficiency of the multidisciplinary team was considered to be of a high standard, as shown in *Table 18.4*, even though 61% of patients needed to contact other specialists: dentist (57%), ophthalmologist (48%), gynaecologist (35%), cardiologist (26%) and others (48%).

Finally, 18.3% of patients believed that professionals should visit the patients on call only, whereas 81.7% of them would prefer receiving home care visit on an established, regular basis. Finally, the need for a permanent programme of home care was reported by 96% of patients.

Table 18.4   Quality and efficiency of service (% of patients expressing satisfaction) in the Rome study.

Usefulness of central telephone number	98.6%
Efficiency of the team	90%
Neurologist	96%
Specialist in rehabilitation	93%
Physiotherapist	90%
Psychologist	89%
Urologist	85%
Social worker	82%
Nurse	80%

CONCLUSIONS

Hospital-at-home schemes are a popular alternative to standard hospital care, but there is uncertainty about their cost effectiveness. Any models of hospital-at-home scheme should be analysed for their effectiveness and efficiency from at least three points of view: the consumers' (patients and caregivers), the policymakers' and the service providers'.

A preliminary analysis of the satisfaction questionnaire sent to the patients or their caregivers in the Rome study indicate that they were quite satisfied and strongly favour the continuation of the home-care service. However, greater levels of patient satisfaction did not lead to improved health outcome. Patients with a strong preference for hospital care may have declined to enter the study and patients could be admitted to the scheme only if they agreed to be randomized.

Some interesting observations stem from looking at the different professionals requested by patients. The neurologist was not the unique 'key actor' in this hospital-at-home scheme, since other specialists also played an important role. It is worth mentioning the role of the social worker, who was often asked to provide information and help about social security, bureaucratic issues and daily life problems. A remarkable amount of work was performed by the psychologist, whose interventions were directed, in some cases, not only towards the patient but to the patient's family as well.

The very small number of requests with 'emergency' characteristics points to another feature of this experience, which may be relevant to future programs: a 24-hour-a-day service is not needed for this patient population, with a remarkable saving in costs.

Hospital-at-home schemes potentially provide care to patients who would otherwise not be receiving health-care services. The authors observed that there were situations in which the hospital-at-home scheme was the only way of reaching chronically severely disabled patients who were no longer used to ask for medical care. In these cases, one should take into account that the availability of the multidisciplinary team is likely to result in a sudden increase in needs for these people and, consequently, in a potentially sharp increase in health-care costs.

ACKNOWLEDGMENTS

We thank Dr G Ristori, A Mancini, C Gasperini, T Koudriavtseva, E Frascaro, D Di Diego, S Gagliarducci, M Ricci, S Leoncini, P Di Giuseppe, T Corliano and F Cipriani, A Bracci of the Roman Home Care Multiple Sclerosis Group for their contribution. The research has been supported by the Italian Federation of MS (Trenta ore per la vita) and the Istituto Superiore di Sanità.

REFERENCES

1. August DA, Faubion WC, Ryan ML et al. A clinician-driven home care delivery system. *Cancer* 1993; **72**: 3542–3547.
2. Shaughnessy PW, Kramer AM. The increased needs of patients in nursing homes and patients receiving home health care. *N Engl J Med* 1990; **322**: 21–75.
3. Hollingworth W, Todd C, Parker M et al. Cost analysis of early discharge after hip fracture. *Br Med J* 1993; **307**: 903–906.
4. Shepperd S, Harwood D, Jenkinson C et al. Randomised control trial comparing hospital at home care with inpatient hospital care. I. Three month follow up of health outcome. *Br Med J* 1998; **316**: 1786–1791.
5. Richards SH, Coast J, Gunnell DJ et al. Randomised control trial comparing effectiveness and acceptability of an early discharge, hospital at home scheme with acute hospital care. *Br Med J* 1998; **316**: 1796–1801.
6. Coast J, Richards SH, Peters TJ et al. Hospital at home or acute hospital care? A cost minimization analysis. *Br Med J* 1998; **316**: 1802–1806.
7. Shepperd S, Harwood D, Jenkinson C et al. Randomised control trial comparing hospital at home care with inpatient hospital care. II. Cost minimisation analysis. *Br Med J* 1998; **316**: 1791–1796.
8. Weinshenker BG, Bass B, Rice GPA et al. The natural history of multiple sclerosis: a geografically based study. *Brain* 1989; **112**: 133–146.

9. Poser S, Kurztke JF, Poser W et al. Survival in multiple sclerosis. *J Clin Epidemiol* 1989; **42**: 159–168.

10. Blumhardt LD, Wood C. The economics of multiple sclerosis: a cost of illness study. *Br J Med Economics* 1996; **10**: 99–118.

11. Spilker B, ed. *Quality of Life Assessment in Clinical Trials*. New York: Raven Press, 1990.

12. Ware JE, Sherbourne CD. The SF-36 health status survey. I. Conceptual framework and item selection. *Med Care* 1992; **30**: 473.

13. Ware JE, Kosinki M, Keller SD. *SF-36 Physical and Mental Health Summary Scales: a User's Manual*. Boston, Massachussetts: The Health Institute, New England Medical Center, 1994.

14. Aronson KJ. Quality of life among persons with multiple sclerosis and their caregivers. *Neurology* 1997; **48**: 74–80.

15. Cella DF, Dineen K, Arnason B et al. Validation of the Functional Assessment of Multiple Sclerosis quality of life instrument. *Neurology* 1996; **47**: 129–139.

16. Lankhorst GJ, Jelles F, Smiths RCF et al. Quality of life in multiple sclerosis: the disability and impact profile (DIP). *J Neurol* 1996; **243**: 469–474.

17. Vickrey BG, Hays RD, Harooni R et al. A health-related quality of life measure for multiple sclerosis. *Quality Life Res* 1995; **4**: 187–206.

18. Hermann BP, Vickrey B, Hays RD et al. A comparison of health related quality of life in patients with epilepsy, diabetes and multiple sclerosis. *Epilepsy Res* 1996; **25**: 113–118.

19. Rothwell PM, McDowell Z, Wong CK et al. Doctors and patients don't agree: cross sectional study of patients and doctors' perceptions and assessments of disability in multiple sclerosis. *Br Med J* 1997; **314**: 1580–1583.

20. Kurtzke J. Rating neurological impairment in multiple sclerosis: an Expended Disability Status Scale (EDSS). *Neurology* 1983; **33**: 1444–1452.

21. Folstein M, Folstein S, McHugh PR. Mini mental state: a practical method of grading the cognitive state of patients for the clinicians. *J Psychiatry Res* 1975; **12**: 189–198.

22. Raven JC. *Standard Progressive Matrices: sets A, B, C, D and E*. London: HK Lewis, 1938.

23. Kidd D, Stewart G, Baldry J et al. The Functional Independence Measure: a comaprative validity and reliability study. *Disability Rehabil* 1995; **17**: 10–14.

24. Krupp LB, La Rocca NC, Muir-Nash J et al. The Fatigue Severity Scale applied to patients with multiple sclerosis and systemic lupus erythematosus. *Arch Neurol* 1989; **46**: 1121–1123.

25. Pilowski I, Spence ND. Patterns of Illness Behaviour in patients with intractable pains. *J Psychosom Res* 1975; **19**: 299.

26. Spielberger CD. *Manual for the Stait-Trait Anger Inventory*. Palo Alto: Consulting Psychologist Press, 1983.

27. Spielberger CD, Vagg PR, Barker LR et al. The factor structure of State-Trait Anxiety Inventory. In: Saranson IG, Spielberger CD, eds. *Stress and Anxiety*, vol 7. New York: Hemisfere–Wiley, 1980.

28. Krugg SE, Scheier JH, Cattell RB. *Handbook for the IPAT Anxiety Scale*. Champaign, Illinois: IPAT, 1976.

29. McNair DM, Lorr M. Droppleman LF. *Manual for the Profile of Mood States*. San Diego, California: ITS Educational and Industrial Testing Service, 1981.

19

The Multiple Sclerosis National Competence Centre: the Norwegian approach to improved multiple sclerosis care and research

Rune Midgard

INTRODUCTION

Professor GH Monrad-Krohn, known for his textbook *The Clinical Examination of the Nervous System*,[1] was born in Bergen in Norway. He was the first head of Department of Neurology in Haukeland Hospital; the department opened in 1952. He proposed the establishment of a multiple sclerosis (MS) research unit in Bergen in 1953, but this idea was never realised. A hospital-based epidemiological study[2] during the late 1940s was the first to describe the geographical distribution of MS in Norway. AG Frøvig and J Presthus conducted the first studies on the epidemiology of MS in western Norway in the 1950s and the 1960s.[3,4]

With the Danish MS Registry[5,6] as a model, three prominent Norwegian neurologists proposed the establishment of a national registry of MS in Norway in 1960. The Director General of Health was positive, but for some unknown reason this registry was never established. Several epidemiological studies[7] in different counties of Norway have been performed since the early studies on MS, and these represent our basic epidemiological knowledge.

Infectious medicine, immunological research and neuroimmunological research have had a strong tradition in Bergen[8] ever since the discovery by Armauer Hansen of the leprosy bacil-

lus in 1884.[9] When a neuroimmunological research laboratory within the Department of Neurology was established in 1972, research took a new step forward; efforts were concentrated on myasthenia gravis and demyelinating diseases.

In 1992, the Norwegian Neurological Association suggested the establishment of two national MS centres in Norway in order to strengthen MS research, treatment and patient management in Norway. The two national MS lay organizations supported this idea, and during the next 4 years the plans gradually materialized and public funding was secured. After evaluating applications from three Norwegian university clinics, the Ministry of Health and Social Affairs concluded, in early July 1996, that the new MS centre should be established at the Department of Neurology, Haukeland Hospital.

WHAT IS A NATIONAL COMPETENCE CENTRE?

According to the Ministry of Health and Social Affairs, the main responsibility of the MS National Competence Centre should be to contribute to research, supervision and education among doctors and other health care profession-

<table>
<tr><td>

Table 19.1 Guidelines from the Norwegian Ministry of Health and Social Affairs for the MS National Competence Centre in Bergen, Norway.

1. Establish clinical guidelines and arrange post-graduate courses for doctors and other health-care professionals in Norway
2. Provide structured and updated information to patients and the public
3. Organize and facilitate national clinical research networks
4. Perform basic research and establish international collaborations

</td></tr>
</table>

als in Norway (*Table 19.1*). Specific patient treatment and management as previously will be given in the neurological wards and outpatient clinics around the country. When establishing the centre, a simple questionnaire was sent to Norwegian neurology departments, MS institutions and lay MS organizations asking their opinion of what the main tasks of a national MS competence centre ought to be. The results of this inquiry are shown in *Table 19.2*.

As an extension of the MS Centre, the Norwegian parliament in June 1996 demanded that the Government establish a national MS registry connected to the MS National Competence Centre. The Ministry of Health and Social Affairs approved this proposal in November 1997, and provided public funding in June 1998. The Data Inspectorate, an independent administrative body under the Ministry of Justice, approved and granted the licence to establish a computerized personal data register containing sensitive personal data in October 1998 (*Table 19.3*). The basic requirement laid down by the parliament, the national health authorities and the Data Inspectorate is that all the patients registered in the MS Registry must give their signed, informed consent.

Table 19.2 Questionnaire sent to Norwegian neurology departments, MS institutions and lay MS organizations, with responses, before the establishment of the MS National Competence Centre in Bergen. The response rate was 18 out of 35 (51.4%).

What is in your opinion the main task for the MS National Competence Centre?	
Continuous education of health care professionals around the country	94.4%
Basic research, clinical research and college research supervision	77.8%
Structured and updated information to patients and the public	33.3%
Traditional clinical work	5.6%
Should the MS Centre initiate systematic registration of patients?	
Yes	94.4%
No	5.6%
In what form should in your opinion information and teaching be given?	
Written material	94.4%
Oral presentations, lectures etc.	5.6%
Should the MS Centre initiate and organize educational meetings, workshops, courses etc.?	
General educational courses and meetings	72.2%
Seminars with specific topics	27.8%

Table 19.3 The National Multiple Sclerosis Registry: form of registration

1–5   1   2   3   4   5
Registration Number
Name (capital letters)
6–16   6   7   8   9   10   11   12   13   14   15   16
11-digit personal number
17   17
Sex (1 = Man, 2 = Woman)
18–21   18   19   20   21
Post code of present address
22–25   22   23   24   25
Municipality code of present address
26–29   26   27   28   29
Post code of place of birth
30–33   30   31   32   33
Municipality code of place of birth
34–37   34   35   36   37
Year of onset of MS
38–41   38   39   40   41
Post code of address at date of onset of MS
42–45   42   43   44   45
Municipality code of address at date of onset of MS
46–49   46   47   48   49
Year of diagnosis of MS
50–53   50   51   52   53
Post code of address at date of diagnosis of MS
54–57   54   55   56   57
Municipality code of address at date of diagnosis of MS
58   58
Education (1 = 9 years of school; 2 = 9–12 years; 3 = 12–15 years; 4 = >15 years
59–62   59   60   61   62
MS in the family*
63–72   63   64   65   66   67   68   69   70   71   72
Symptoms at onset (maximum 5)†
73–76   73   74   75   76
Diagnostic procedure (1 = clinical examination; 2 = magnetic resonance imaging; 3 = cerebrospinal fluid examination;
4 = evoked responses; 9 = not done)
77   77
MS category (1 = CD-MS; 2 = LSD-MS; 3 = CP-MS; 4 = LSP-MS; 5 = possible)
78   78
Course of disease (1 = RR; 2 = SP; 3 = PP)
Who made the diagnosis (capital letters)?
79–82   79   80   81   82
Where was the diagnosis made (institution code)?
83   83
Diseases in the family (1 = cerebrovascular disease; 2 = autoimmune disease; 3 = allergic conditions)
84   84
Written report (1 = Yes; 2 = No)
85–91   85   86   87   88   89   90   91
EDSS (month and year)   ,
92   92
Immunomodulating treatment (1 = Yes; 2 = No)
Which drug (capital letters)?
93–98   93   94   95   96   97   98
When was treatment started (month and year)?

* First digit: 1 in first generation (parents of the afflicted); 2 in second generation (afflicted and siblings); 3 in third generation (children of the afflicted). Second digit: 1 afflicted; 2 not afflicted. Third and fourth digits: lowest non-paired number is the older man, lowest paired number is the older woman.
† 01 = Optical neuritis; 02 = Diplopia; 03 = Vertigo; 04 = Facial paresis; 05 = Sensory symptoms; 06 = Limb paresis; 07 = Bladder dysfunction; 08 = Trigeminal neuralgia; 09 = Ataxia; 10 = Dysarthria; 11 = Other (specify).

EVIDENCE-BASED MEDICINE, CRITICAL ANALYTICAL APPROACH AND THE COCHRANE COLLABORATION

The centre intends to include a critical analytical approach[10] in its strategy. This is especially important at a time when governments in many of the world's developed countries are contemplating changes in the delivery of health care. More than ever, physicians and medical scientists need to cultivate a critical approach to medicine.

Both established clinical practice and new investigative or therapeutic procedures require repeated appraisal of their utility by analytic studies that employ appropriate end-points or objectives. A critical approach to the subject, however, does more than encourage safe, effective and cost-efficient medical practice; it is central to the advance of medicine in general and of neurology in particular.

An important part of critical and evidence-based medicine is the work of the many volunteers taking part in the international Cochrane Collaboration under the motto *Preparing, maintaining and disseminating systematic reviews of the effects of health care.*

THE COCHRANE MS REVIEW GROUP

Health-care professionals, consumers, researchers and policy makers are overwhelmed with unmanageable amounts of information. In an influential book published in 1972,[11] Archie Cochrane, a British epidemiologist, drew attention to our great collective ignorance about the effects of health care. He recognized that people who want to make more informed decisions about health care do not have ready access to the available evidence. In 1979, he wrote:[12] 'It is surely a great criticism of our profession that we have not organized a critical summary, by specialty or subspecialty, adapted periodically, of all relevant randomized controlled trials.'

The Cochrane Collaboration has evolved rapidly since it was inaugurated at the 1st colloquium organized as a meeting by the New York Academy of Sciences,[13] but its basic objectives and principles have remained the same as they were at its inception. It is an international organization that aims to help people to make well-informed decisions about health care by preparing, maintaining and ensuring the accessibility of systematic reviews of the effects of health-care interventions. The Collaboration is built on eight values: collaboration, building on the enthusiasm of individuals, avoiding duplication, minimizing bias, keeping up to date, ensuring relevance, ensuring access and continually improving the quality of its work.

After a few preparatory meetings at congresses around the world, a Cochrane MS Review Group was established, and the application for participation in the international Cochrane Collaboration was approved in December 1997. The editorial base has been set up at the Laboratory of Neuroepidemiology, Istituto Nazionale Neurologico Carlo Besta in Milan, Italy; the editorial group consists of Graziella Filippini, Massimo Filippi, George Rice, Alan J Thompson and Bernhard Uitdehaag.

The members of the review group are presently working on systematic review protocols on interferons, corticosteroids and 4-aminopyridine in MS. The first Cochrane protocol dealing with MS and corticosteroids has been published.[14] The systematic review is underway. All the reviews will eventually appear in the Cochrane Library, which is published quarterly on CD-ROM and on the Internet. One of the neurologists at the MS National Competence Centre participates in the Cochrane MS Review Group as a reviewer. The MS Centre will apply evidence-based medicine as a general principle for the approach towards interventions in MS in the future.

THE WORLD WIDE WEB

In order to fulfil the demands from the Ministry of Health, Norwegian website[15] for professionals, patients and the public has been established. This includes updated practical guidelines for newly diagnosed patients. On this home page are included links to inter-

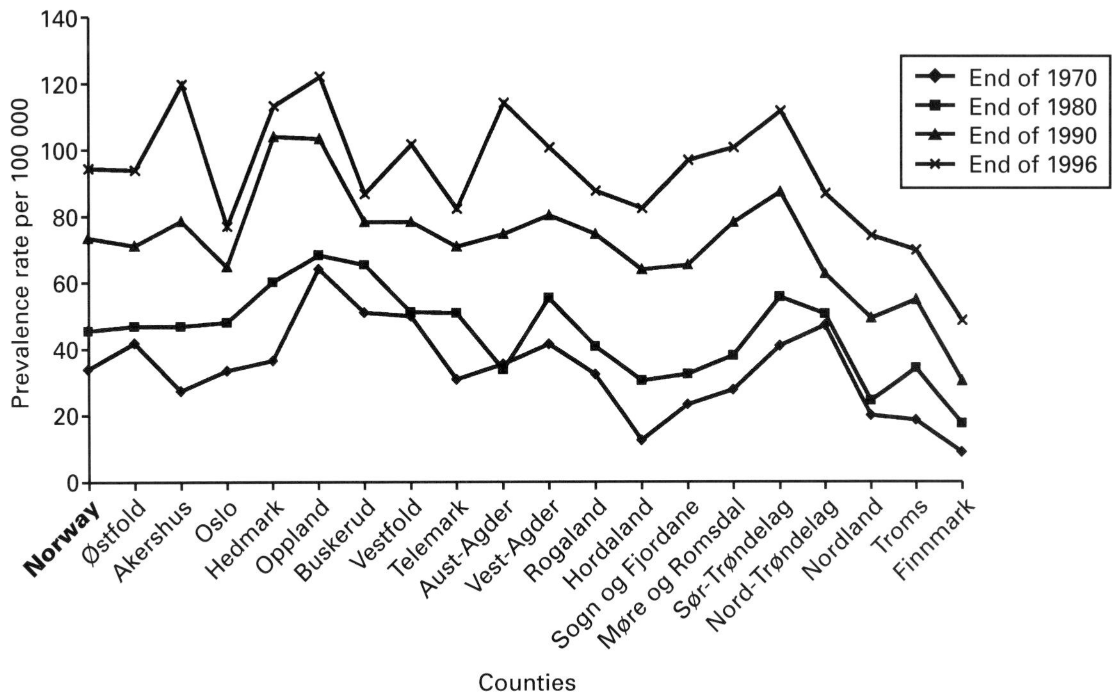

Figure 19.1 MS-specific disability pension prevalence rates per 100 000 in Norway by county (1970, 1980, 1990 and 1996).

national websites in different languages, with a particular link to the much awarded website of the International Federation of MS Societies (*The World of MS*),[16] which even features Norwegian translations among many other languages. This website is updated on a weekly basis, and it is also possible to subscribe to regular weekly news bulletins from the webmaster of this site.

MAIN RESEARCH AREAS

National epidemiology and population-based clinical research

The lack of understanding of the nature of possible environmental factors demands an open mind. Increasing rates in prevalence,[17,18] incidence[19] and mortality[20] in Norway have been observed, and the implications of these observations are too important to ignore.

MS-specific disability pension prevalence rates and MS-specific crude annual mortality rates in Norway are shown in *Figs 19.1* and *19.2*, illustrating the trend in the period from 1966 to 1996. The distribution pattern is fairly consistent throughout this period, with a steadily increasing tendency with time in the country as a whole and in each county separately.

Studies[19,21] indicate that the disability and mortality statistics capture approximately 60% of all people with MS in a society. Thus, with 4157 disability pension recipients by the end of 1996, the total MS population in Norway may actually be somewhere between 7000 and 8000 people.

Therefore, the most useful strategy is to develop reference populations, especially in Caucasian-predominant countries, which have stable spider networks and large established populations with a high risk of MS.[22] A continuous

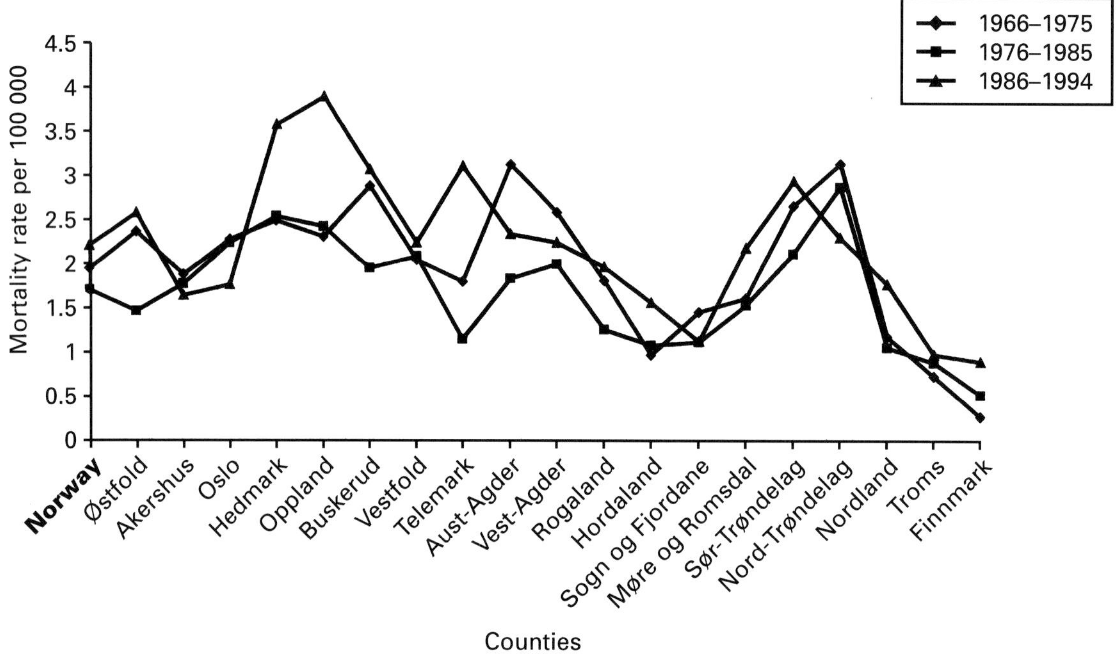

Figure 19.2 MS-specific crude annual mortality rates per 100 000 in Norway by county (1966–1975, 1976–1985, 1986–1994).

surveillance of the incidence of MS in Norway, through the establishment of a national MS registry, is likely to be the most effective of identifying trends of possible importance to the aetiology of MS. When fully developed, a national MS registry will serve as a population base for all kinds of epidemiological and clinical research. The design of prospective studies comprising different kinds of intervention will be possible, and the registry will also be well suited for natural history studies.

International epidemiology

In collaboration with colleagues from Sweden, Russia and Italy the MS Centre has developed an international research project that is partly epidemiological, partly genetic. The main objective of the study—'Genetic and exogenous factors of multiple sclerosis susceptibility: from Scandinavia and Mediterranean to Central Russia and Siberia'—is to analyse both genetic and environmental factors contributing to a susceptibility to MS in populations living in geographically different regions of Europe and Asia (Scandinavia, the Apennines, Central Russia, the Ural Mountains and western Siberia). An application for funding has been sent to the International Association for the Promotion of Co-operation with Scientists from the New Independent States of the former Soviet Union.

In collaboration with the Centre for International Health at the University of Bergen the researchers at the MS Centre are working on a project with professor Redda Tekla-Haimanot at the University of Ethiopia, Addis Ababa entitled 'Comparative studies on genetics and environmental factors in Ethiopia and Norway'.

Basic seroepidemiological studies on blood donors in Norway and Ethiopia are performed to look at various immunological and genetic aspects of MS. At the same time a project on MS epidemiology is being developed, based on the fact that MS is a very rare disease in Ethiopia. Professor Haimanot has seen four or five cases during the past 15 years of working in a large referral hospital.

The population in Ethiopia is approximately 58 million with a pyramidal age distribution and a life expectancy lower than 50 years. In a door-to-door survey of 60 000 people in rural Ethiopia south of Addis Ababa based on a random sample of a total of 250 000 people, no MS cases were found.[23,24] The main findings in this survey looking for neurological disorders in rural Ethiopia were epilepsy, followed by polio and several diseases with spastic paraspareses. The main aetiologies behind the parapareses were neurolathyrism,[25] tropical spastic paraparesis (associated with human T leukaemia virus type 1) and cervical myelopathies secondary to fluorosis (with toxic or mechanical aetiologies). The population pyramid based on the 1989 Ethiopian census shows almost 1 million men and 1 million women in each age segment from 20 to 50 years; thus there should be a possibility of finding some MS patients in this population. One approach might be to take a closer clinical look, including cerebrospinal fluid analyses, at the selection of patients with paraparesis of various aetiologies. There may be some MS patients wrongly diagnosed in this cohort.

An authorized Locus on Registry Epidemiology

The MS National Competence Centre and the National MS Registry are part of an authorized Locus on Registry Epidemiology within the Faculty of Medicine, University of Bergen. The Locus authorization carries the following institutional commitments:

(a) to provide the best possible conditions for a research group to concentrate on advanced, comprehensive scientific work within a specified research area;

(b) to provide stability for the group over a 10-year period, including expansion and replacement of scientific staff and other personnel.

(c) to facilitate applications for funding, and secure the receipt of research grants, national and international, in accordance with conditions set forth by the financing institutions (this includes formal negotiations and contracts, if required);

(d) to enjoy basic funding and other assistance, including salaries for key personnel, equipment and running costs;

(e) to provide proper working space in collaboration with the University of Bergen and the Haukeland University Hospital; and

(f) to assist in problem solving when considered necessary or when required by a relevant party, which may approach the Faculty of Medicine on such matters.

Present partners are the Medical Birth Registry, the Norwegian Arthroplasty Register, the Norwegian Kidney Biopsy Register, The Health Surveillance in Hordaland, the Patient Registry for Cardiovascular and Cerebrovascular Diseases in Health Region III, the Norwegian Centre for Securing Quality of Laboratory Analyses outside Hospitals, and the Division for Occupational Medicine in Department of Public Health and Primary Health Care at the University of Bergen.

Neuropathology

In a recent publication,[26] which was subject to much attention at scientific conferences on MS in 1998, axonal transection in acute demyelinating lesions in multiple sclerosis is described. It is proposed that axonal transection may be the pathological correlate of the irreversible neurological impairment in this human disease. Although this knowledge is not entirely new,[27] this study, which is based on the access to human brain material, modern immunohistochemical staining techniques and confocal microscopy, sheds new light on the basic pathogenic mechanisms in MS.[28] The axonal loss visualized in this study challenges the traditional view that T-cell-mediated inflammation is the primary event in the pathogenesis of MS. The study thus contributes to a more heterogeneous, complementary picture of a complex process, recognizing that MS is in part an axonal disease (as mentioned by Charcot in his early descriptions[29,30]).

Two of the authors of this paper[26] (Sverre Mørk and Lars Bø) are closely associated with the MS National Competence Centre. They are presently applying the above-mentioned techniques on new brain material, pursuing the concept of axonal loss. By the use of these methods, early demyelination in the rather marginal amount of myelin in the cerebral cortex has been observed recently. A local brain bank established at the Department of Pathology provides the researchers with the necessary human material.

Neuroimmunology and genetics

The clinical and laboratory research in Bergen has covered many different aspects of MS research. The researchers have thus participated in building up the many-faceted research competence available in Bergen, and all of them are part of the Haukeland MS network.

The basic neuroimmunological research in this network and through several international collaboration projects has focused on numerous immunological[31–35] and serological[36–38] parameters over the years. The published papers comprise studies on Fc receptors, complement factors and receptors, and viral serology. Several studies are under way, and in connection with the establishment of the MS Centre, more public funding for basic research has become available. Approximately 500 000 Norwegian kroner were spent on equipment and reagents to update and optimize the research laboratory facilities during 1997.

In the future the established research projects will be pursued, with an emphasis on the immunoglobulin receptor research owing to the wide variety of functions that these receptors have in the pathogenesis of the disease. Their potential role in future therapy is also a motivation for this research focus.

Neuroimaging and functional MRI magnetic resonance imaging

A recently published study[39] on serial monthly magnetization transfer suggested that changes in the normal-appearing white matter of patients with MS occur before lesions become evident on conventional magnetic resonance imaging (MRI) scans. Using modern imaging sequences, some researchers[40] have also reported a weak but statistically significant correlation between cortical lesions as visualized in the FLAIR (fluid-attenuated inversion recovery) sequence and cognitive dysfunctions as evaluated with a standardized battery of neuropsychological tests. Early results also suggest that functional MRI is a method that can be used to study cognitive function in MS.[41] An MRI sequence comprising diffusion-weighted images[42] is also a tool developed to improve our understanding of diffusion processes in MS lesions. Prospective studies on newly diagnosed MS patients are being developed in which it is intended to include sequential imaging studies focusing on the events at the blood–brain barrier.

The dietary approach

Through collaboration with the Norwegian University of Science and Technology in Trondheim, a small, open, uncontrolled pilot study consisting of dietary advice and intervention with cod liver oil (omega-3 fatty acids) has been performed. After 2 years of observations, the effects seem rather promising clinically and biochemically. Researchers at the MS Centre are therefore in the process of expanding the approach with dietary intervention to a randomized, placebo-controlled double-blind study with clinical status, sequential MRI and serum analyses of omega-3 and omega-6 fatty acids as outcome measures.

Health economics

In the current economic climate the cost effectiveness of a treatment is almost as important as its clinical efficacy. The cost of any treatment should be considered against the total cost of the disease. The studies looking at the cost of MS conclude that the indirect costs far outweigh the direct costs.[43,44] The reduction of the quality of life is always difficult to estimate in terms of cost. Based on the available figures, the cost of illness for MS in Norway in 1994 was calculated to be higher than 1 billion Norwegian kroner.[45] The cost of saving 1 quality-adjusted life year for a Norwegian MS patient is (according to a cost–utility analysis) more than 240 000 Norwegian kroner. Any new treatment needs to be evaluated against such figures and the effects on the disability and prognosis of MS must be documented.

In collaboration with the Department of Finance and Management Science at the Norwegian School of Economics and Business Administration in Bergen, researchers at the MS Centre will continue the health economy research, focusing on cost of illness and cost–utility analyses, thereby trying to penetrate the true cost of MS.

THE NATIONAL NETWORK AND QUALITY STANDARDS

The MS Centre has recently established a network of neurologists experienced in the management of MS patients and devoted to different kinds of MS research. The members of the group have started working on a booklet (*Guidelines in the Diagnosis, Treatment and General Management of MS*). This booklet will be distributed among neurologists and specialist candidates in Norway, and will be available to other health care professionals in the country. The Norwegian Neurological Association con-

tributes to the financing of the booklet. The intention is also to develop a basic information brochure on MS aiming at general practitioners. It is of utmost importance to maintain and strengthen this network of neurologists in the future.

In addition researchers at the MS Centre would like to make connections with other research groups in Norway and abroad working with MS, and in this way contribute to the advance of research and scientific development. The MS Centre is in the process of planning an electronic Norwegian MS Network.

THE PRESENT STAFF

The present staff at the MS centre includes two doctors, a sociologist, a registered nurse and a research laboratory technician. There is one more position, which will be used to employ different kinds of professionals, full time or part time, depending on the ongoing projects. There is an annual budget of approximately 2.7 million Norwegian kroner. The National MS Registry was granted a starting budget in 1998 of 1.4 million Norwegian kroner. This sum includes money for the salaries of key personnel and for equipment and running costs. The key personnel will include an epidemiologist or statistician, a computer engineer and clerical staff.

REFERENCES

1. Monrad-Krohn GH. *The Clinical Examination of the Nervous System*, 1st edn. London: HK Lewis, 1921.
2. Swank RL, Lerstad O, Strøm A, Backer J. Multiple sclerosis in rural Norway. *N Engl J Med* 1952; **246**: 721–728.
3. Frøvig AG, Presthus J, Sponheim N. The significance of allergy in the etiology and pathogenesis of multiple sclerosis. A clinical study. *Acta Neurol Scand* 1967; **43**: 215–227.
4. Presthus J. Report on the multiple sclerosis investigations in West Norway. *Acta Psychiatr Neurol Scand* 1960; **35**(suppl 147): 88–92.

5. Koch-Henriksen N, Hyllested K. Epidemiology of multiple sclerosis: incidence and prevalence rates in Denmark 1948–64 based on the Danish Multiple Sclerosis Registry. *Acta Neurol Scand* 1988; **78**: 369–380.

6. Koch-Henriksen N, Brönnum Hansen H, Hyllested K. Incidence of multiple sclerosis in Denmark 1948–1982: a descriptive nationwide study. *Neuroepidemiology* 1992; **11**: 1–10.

7. Midgard R, Riise T, Svanes C, Kvåle G et al. Incidence of multiple sclerosis in Møre and Romsdal, Norway from 1950 to 1991. An age–period-cohort analysis. *Brain* 1996; **119**: 203–211.

8. Aarli JA, Behan WMH, Behan PO, eds. *Clinical Neuroimmunology.* Oxford: Blackwell Scientific, 1987.

9. Hansen GA. Die Aetiologie und Pathologie der Lepra. *Vierteljahresschr Dermatol Syphil* 1884; **11**: 317–336.

10. Aminoff MJ. Criticism in neurology and Medicine. *Neurology* 1994; **44**: 1781–1783.

11. Cochrane AL. *Effectiveness and Efficiency. Random Reflections on Health Services.* London: Nuffield Provincial Hospitals Trust, 1972.

12. Cochrane AL. 1931–1971: a critical review, with particular reference to the medical profession. In: *Medicines for the Year 2000.* London: Office of Health Economics, 1979, 1–11.

13. Chalmers I. The Cochrane Collaboration: preparing, maintaining and disseminating systematic reviews of the effects of health care. In: Warren KS, Mosteller F, eds. Doing more good than harm: the evaluation of health care interventions. *Ann N Y Acad Sci* 1993; **703**: 156–163.

14. Filippini G, Brusaferri L, Sibley WA et al. Corticosteroids or ACTH for acute exacerbations in multiple sclerosis (Protocol for a Cochrane Review). Cochrane Library Issue 2. Oxford: Update Software, 1999.

15. Website: http://www.uib.no/med/ms/

16. Website: http://www.ifmss.org.uk

17. Larsen JP, Aarli JA, Nyland H, Riise T. Western Norway, a high-risk area for multiple sclerosis: a prevalence/incidence study in the county of Hordaland. *Neurology* 1984; **34**: 1202–1207.

18. Midgard R, Riise T, Nyland H. Epidemiologic trends in multiple sclerosis in Møre and Romsdal, Norway: a prevalence/incidence study in a stable population. *Neurology* 1991; **41**: 887–892.

19. Riise T. Is the incidence of multiple sclerosis increasing? In: Thompson AJ, Polman C, Hohlfeld R, eds. *Multiple Sclerosis. Clinical Challenges and Controversies.* 1–12. Martin Dunitz Ltd: London, 1997.

20. Midgard R, Riise T, Kvåle G, Nyland H. Disability and mortality in multiple sclerosis in Western Norway. *Acta Neurol Scand* 1996; **93**: 307–314.

21. Larsen JP, Kvåle G, Aarli JA. Multiple sclerosis and mortality statistics. *Acta Neurol Scand* 1985; **71**: 237–241.

22. Weinshenker BG. Epidemiologic strategies to detect an exogenous cause of MS. *Acta Neurol Scand* 1995; **92**(suppl 161): 93–99.

23. Haimanot RT, Abebe M, Mariam AG et al. Community-based study of neurological disorders in rural central Ethiopia. *Neuroepidemiology* 1990; **9**: 263–277.

24. Haimanot RT, Abebe M, Mariam AG et al. Community-based study of neurological disorders in Ethiopia: development of a screening instrument. *Ethiop Med J* 1990; **28**: 123–137.

25. Haimanot RT, Kidane Y, Wuhib E et al. Lathyrism in rural northwestern Ethiopia: a highly prevalent neurotoxic disorder. *Int J Epidemiol* 1990; **19**: 664–672.

26. Trapp B, Ransohoff R, Rudick R et al. Axonal transection in multiple sclerosis. *N Engl J Med* 1998; **338**: 278–285.

27. McDonald WI, Miller DH, Barnes D. The pathological evolution of multiple sclerosis. *Neuropathol Appl Neurobiol* 1992; **18**: 319–334.

28. Waxman SG. Demyelinating diseases—new pathological insights, new therapeutic targets (editorial). *N Engl J Med* 1998; **338**: 323–325.

29. Charcot JM. Histologie de la sclerose en plaques. *Gazette des Hospitaux Civils et Militaires* 1868; **41**: 554–556.

30. Charcot JM. *Lectures on the Diseases of the Nervous System*, 1st series (translated by G. Sigerson). London: New Sydenham Society, 1877.

31. Nyland H, Matre R, Mørk S. Fc receptors of microglial lipophages in multiple sclerosis. *New Engl J Med* 1980; **302**: 120–121.

32. Vedeler C, Ulvestad E, Nyland H et al. Receptors for gammaglobulin in the central and peripheral nervous system. *J Neurol Neurosurg Psychiatry* 1994; **57**(suppl): 9–10.

33. Vedeler C, Matre R, Sadallah S, Schifferli J. Soluble complement receptor type 1 in serum and cerebrospinal fluid of patients with Guillain–Barré syndrome and multiple sclerosis. *J Neuroimmunol* 1996; **67**: 17–20.

34. Vedeler C, Ulvestad E, Grundt IK et al. Fc-

receptors for IgG (FcR) on rat microglia. *J Neuroimmunol* 1993; **49**: 19–24.

35. Ulvestad E, Williams K, Bø L et al. Fc-receptors for IgG on cultured human microglia mediate cytotoxicity and phagocytosis of antibody-coated targets. *J Neuropathol Exp Neurol* 1994; **53**: 27–36.

36. Myhr KM, Frost P, Grønning M et al. Absence of HTLV-I related sequences in MS from high prevalence areas in Western Norway [Published erratum appears in *Acta Neurol Scand* 1994; **90**: 143]. *Acta Neurol Scand* 1994; **89**: 65–68.

37. Myhr KM, Riise T, Barrett-Connor E et al. Altered antibody pattern to Epstein–Barr virus but not to other herpesviruses in multiple sclerosis: a population based case-control study from western Norway. *J Neurol Neurosurg Psychiatry* 1998; **64**: 539–542.

38. Vaughan JH, Riise T, Rhodes GH et al. An Epstein–Barr virus-related cross reactive autoimmune response in multiple sclerosis in Norway. *J Neuroimmunol* 1996; **69**: 95–102.

39. Filippi M, Rocca MA, Martino G et al. Magnetization transfer changes in the normal appearing white matter precede the appearance of enhancing lesions in patients with multiple sclerosis. *Ann Neurol* 1998; **43**: 809–814.

40. Lazeron RHC, Langdon D, Filippi M et al. Cortical lesions on FLAIR and neurophysiological impairment (The Magnims A.1.2 Study) (abstract). *Multiple Sclerosis* 1998; **4**: 298.

41. Lazeron RHC, Rombouts SARB, Machielsen WCM et al. Functional MRI of two neuropsychological tasks in MS patients; first results (abstract). *Multiple Sclerosis* 1998; **4**: 298.

42. Werring DJ. Diffusion MRI in multiple sclerosis (abstract). *Multiple Sclerosis* 1998; **4**: 281.

43. Jönsson B. The economic cost of multiple sclerosis in Sweden. *EFI Research Paper* no 6551, 1995.

44. Midgard R, Riise T, Nyland H. Impairment, disability and handicap in multiple sclerosis. A cross-sectional study in an incident cohort in Møre and Romsdal County, Norway. *J Neurol* 1996; **243**: 337–344.

45. Fuglset SB, Meling OH. *Kostnader ved multippel sklerose i Norge. En 'cost-of-illness' studie* (dissertation). Bergen: Norges Handelshøyskole, 1996.

20

The characteristics of multiple sclerosis in southern China

Chuan-Zhen Lu

Multiple sclerosis (MS) is a well-known demyelinating disease. In China, MS used to be considered a rare disease, while several cases of optic neuromyelitis (Devic's disease) have presented every year (*Table 20.1*). However, the situation has greatly changed since the 1970s. MS is no longer a rare disease in China, particularly in certain parts of the country. The reason for the increase in the diagnosis of MS may be partly because:

(a) the number of trained neurologists, who are aware of the diagnosis of MS, has greatly increased, because of the many training courses held by neurological centres for doctors from various parts of the country;

(b) newer diagnostic tools, such as magnetic resonance imaging (MRI), cerebrospinal fluid (CSF), electrophoreses or isoelectric focusing, and evoked potentials, have become widely available in China, not only in large city hospitals, but also in county hospitals and district hospitals;

(c) the prevalence of MS has actually been increasing during the past 20 years.

Questions about MS in China include:

(a) Are there any differences in the clinical pictures between Chinese patients and Caucasian patients?

(b) Is the increased prevalence of MS in China associated with any viral infection, particularly with hepatitis B or A virus?

(c) What does the acute form of MS in China represent? Is there any relationship between so called sporadic encephalitis and acute MS?

THE CLINICAL CHARACTERISTICS OF MS IN CHINA

The association between optic neuritis and MS in China is weak. After 10 years of following up 1207 cases with optic neuritis, the author found that 12% (117 patients) developed signs and symptoms from other parts of CNS or recurrent optic neuritis (maybe MS). In comparison with Western countries, the frequency of optic neuritis presenting as the first manifestation of MS is low.

Acute myelitis may also be related to MS. The author followed 230 patients with acute myelitis at the Huashan Hospital for 25 years and found that 10% (24 patients) suffered from recurrent disease and went on to develop neuromyelitis optica. Eleven patients developed typical MS. Transverse myelitis may be another type of demyelinating disease, and not a first symptom of MS or neuromyelitis optica.

Table 20.1   The number of patients with MS and the number of patients with neuromyelitis optica in Huashan Hospital.

Years	Number of patients with MS	Number of patients with neuromyelitis optica
1951–1960	11	17
1961–1970	23	20
1971–1980	41	19
1981–1990	85	16
1991–1997	108	16

Devic's disease is a common form of CNS demyelinating disease in China. However, its prevalence in the last 20 years has not increased. The author analysed the patients who were hospitalized at Huashan Hospital since the 1950s and found that the number of cases of Devic's disease was stable at around 1.5–2.0 cases per year. The number of cases of MS, on the other hand, increased rapidly from one patient per year in the 1950s to 10 patients per year in the 1990s.

Oligoclonal bands of the IgG class were detected in the CSF from only 40–50% of patients with MS. The Neuroimmunology Research Laboratory of the Institute of Neurology. Shanghai Medical University has analysed 290 pairs of CSF and serum samples for oligoclonal bands. IgG bands in CSF were demonstrated in only 40–50% of the patients with MS who were diagnosed on the basis of the Poser criteria[1] and Schumacher criteria.[2] When the IgG index and IgG synthesis rate in the central nervous system (CNS) were analysed, evidence was found for IgG synthesis within the CNS in MS and Guillain–Barré syndrome, but not in neuromyelitis optica. The reasons for these neuroimmunological features remain to be defined.

IS MS ASSOCIATED WITH HEPATITIS VIRUS INFECTION?

As mentioned above, the prevalence of MS in China has increased during the past 20 years. It is also known that about 150 million people in China are carriers of hepatitis B virus (HBV) infection. This virus infection was also first recognized in the 1960s. The amino acid sequence of one fraction of bovine myelin basic protein shares the amino acid sequence with one part of polymerase of HBV. So it may be that MS is related to HBV infection. Therefore, antibodies to hepatitis B surface antigen, hepatitis B_e antigen and hepatitis B core antigen were measured, as were the titres of each of these antigens in the CSF and sera of 23 patients with clinically definite MS, 23 patients with probable MS, 43 patients with other neurological diseases and 34 controls. It was found that antibodies to HBV were present in 78% of patients with definitive MS, in 56% of patients with probable MS and in 30% of controls. The HBV antigens did not show any difference between MS patients and patients with other neurological diseases. The author suggests that MS may be associated with HBV infection.

SOME CASES OF 'SPORADIC ENCEPHALITIS' MAY BE A SPECIAL FORM OF MS

The author has found that 20% of patients with sporadic encephalitis suffer from coma or various degrees of unconsciousness in the acute stage. MRI shows typical features of MS. After 1–2 years of follow-up, patients recover completely, irrespective of whether the MRI still shows the characteristic changes of MS.

Based on these findings, the author suggests several projects comparing MS in Western countries and in China, including the occurrence of clinical features and the relationship with infections, as well as basic research into the neuroimmunological features and a clinical trial including MS patients from multiple centres.

REFERENCES

1. Poser CM, Paty DW, Scheinberg L et al. New diagnostic criteria for multiple sclerosis. *Ann Neurol* 1983; **13**: 227.
2. Schumacher GA, Berbe G, Kibler RF et al. Problems of experimental trials of therapy in multiple sclerosis: Report by the panel on the evaluation of experimental trials of multiple sclerosis. *Ann NY Acad Sci* 1965; **122**: 552.

21

International perspectives on the treatment and care of multiple sclerosis

Jürg Kesselring

The management of patients with multiple sclerosis (MS) has always been a formidable challenge for physicians, therapists and nurses. For a long time, even when the author started to get interested in MS 17 years ago,[1] management of MS consisted mainly of trying to establish the diagnosis as accurately as possible, and after that the patients were left more or less on their own in the care of their relatives. Bed rest, the often-prescribed treatment for exacerbations, could be provided in every hospital and too often just in nursing homes.

The management of MS has changed dramatically in recent years, not least because of the active engagement of patients themselves and their relatives in national and international MS societies: their calls for guidelines concerning diagnosis, treatment and long-term care could not be ignored any more. The development of clinical practice guidelines has become a science of its own[2] and it is very important that they be formulated very carefully and by truly neutral and independent experts,[3] since they should serve not only the patients and their doctors but also third-party payers and insurers.

Using the traditional list of priorities in neurology, criteria for the diagnosis were established first, following various individual attempts. In 1983, the Poser Committee[4] proposed research criteria that are still widely accepted and have been proven to be useful by various studies comparing their relevance to post mortem findings. Recently, Don Paty, who was in the Poser Committee, has added magnetic resonance imaging criteria for the diagnosis, which will prove to be very useful.[5] No one would doubt his authority, but it raises the question as to who is accepted as being an expert and an authority to produce guidelines. Time and the market will determine this.

For more than 15 years the International Federation of Multiple Sclerosis Societies (IFMSS) has had a Medical Management Committee, which has produced a booklet (*Therapeutic Claims in MS*).[6] More than 150 treatment regimens are covered: for each there is a description, a discussion of the rationale for its use and an evaluation of its efficacy, and cost effectiveness and recommendations are given. This publication is widely used, has been constantly updated and has been translated into many languages. The Medical Management Committee of the IFMSS is now under the Chairmanship of Professor Alan Thompson and it was commissioned at the latest meeting of the Medical Advisory Board of the IFMSS in Buenos Aires in 1997 to update its booklet again and also to make the new edition available on the Internet.

The various clinical patterns and the course of MS have been defined at a conference of international experts convened by the National MS Society of the United States, and their publication[7] has made them widely available.

In May 1998, after a state-of-the-art conference jointly organized by the IFMSS and the World Health Organization (WHO),[8] the WHO decided to make multiple sclerosis one of the priorities of its Division of Mental Health and so it set up a Working Group on MS, which has the task of producing guidelines about diagnosis, treatment and long-term care. The members of the Working Group serve on several Committees of the Medical Advisory Board of the IFMSS and thereby guarantee that these guidelines of the WHO Working Group will correspond with the ones of the Medical Management Committee of the IFMSS. The close collaboration with the Division of Mental Health of the WHO has the aim of applying the thoroughly revised version of the International Classification on Impairment, Disability and Handicap (ICDH-2).[9] This implies a major shift of paradigms concerning the consequences of diseases and will require a long-term commitment in research on education on these aspects of MS.

Over the past year, a group of experts with the help of the Lewin Group, a professional organization for elaborating guidelines for various diseases, have produced (by the formal consensus method) guidelines on diagnosis and treatment of relapsing–remitting MS.[10] These guidelines will be considered as forming a basis for the guidelines to be produced by the IFMSS Medical Management Committee and the WHO Working Group, since the exchange of knowledge between them is very generous and unhindered.

In the USA, the MS Council for Clinical Practice Guidelines is supported by the Paralyzed Veterans of America, which has set up several task forces to elaborate guidelines for the management of the common symptoms encountered in MS (e.g. fatigue, spasticity, pain). These guidelines will be published soon and will be widely distributed. The Consortium of MS Centers and its growing European counterpart, Rehabilitation in MS (RIMS), are in close collaboration with the US Council for Clinical Practice Guidelines and are much involved in the preparation of these guidelines.

It seems to be more difficult to provide guidelines about long-term care and rehabilitation for MS patients, since the standards differ more widely between countries. One set of guidelines about rehabilitation in MS has been produced by the Medical Advisory Board of the Swiss MS Society, and it has been distributed in German- and French-speaking countries and will soon be available in English.[12]

It will be a major task for the IFMSS, the WHO Working Group, the Consortium and RIMS to produce such guidelines on long-term management and patient care in MS. The next European Committee for Treatment and Research in MS (ECTRIMS) Congress will be a joint conference with the IFMSS, the American Committee for Treatment and Research in MS (ACTRIMS), RIMS and the Consortium, and will be held in Basel, Switzerland on 12–16 September 1999. This conference should provide a forum for the discussion of such international endeavours under the main heading of this Conference, which will be 'Standards of Care in MS'.

REFERENCES

1. Davison AN, Humphreys JH, Liversedge AL et al. *Multiple Sclerosis Research.* London: Her Majesty's Stationery Office, 1975.
2. Audet AM, Greenfield S, Field M. Medical practice guidelines: current activities and future directions. *Ann Intern Med* 1990; **113**: 709–714.
3. Woolf SH. Practice guidelines, a new reality in medicine. II. Methods of developing guidelines. *Arch Intern Med* 1992; **152**: 946–952.
4. Poser CM, Paty DW, Scheinberg LC et al. New diagnostic criteria for multiple sclerosis: guidelines for research protocols. *Ann Neurol* 1983; **13**: 227–231.
5. Paty DW, Li DKB. Diagnosis of multiple sclerosis 1998: do we need new diagnostic criteria? In: Siva A, Kesselring J, Thompson AJ, eds. *Frontiers in Multiple Sclerosis*, volume 2. London: Martin Dunitz, 1999, 47–50.
6. Sibley WA, the Therapeutic Claims Committee of the IFMSS. *Therapeutic Claims in MS*, 4th edn. The National Multiple Sclerosis Society. New York: Demos, 1996.

7. Lublin FD, Reingold SC. Defining the clinical course of multiple sclerosis. Results of an international survey. *Neurology* 1996; **46**: 907–911.
8. Kesselring J, ed. State of the art conference: key issues in multiple sclerosis today. *Eur J Neurol* 1998; **5**(suppl 2): S1–S51.
9. World Health Organization. *International Classification of Impairments, Activities and Participation 1997.* Geneva: World Health Organization, 1997.
10. Hartung HP, Paty DW, Ebers GC et al. Development of clinical practice guidelines for the management of relapsing–remitting multiple sclerosis. *Multiple Sclerosis* 1998; **4**: 274.
11. Messmer Uccelli M, Shindell S, Miller D. Multiple sclerosis clinical practice guidelines. *Multiple Sclerosis* 1998; **4**: 279.
12. Medical Advisory Board Swiss MS Society. *Rehabilitation und Multiple Sklerose 1997.* Zürich: Schweizerische Multiple Sklerose Gesellschaft, 1997, 1–23.

22

The Canadian experience: Multiple sclerosis clinics versus traditional medical care, and what made multiple sclerosis research flourish in Canada?

Donald W Paty on behalf of the Canadian Network of Multiple Sclerosis Clinics

THE CANADIAN NETWORK OF MULTIPLE SCLEROSIS CLINICS (FROM WEST TO EAST)

Vancouver, British Columbia: Duncan Anderson, Virginia Devonshire, Kathy Eisen, Stan Hashimoto, John Hooge, Lorne Kastrukoff, Janette Lindley, Joël Oger, Donald Paty, Elaine Price, Dessa Sadovnick
Calgary, Alberta: Robert Bell, David Patry, Donald McGowan, Luanne Metz, William Murphy, Michael Yeung (previously Peter Seland)
Edmonton, Alberta: Kenneth Warren, Sharon Warren
Saskatoon, Saskatchewan: Walter Hader
Winnipeg, Manitoba: Anthony Auty, Christopher Power
Ottawa, Ontario: Mark Freedman, Robert Nelson
Toronto, Ontario: Trevor Gray, Paul O'Connor
Kingston, Ontario: Donald Brunet
Hamilton, Ontario: Rick Paulseth
London, Ontario: George Ebers, George Rice (previously John Noseworthy, Brian Weinshenker, Tom Feasby)
Montreal, Quebec (Montreal Neurological Institute): Jack Antel, Doug Arnold, William Barkas, Gordon Francis, Yves Lapierre, Dianne Lowden
Montreal, Quebec (Hôpital Notre Dame): Pierre Duquette, Renée Dubois, Josée Poirier
Quebec City, Quebec: Jean-Pierre Bouchard, Manon Thibault
Halifax, Nova Scotia: Verinder Bhan, Chuck Maxner, Jock Murray
St John's, Newfoundland: William Pryse-Phillip

HISTORY OF MULTIPLE SCLEROSIS CLINICS IN CANADA

The first Canadian multiple sclerosis (MS) clinic was established in 1954 or so by Dr Bert Cosgrove and Dr Roy Swank at the Montreal Neurological Institute (MNI). For years Dr Cosgrove ran the clinic by himself, and he helped to establish a focus of interest in MS research at the MNI.[1]

In 1972, Don Paty started an MS clinic in London, Ontario, recognizing the need for a well-documented, prospectively followed group of patients that could be used for clinical research. In addition, an advisory committee on MS research[2] recommended that there was an urgent need for additional clinical MS centres. These recommendations envisaged the development of clinical centres in order to gain meaningful data on a large number of patients. The plan to develop clinical centres was supported as follows: 'to accomplish these purposes, it is proposed that clinical centres, geographically dispersed, be established'. Another comment of the advisory committee was that this concept was of particular 'importance' that could not be overstressed.

George Ebers joined the MS clinic in London, Ontario in 1977. George Rice joined him in 1984. Since that time, both of these neurologists have had a major influence on the conduct of MS research in Canada. Others involved were Tom Feasby, John Noseworthy and Brian Weinshenker.

During the 1970s and 1980s there were a number of meetings sponsored by the MS Society of Canada concerning the organization of clinics (McIlroy W; personal communication, 1998). There was a nation-wide meeting in Calgary, Alberta on 10 December 1974 regarding the need for a clinical registry of MS patients. The concept of a common protocol for future clinical studies was discussed at that time.

On 8 July 1976, the MS Research Clinic in Calgary (Peter Seland) was supported with a start-up grant from the MS Society of Canada. That grant was made on the basis of 'Guidelines recommended by the Society Symposium on Clinics' held in 1976. On 7 June 1979, the MS Society of Canada committed itself to supporting both basic and clinical research activities with the following statement: [We supported] 'the establishment of a limited number of research-oriented MS clinics at Canadian university teaching hospitals across the country in order to provide a pool of well-documented MS patients for use in future clinical trials, to provide various body tissues and fluids for current MS research, and to provide ongoing care and services for MS patients in those communities'. There are now 15 clinics based in universities or teaching hospitals across the country (*Fig. 22.1*, *Table 22.1*).

THE CONCEPT OF THE MULTIDISCIPLINARY MS CLINIC

The purpose of the specialty multidisciplinary MS clinic, as it has evolved in Canada, is primarily to provide expert clinical care in a setting that allows for systematic documentation of clinical data for both clinical and basic research purposes. The overall plan was to document prospectively a representative portion of the population of MS in a region. Expert multidisciplinary medical care could be delivered to those patients in a setting that allowed for a systematic and defined collection of various aspects of clinical data. In addition, the concept of MS clinics has broadened to include the support of more basic research directed toward MS by bringing together a critical mass of clinical and basic science investigators focused upon the disease.

In addition to the systematic collection of clinical data for natural history[8–11] using agreed upon standards for collection of data at London, Ontario, the organization of such clinics directly supports activities in clinical trials. Moreover, such a clinic can provide expert medical education for the MS clinic staff, medical students, residents, practising physicians, nurses, therapists and other health-care staff.

In Canada the means for developing such a multidisciplinary clinic have come from many

Table 22.1 Milestones in the development of MS clinics in Canada.

1954	First MS clinic at Montreal Neurological Institute
1972	MS Clinic at University of Western Ontario, London, Ontario
1976	MS Clinic at University of Calgary, Alberta
1970s	Collaborative studies started: (a) Genetics[3,4] (b) Amantadine[5] (c) Childhood MS[6] (d) Native Americans and MS[7]
1998	Canadian Network of MS Clinics established

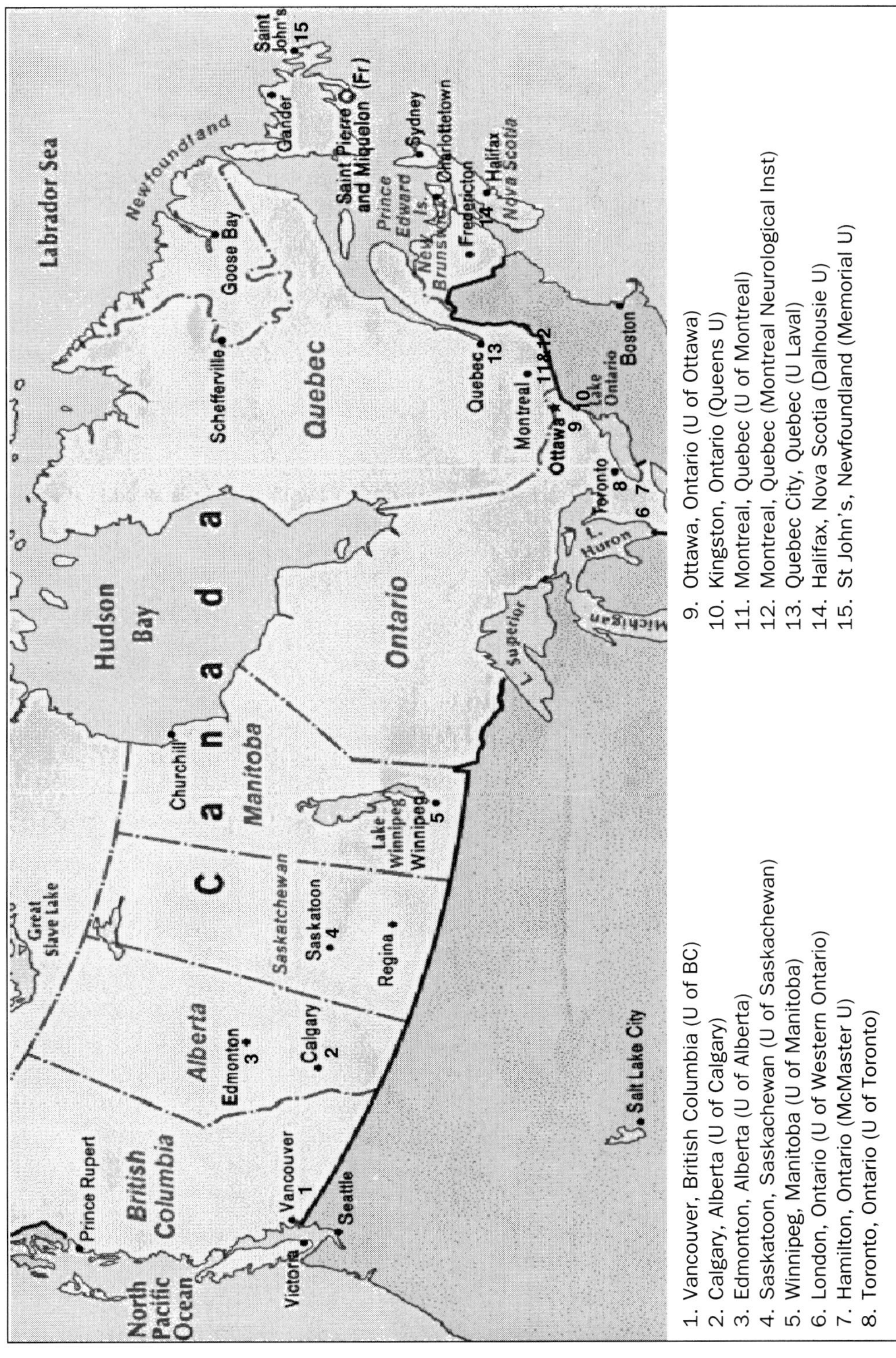

1. Vancouver, British Columbia (U of BC)
2. Calgary, Alberta (U of Calgary)
3. Edmonton, Alberta (U of Alberta)
4. Saskatoon, Saskachewan (U of Saskachewan)
5. Winnipeg, Manitoba (U of Manitoba)
6. London, Ontario (U of Western Ontario)
7. Hamilton, Ontario (McMaster U)
8. Toronto, Ontario (U of Toronto)
9. Ottawa, Ontario (U of Ottawa)
10. Kingston, Ontario (Queens U)
11. Montreal, Quebec (U of Montreal)
12. Montreal, Quebec (Montreal Neurological Inst)
13. Quebec City, Quebec (U Laval)
14. Halifax, Nova Scotia (Dalhousie U)
15. St John's, Newfoundland (Memorial U)

Figure 22.1 Map of Canada.

different sources. An important thrust of support for the concept has come from the Multiple Sclerosis Society of Canada by referral of patients to individual clinics and monetary support for some of the clinics. The degree of monetary support has varied from region to region and from time to time. A major consideration that has allowed for the success of such a multidisciplinary approach to MS care is the consistent nature of the health-care system applied across the country, province to province. Support for MS clinics has come from medical schools, hospitals (e.g. in the case of the Vancouver Clinic, Vancouver Hospital and Health Sciences Centre has provided continuing support from the beginning), various insurance carriers, granting agencies and, more recently, from the pharmaceutical industry.

In addition, enthusiastic support from neurological colleagues across the country has been a major factor in which sharing of patients has been willingly accomplished. There seems to be plenty of work for all that are interested, and intrinsic to the Canadian medical care system is the concept that everyone is eligible for government-insured medical care—the concept of universalty).

Another consideration that has been very important is the fact that there is a high prevalence of MS in Canada,[12–14] and when compared to other countries the number of specialists available to deliver care to the relatively high number of MS patients in the population has been relatively low.

In some regions, satellite clinics have been set up, and these are able to feed data into and get guidance from the regional provincial centres. In addition, the advent of new therapies (interferon-β agents and COP-1) has stimulated the development of several province-wide systems linked to MS clinics for approval, funding, follow-up and management of patients receiving the new therapies.

STRUCTURE AND PERSONNEL OF THE MS CLINIC

The following discussion uses the MS clinic in Vancouver as an example.

Central to the concept of an MS clinic is a co-ordinator. The co-ordinator has usually been a nurse, but it could just as well be another health-care professional. It is most important that the co-ordinator should work with the multidisciplinary team in order to provide a smooth and seamless system for provision of medical care and for clinical research.

Medical care in the clinic is usually delivered by neurologists. However, as a part of the Canadian system, each patient has a general practitioner, and some of the patients retain a local neurologist while still attending the clinic on a regular basis. Exchanges of clinical notes and other communications are of vital importance in this system. None of the neurologists is a full-time MS expert, but many of them are full-time university academics. In addition, community neurologists have been recruited into the clinics and fill a most important role in the delivery of medical care at MS clinics and in the neurological aspect of clinical trials.

Other medical experts that have been recruited into the clinic organization include neuro-ophthalmologists, neuro-urologists, geneticists, psychiatrists, psychologists, sexual therapists, and rehabilitation specialists. Other areas of importance are pain and surgical consultants.

Moreover, patients are seen quite regularly when appropriate by a clinical geneticist, a reproduction counsellor, a social worker, nurses, an occupational therapist, a physiotherapist and other health-care professionals. The range of therapists available varies among clinics.

For the convenience of patients, one of the aspects of multidisciplinary clinics that is most helpful is the concept of 'one-stop shopping'. Under this system, referrals can be made to other health-care professionals in a direct and accelerated way, often on the same day as the patient is seen in the MS clinic. In some of the larger clinics, separate but communicating systems have been set up for the following functions:

(a) General clinic function (yearly visits): a computerized medical record and database system[15] that is accessible to all personnel helps in documentation, scheduling and planning in the Vancouver Clinic.

(b) Acute relapse care: only one person receives acute relapse calls and organizes the most appropriate intervention and documentation. This function can be a rotating responsibility among nurses and physicians.

(c) Clinical trials: a team of nurses, neurologists and administrators deals with clinical trial patients. Ideally, the clinical trial personnel rotate through the various routine clinic operations as well. The data from clinical trials is eventually also incorporated into the overall clinic database.

(d) Research co-ordination and database function: a separate group of expert personnel enter data and maintain the computer system.[10] In ideal circumstances, each arm of the clinic organization has access to data and responsibility for data entry in order to keep the system up to date. At any time the computer system can be searched for important individual patient data or for grouped data for clinical research purposes.

In Vancouver, this type of regular on-site interaction has been most helpful in the case of neuro-ophthalmology. The presence of on-site psychiatry and psychology services has also been of major help. Areas such as genito-urinary medicine, sexual medicine and rehabilitation have generally been off-site referrals.

COMPARISON BETWEEN MULTIDISCIPLINARY CLINIC PRACTICE AND TRADITIONAL NEUROLOGICAL CARE

Traditional neurological care—positive features

The positive features of neurological follow-up in the neurologist's office can be described as follows:

(a) there is a one-to-one relationship between the doctor and the patient;

(b) scheduling and availability is more flexible than in a large organization; and

(c) the medical care, dependent as it is on the individual, is more readily holistic by nature than multidisciplinary care, which is somewhat fragmented into many different subspecialities.

Traditional neurological care—negative features

The negative features of traditional neurological care can be summarized as follows:

(a) there is no ability to have 'one-stop shopping' and expedited referrals designed specifically for MS patients;

(b) it is not, by nature, multidisciplinary expert medical care;

(c) there is no subspecialist expert medical care except by referral, and even then the referrals do not necessarily go to an MS expert; and

(d) very little clinical research is undertaken in this setting.

The multidisciplinary clinic—positive features

The positive features of the multidisciplinary clinic setting can be summarized as follows:

(a) the multidisciplinary clinic provides expert care with multiple views on problems, and therefore is more likely to identify solutions to those problems readily;

(b) the system allows expeditious subspecialist referrals for specific problems, and referrals can also be made to specific MS specialists that may not be on site; and

(c) the localization of specialists in one physical area also concentrates the patients from that region into one standardized unit for the provision of medical care and the development of clinical research.

The multidisciplinary clinic—negative features

The negative features of the multidisciplinary clinic setting can be summarized as follows:

(a) there is less one-to-one contact, and contact may include multiple health-care professionals, students and trainees; furthermore, the process is also time consuming for both professionals and patients, and therefore expensive;

(b) the demand for resources in these circumstances may outstrip the ability to provide those resources, and one must be very careful not to inflate the expectations of the patients in this regard;

(c) a large organization such as a regional MS clinic can develop a rigid structure that sometimes is not flexible enough for provision of the rapid responses to patients' requests that may be required; and

(d) a major problem could be that patients become overly dependent on the clinic and develop unrealistic expectations; in such cases the patients can be disappointed and attendance at the clinics can drop off—when attendance at the clinic becomes sporadic there is no longer a systematic data set collected.

THE CANADIAN NETWORK OF MS CLINICS

The enthusiastic organizational support of the Multiple Sclerosis Society of Canada had a great deal to do with the momentum to develop MS clinics across the country. Not only was limited start-up monetary support made available to some of the clinics, but collaboration was also encouraged. The frequency of meetings of the clinic and research directors across the country has gradually increased since that time, especially in regard to the nationwide genetics collaborative study.

In June 1998, it was decided to organize formally a loosely regulated entity—The Canadian Network of MS Clinics (CNMSC). The CNMSC has an e-mail distribution source located at the University of Calgary. Pilot initiatives in clinical research that begin locally are encouraged to become national collaborative studies. In general, the clinics have expressed a willingness to contribute data and comments on proposed collaborative studies using the communication system of the CNMSC and through annual meetings of clinic directors.

The clinics are all university- and teaching hospital-based. It is critical for the clinic concept that MS clinics should be involved in clinical care, in education of patients, the public and families, and in research activities. Some clinics have developed regional satellites and recruited regional clinical neurologists to develop their own multidisciplinary clinic that operates under the mandate of the university-based clinic.

COLLABORATIVE STUDIES

The most major collaborative project so far has been the nation-wide genetics project headed by Ebers[3] and Sadovnick.[4] Yearly meetings of the MS clinic directors have been necessary in order to maintain the collaboration that is intrinsic to the success of the project. However, collaboration across the country has always been voluntary and interest-driven. No one is excluded from participation in studies, but the data provided must reach the standards of the principal investigators for each individual study.

Some of the collaborative studies that have been successful across the country include:

(a) genetic and epidemiological studies that were conceived in the late 1970s by George Ebers;[3,4]

(b) the Canadian co-operative twin study that was organized by George Ebers in 1984;[4]

(c) the childhood MS[6] study that was organized by Pierre Duquette and published in 1987;

(d) therapeutic trials—the first collaborative therapeutic trial was with amantidine[5] and was organized by Jock Murray in 1985 and published in 1987; subsequent therapeutic trials have been organized, most notably the Canadian co-operative cyclophosphamide study organized by John Noseworthy and published in 1991;[16] many of the more recent trials have been run by pharmaceutical sponsors aided by the interest in collaboration among the various MS clinics across the country.[17–23]

Factors that have allowed and encouraged collaboration

Factors that have allowed and encouraged collaboration across the country include the availability of financial support, the nature of Canadian neurological practice and the nature of Canada itself.

Financial support

The Multiple Sclerosis Society of Canada started things off by supporting some clinics, projects and both general and focused meetings of investigators. Some neurologist research training has also been supported. Funding has also been available through various other granting agencies (e.g. the Canadian Medical Research Council and provincial grants).

In recent years, industry funding of clinical trials has taken a major position of importance. Additional communications with annual research meetings at the Canadian Congress of Neurological Sciences, an e-mail communication system and other collaborative studies have been undertaken.

The nature of Canadian neurological practice

There have been individual areas of leadership both overall and for individual projects. The overall quality of the research leadership has been high. During the formative years the contributions of Pierre Duquette, George Ebers, Gordon Francis, Walter Hader, Jock Murray and Peter Seland were instrumental in getting the project off the ground. The non-competitive aspect of Canadian neurological practice has contributed greatly toward the ability to do collaborative studies and to develop population-based regional pools of MS patients for clinical research.

The nature of Canada itself

Canada is a physically large country (see *Fig. 22.1*), but its population is relatively small, allowing the concept of regional collaboration (both clinical and research-based) to develop without a great deal of regional conflict. In addition, each of the clinics has been greatly enhanced by a highly motivated staff at each level, most importantly at the co-ordinator level. The health-care system across the country is uniform and of high quality. There is a high prevalence of MS, so there are plenty of patients to be shared across the country.

In addition, it is in the interest of patients to become involved in MS clinics because they can be exposed to multidisciplinary experts for their medical care and education. Moreover, the patients have been extremely compliant and supportive of the research endeavours of the clinics. One potential problem, however, is that the high level of compliance from our patients puts major responsibilities on the shoulders of the investigators to make sure that the patients' willing compliance is not exploited in such a way as to put them in jeopardy by being placed in potentially harmful clinical studies.

SUMMARY

In Canada, a large percentage of the medical care for MS patients is provided by university-affiliated multidisciplinary clinics. This kind of organization can provide expert medical care in a setting of systematic approaches to data collection, which in turn stimulates research. This concept has resulted in the development of 15 MS clinical centres and a number of collaborative studies.

The MS clinic system in Canada has evolved from a few isolated units into a network that is determined to enhance collaboration. The factors that came together to foster collaboration were:

(a) individual and group leadership and motivation;
(b) encouragement from the lay body (the Multiple Sclerosis Society of Canada); and
(c) the unique Canadian nationwide health care system.

ACKNOWLEDGEMENTS

We would like to thank our patients, without whose support we would not have been able to make this report.

REFERENCES

1. Baxter DW, Andermann F. In memoriam: Bert Cosgrove. *Can J Neurol Sci* 1984; **11**: 483–484.
2. National Advisory Commission on Multiple Sclerosis. *Report and Recommendations.* 74–534 US Department of Health, Education, and Welfare: Washington DC, 1974.
3. Ebers GC, Kukay K, Bulman DE et al. A full genome search in multiple sclerosis. *Nature Genet* 1996; **13**: 472–476.
4. Sadovnick AD, Risch NJ, Ebers GC et al. Canadian Collaborative Project on Genetic Susceptibility to MS, Phase 2: rationale and method. *Can J Neurol Sci* 1998; **25(3)**: 216–221.
5. Murray TJ. Amantadine therapy for fatigue in multiple sclerosis. *Can J Neurol Sci* 1985; **12**: 251–254.
6. Duquette P, Murray TJ, Pleines J et al. Multiple sclerosis in childhood: clinical profile in 125 patients. *J Pediatr* 1987; **111**: 359–363.
7. Hader WJ, Feasby TE, Noseworthy JH et al. Multiple sclerosis in Canadian Native people. *Neurology* 1985; **35**: 300.
8. Weinshenker BG, Bass B, Rice GP et al. The natural history of multiple sclerosis: a geographically based study. I. Clinical course and disability. *Brain* 1989; **112**: 133–146.
9. Weinshenker BG, Bass B, Rice GP et al. The natural history of multiple sclerosis: a geographically based study. II. Predictive value of the early clinical course. *Brain* 1989; **112**: 1419–1428.
10. Weinshenker BG, Rice GPA, Noseworthy JH et al. The natural history of multiple sclerosis: a geographically based study. III. Multivariate analysis of predictive factors and models of outcome. *Brain* 1991; **114**: 1045–1056.
11. Weinshenker BG, Rice GPA, Noseworthy JH et al. The natural history of multiple sclerosis: a geographically based study. IV. Applications to planning and interpretation of clinical therapeutic trials. *Brain* 1991; **114**: 1057–1067.
12. Sweeney VP, Sadovnick AD, Brandjes V. Prevalence of multiple sclerosis in British Columbia. *Can J Neurol Sci* 1986; **13**: 47–51.
13. Hader WJ, Elliot M, Ebers GC. Epidemiology of multiple sclerosis in London and Middlesex County, Ontario, Canada. *Neurology* 1988; **38**: 617–621.
14. Warren S, Warren KG. Multiple sclerosis and associate diseases: a relationship to diabetes mellitus. *Can J Neurol Sci* 1981; **8**: 35–39.
15. Studney D, Lublin F, Marcucci L et al. MS COSTAR: a computerized record for use in clinical research in multiple sclerosis. *J Neurol Rehabil* 1993; **7**: 145–152.
16. Noseworthy JH. The Canadian Co-operative trial on cyclophosphamide and plasma exchange in progressive multiple sclerosis. *Lancet* 1991; **337**: 441–446.
17. IFNB Multiple Sclerosis Study Group. Interferon beta-1b is effective in relapsing–remitting multiple sclerosis. I. Clinical results of a multi-center, randomized, double-blind, placebo-controlled trial. *Neurology* 1993; **43**: 655–661.
18. Paty DW, Li DKB, UBC MS/MRI Study Group, the IFNB Multiple Sclerosis Study Group. Interferon beta-1b is effective in relapsing–remitting multiple sclerosis. II. MRI analysis results of a multicenter, randomized, double-blind, placebo-controlled trial. *Neurology* 1993; **43**: 662–667.
19. IFNB Multiple Sclerosis Study Group, the University of British Columbia MS/MRI Analysis Group. Interferon beta-1b in the treatment of multiple sclerosis: final outcome of the randomized controlled trial. *Neurology* 1995; **45**: 1277–1285.
20. PRISMS (Prevention of Relapses and Disability by Interferon β-1a Subcutaneously in Multiple Sclerosis) Study Group. Randomized double-blind placebo-controlled study of interferon β-1a in relapsing/remitting multiple sclerosis. *Lancet* 1998; **352**: 1498–1504.
21. The once weekly interferon for multiple sclerosis OWIMS Study Group. Dose-dependent clinical and magnetic resonance imaging efficacy of interferon β-1a in multiple sclerosis (abstract). Presented at the Annual Meeting of the American Neurological Association, Montreal, October 1998. *Ann Neurol* 1998; **44**: 992.
22. Li DKB, Cover K, Paty DW et al. Further evidence of dose-response effects of interferon β-1a in relapsing–remitting multiple sclerosis: results of low dose therapy. *Ann Neurol* 1999; in press.
23. The Lenercept Multiple Sclerosis Study Group and the UBC MS/MRI Analysis Group, presented by Paty DW. TnF neutralization induces an increase in relapses in patients with multiple sclerosis (abstract). *Can J Neurol Sci* 1998; **25(Suppl 1)**: S31. *Ann Neurol* 1999; in press.

MS-COSTAR: a computerized medical record adapted for multiple sclerosis clinical research

Donald W Paty, Donald Studney, Virginia Devonshire and Kin Ho

INTRODUCTION

Clinical research requires standardization of data, and if possible the prospective collection of data. In the early 1980s in Vancouver, the authors decided to collect such data into an existing computerized medical record system[1] and renamed the system MS-COSTAR.[2]

METHODS

The purpose of the system was to increase the power of data collection, to facilitate the analysis of data and possibly, in the future, to create a new pool of data for research studies by multisite pooling.

MS-COSTAR is an integrated computer software system written in the MUMPS computer language. It is designed to facilitate both clinical care and clinical research. It provides functions for storing, retrieving, analysing and displaying the demographic, clinical and test data that accrue as patients are seen and cared for over time in a typical multiple sclerosis (MS) clinic. The original program was a computer stored ambulatory record (COSTAR).[1] This electronic medical record is used in many general clinic settings across North America.

The MS-COSTAR system includes a natural time base, comprehensive encoding and the systematic quantitation of clinical and test data designed for precise retrieval and analysis. It is written in a broadly compatible format designed to facilitate data exchange and pooling among both MS-COSTAR users and other databases such as the European EDMUS system.[3] The system software is regularly updated to keep it current with advances in hardware and software. It is also designed to be responsive to user requirements for various enhancements and particularly for new codes needed to describe evolving diagnostic, therapeutic and evaluation concepts in MS.

Entry of coded data, both general neurological data and MS-specific data (e.g. onset of disease, relapses and their characteristics, and disability as measured by the expanded disability status scale) is made at each patient visit. In addition, there is entry of general medical data (mostly uncoded), which can be searched to provide background information. Time-related data can be captured and analysed for variables such as demographics, background medical information, number of relapses, degree of disability over time, diagnostic procedures and various therapies.

Thus, MS-COSTAR can be used for maintaining an up-to-date description of the demographics of patients seen locally. It also can be searched for coded data in history (relapses), physical examination findings and coded clinical outcome measures. In addition, diagnostic procedures and medications are able to be accessed separately.

The primary display of MS-COSTAR data is organized for its use as a computerized medical record. The authors currently have over 5000 patients in the database. Most of the data on these patients has been entered prospectively, visit-by-visit. If necessary, the clinic could operate completely without paper except for the data entry forms, which are coded by the neurologists and other users. Data entry is then done by professionals, with intermittent monitoring for checks of accuracy.

Uses at the Vancouver clinic

Uses of the database at the Vancouver clinic are:

(a) management of patient appointments in the clinic;
(b) identification of patients for clinical trials— patients are prospectively coded as to the type of MS (e.g. relapsing–remitting, secondary progressive, primary progressive), and the number and timing of relapses is also coded; the disability status is also recorded at all visits. Therefore patients can be selected for appropriate variables in order to identify those who can qualify for various clinical trials;
(c) searching natural history data;[4] and
(d) calculation of a computer-assisted disability scale.[5]

SUMMARY

The authors chose COSTAR because of its flexibility as an electronic medical record. They have also chosen to limit the job of data entry to data entry professionals. Users (physicians, nurses and other health-care professionals) fill out an encounter form, from which the data is transferred into MS-COSTAR by a professional data entry person. However, any user in the system can seek information both for individual patients and for groups of patients. Files can be downloaded into standard databases for sophisticated statistical analysis.

The authors have found MS-COSTAR to be very helpful in the day-to-day operation of the clinic as well as in various clinical research programs.

ACKNOWLEDGEMENTS

Thanks to Ken Redekop and Erin Black for their invaluable help over the years.

REFERENCES

1. Barnett GO, Justice NS, Somand ME et al. COSTAR: a computer-based medical record system for ambulatory care. *Proc IEEE* 1979; **67**: 1226–1237.
2. Studney D, Lublin F, Marcucci L et al. MS COSTAR: a computerized record for use in clinical research in multiple sclerosis. *J Neurol Rehabil* 1993; **7**: 145–152.
3. Confavreux C, Compston DAS, Hommes OR et al. EDMUS, a European database for multiple sclerosis. *J Neurol Neurosurg Psychiatry* 1992; **55**: 671–676.
4. Redekop WK. *Prognosis in Multiple Sclerosis: the Predictors and Prediction of Specified Functional Impairments* (PhD dissertation). University of British Columbia, Vancouver, 1995.
5. Redekop WK, Paty DW. Computerized scoring of neurological impairment in multiple sclerosis. *Ann Neurol* 1991; **30**: 255.

Index